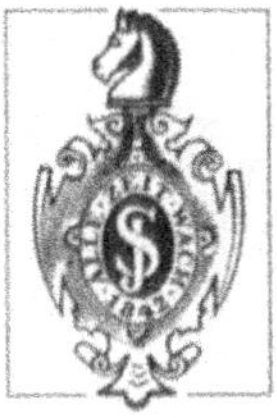

Michel Osteaux (Ed.)
A.R. Bakker, D. Bell, R. Mattheus, D. Meyer-Ebrecht,
S. Orphanoudakis, R. Van de Velde, Th. Wendler (Co-editors)

Hospital Integrated Picture Archiving and Communication Systems

A Second Generation PACS Concept

With 112 Figures and 23 Tables

Springer-Verlag
Berlin Heidelberg New York
London Paris Tokyo
Hong Kong Barcelona
Budapest

Prof. Dr. Michel Osteaux
Head Radiology Department
Director: Pluridisciplinary Research Institute
for Medical Imaging Science, Academic Hospital,
Vrije Universiteit Brussel, Laarbeeklaan 101,
B-1090 Brussel, Belgium

ISBN-13: 978-3-642-76965-8 e-ISBN-13: 978-3-642-76963-4
DOI: 10.1007/978-3-642-76963-4

Library of Congress Cataloging-in-Publication Data
Hospital integrated picture archiving and communication systems: a second generation PACS concept/Michel Osteaux (ed.). p. cm. Includes bibliographical references and index. ISBN 0-387-54592-1 (U.S.) 1. Picture archiving and communication systems in medicine—Congresses. I. Osteaux, M. (Michel), 1944- . R857.P52H671992 616.07'54'0285—dc20 91-37203 CIP

Softcover reprint of the hardcover 1st edition 1992

Typesetting: Best-set Typesetter Ltd., Hong Kong

21/3130-5 4 3 2 1 0 – Printed on acid-free paper

Foreword

The term picture archiving and communications system (PACS) was initiated during the first International conference and workshop on the topic sponsored by The International Society for Optical Engineering (SPIE) in Newport Beach, California in 1982. The research and development (R&D) progress for PACS has been slow until 1988. The earlier PACS modules were mostly off the shelf components connected together to solve a very specific clinical problem. The three major players in PACS R&D are the European countries, United States of America, and Japan. For various reasons, the European countries concentrated in modeling and simulation, U.S.A. preferred in-house development or purchased PACS modules from a manufacturer, whereas Japan organized the PACS as a national project.

Between 1989 and 1990 PACS R&D took a dramatic positive turn. Large scale PACS projects were planned and some are at various stages of implementation, especially in newly constructed hospitals. Examples are the Hokkaido University, Japan; Hammersmith Hospital, United Kingdom; Social and Medical Center East (SMZO), Vienna, Austria; the U.S. Armed Force Medical Diagnostic Imaging Support (MDIS) project; and the UCLA Medical Plaza ambulatory care center. Another phenomenon is the organization of the EC-countries which provides a tremendous impetus for the European PACS R&D efforts. This book "Hospital Integrated Picture Archiving and Communication Systems: edited by Professor M. Osteaux and others is a direct product from these efforts.

In addition to this book, there are currently three other references available: *PACS Handbook, 89*, Japanese PACS Research Association, Japan; *Picture Archiving and Communication Systems (PACS) in Medicine* NATO ASI Proceedings, Springer-Verlag, 1991; *Integrated Diagnostic Imaging-Digital PACS in Medicine*, Elsevier, 1991. Also, there is a special PACS issue in the Journal of Computerized Medical Imaging and Graphics, November, 1991. Each of these references has a different emphasis, the *PACS Handbook, 89* and the *Digital*

PACS in Medicine are a collection of PACS papers of various topics. The PACS in Medicine is a proceedings resulted from a two week NATO Advanced Study Institute. Professor Osteaux's book, on the other hand, is a systematic treatment of a new concept on Hospital Integrated PACS. Its theme is to stress that PACS can no longer be treated as an imaging system alone. It has to be integrated to other hospital information systems in order for it to be useful and recognized. This concept along with another new concept "PACS infrastructure" will, no doubt, lay the foundation for a new era of PACS research and development.

H.K. Huang, D.Sc.
Professor
Department of Radiological Sciences
University of California, Los Angeles

Preface

This book presents the results of a multidisciplinary, cooperative project which was jointly undertaken by research teams from universities, industry, and university hospitals in five European Community countries. The research consortium was founded within the Advanced Informatics in Medicine (AIM) program issued by the Directorate XIII of the Commission of the European Communities (Research and Technological Innovation).

The name of the research project, Hospital Integrated Picture Archiving and Communication System, (HIPACS), indicates the objective of the study, namely, to make the digital management of diagnostic imaging pictures effective in the clinical environment. We deal in detail with the distinct issues of PACS integration such as medical requirements, communication with other systems, networking, workstations, data bases, indexing methods, and standards. We then synthesize a clear collective view on the architective required of a second-generation PACS, taking into account the diverse features of the present state of the art and expected future enhancements of PACS technology.

The authors wish to thank the AIM team of the Commission of the European Communities, which, under the leadership of Dr. Niels Rossing, initiated the formation of a real European medical informatics community in a friendly and relaxed, but highly effective manner. This program as a whole induced fruitful contacts, communication, and collaboration. We thank "our" HIPACS-AIM officer, Mr. M. Wilson, for his support and positive advice in our project. We would also like to thank all other officers of the AIM office, who were always supportive and gave concrete help when it was needed. The input of AIM to achieve European standardization—under the leadership of Mr. J. Noothoven van Goor—was particularly important for the future of our work. We also thank our colleagues from the other AIM projects for their spirit of collaboration and useful suggestions which were indeed incorporated into our general philosophy. HIPACS is only a small part of the

AIM accomplishments, which are already very substantial.

Finally, it would be unfair not to acknowledge the far-reaching influence of the knowledge and wide experience acquired by our colleagues from the United States and Japan on the work reported here. We wish to express our particular gratitude to Dr. M. Greberman (CDRH, Food and Drug Administration), Dr. Seong K. Mun (Georgetown University Medical Center), and Prof. M. Akisada, chairman of the Japan Association of PACS for their international spirit of collaboration.

MICHEL OSTEAUX

Contents

Contributors

Bakker, A.R., Prof. Eng.
Director, BAZIS Leiden, Shipholweg 97, NL-2316 Leiden, The Netherlands

Bell, D., Prof. Eng.
Institute of Informatics, University of Ulster, Newton Abbey, co. Antrim BT37 0QB, United Kingdom

Elsakkers, P.H., Ph.D.
Manager Radiology Department, University Hospital, NL-2316 XA Leiden, The Netherlands

Keizers, A., Eng.
Lehrstuhl für Messtechnik, Rheinisch-Westfälische Technische Hochschule Aachen, W-5100 Aachen, FRG

Koens, M.L.
Product Manager, BAZIS Leiden, Shipholweg 97, NL-2316 XA Leiden, The Netherlands

Kofakis, P., Ph.D.
Institute of Computer Science, Foundation of Research and Technology, Daedalou 36, GR-71110 Heraklio, Greece

Kouwenberg, J.M.L., M. Eng.
VP system development, BAZIS Leiden, Shipholweg 97, NL-2316 XA Leiden, The Netherlands

Ling, D.H.O., Ph.D.
University of Ulster, Newton Abbey, co. Antrim BT37 0QB, United Kingdom

Lodder, H., M. Sc.
BAZIS Leiden, Shipholweg 97, NL-2316 XA Leiden, The Netherlands

Mattheus, R., M. Sc.
Senior scientist, Vrije Universiteit Brussels, Laarbeeklaan 101, B-1090 Brussel, Belgium

Meyer-Ebrecht, D., Prof. Eng., Ph.D.
Lehrstuhl für Messtechnik, Rheinisch-Westfälische Technische Hochschule, W-5100 Aachen, FRG

Mönnich, K.J.
Philips GmbH, Forschungslaboratorium Hamburg, Vogt Koelnn Strasse 30, W-2000 Hamburg 54, FRG

Orphanoudakis, S., Prof. Ph.D.
Institute of Computer Science, Foundation of Research and Technology, Daedalou 36, GR-71110 Heraklio, Greece

Osteaux, M., Prof. M.D. Ph.D.
Head Radiology Department, Academic Hospital, Vrije Universiteit Brussel, Laarbeeklaan 101, B-1090 Brussel, Belgium

Ottes, F.P., Ph.D.
IMAGIS project leader, BAZIS Leiden, Shipholweg 97, NL-2316 XA Leiden, The Netherlands

Schilling, C., Eng.
Department of Electrical Engineering, University of Aachen, W-5100 Aachen, FRG

Schmidt, J.
Philips GmbH, Forschungslaboratorium Hamburg, Vogt Koelnn Strasse 30, W-2000 Hamburg 54, FRG

Stut, W.J.J. Jr., M. Sc.
BAZIS Leiden, Shipholweg 101, NL-2316 XA Leiden, The Netherlands

Temmerman, Y., M.D.
Department of Radiology, Academisch Ziekenhuis, Vrije Universiteit Brussel, Laarbeeklaan 101, B-1090 Brussel, Belgium

Tiberghien, J.G., Prof. Eng., Ph.D.
Applied Sciences, Vrije Universiteit Brussel, Pleinlaan 2, B-1040 Brussel, Belgium

Van den Broeck, R.
Chief Technologist, Department of Radiology, Academisch Ziekenhuis, Vrije Universiteit Brussel, Laarbeeklaan 101, B-1090 Brussel, Belgium

Van de Velde, R., Eng.
Head Information Department, Academisch Ziekenhuis, Vrije Universiteit Brussel, Laarbeeklaan 101, B-1090 Brussel, Belgium

Van Poppel, B.M., M. Sc.
BAZIS Leiden, Shipholweg 97, NL-2316 XA Leiden, The Netherlands

Vossebürger, F., Eng.
Lehrstuhl für Messtechnik, Rheinisch-Westfälische Technische Hochschule Aachen, W-5100 Aachen, FRG

Wein, B., M.D.
Klinik für Radiologische Diagnostik, Rheinisch-Westfälische Technische Hochschule Aachen, Pauwelstrasse 1, W-5100 Aachen, FRG

Wendler, Th., Ph.D.
Philips GmbH, Forschungslaboratorium Hamburg, Vogt Koelnn Strasse 30, W-2000 Hamburg 54, FRG

Young, I.R.
University of Ulster, Newton Abbey, co. Antrim BT37 0QB, United Kingdom

1 Introduction, Definition, and Historical Background of Picture Archiving and Communication Systems*

F.P. OTTES, A.R. BAKKER, and J.M.L. KOUWENBERG

1.1 Background

Since the discovery of X-rays and the demonstration of their application in health care by WK Roentgen in 1895, X-ray images have become increasingly important in health care. Since the 1970s, various new techniques that produce images in a digital representation have been introduced into hospitals. In the conventional projection, X-ray film is currently used for detection, for presentation, for archival purposes, and for distribution. Even for the digital modalities, film is used for presentation, archiving and distribution. Because of the great number of radiological examinations (in the order of 100000 per year for one hospital) film consumption in hospitals is extremely high. For instance, a 900-bed Netherlands University Hospital uses about 30000 m^2 of film per year.

Film provides an extremely high-quality image. However, there are limitations in its use, especially with respect to handling and archiving. The most important problems are:

- Each image is stored on only one, unique sheet of film. It would be very expensive and would involve a reduction in the quality of conventional projection X-ray images if copies of each film were to be made. The existence of only one copy means that if this film is damaged or missing, irreplaceable information is lost for good. If new images are lost, retakes can be made, but the repeated radiation dose implies an extra risk for the patient.
- With the huge number of films in circulation in a hospital and the large number of professionals who need the films for their work, storage and lending of films require much space and manpower. Except in situations where the lending of films is well organized, e.g., by means of a bar code-based tracking system, medical professionals will waste much of their valuable time waiting for mislaid films to be traced.
- The acquisition of radiological images on film requires a lot of processing chemicals and handling, which again implies a lot of costs.

* The authors of this chapter gratefully acknowledge the financial support of the National Facility Informatics / Netherlands Organization for the Advancement of Research for the participation in many of the conferences and in study tours to many of the mentioned PACS sites.

- Currently, image information is stored in a physical film archive, whereas the related textual patient information is stored in one or more information systems. This means that to retrieve the complete patient record, i.e., images *and* alphanumerical data, the images must be traced using a completely different procedure from the one used to retrieve the alphanumerical data.
- Images on film can not be manipulated or analyzed by means of the existing or future digital image processing techniques.
- For medical facilities in rural areas, which are less well equipped for primary diagnosis, it is difficult to consult a larger hospital, because films need to be transported physically.

The introduction of a digital system to support image handling in a hospital could largely solve all the above problems. Such a computer system is called a picture archiving and communication system (PACS). A PACS is defined to include a comprehensive set of facilities which handle digital radiological images. The images can be entered into the system in digital form, archived in the PACS, and distributed and presented, together with the related alphanumerical patient data, to all authorized users. The PACS is not restricted to the radiology department, but explicitly also provides access to the images at the request of the physician who referred the patient from another department.

The initiation of the PACS concept was mainly triggered by three new developments. Firstly, the introduction of the new digital techniques for radiological imaging such as computed tomography (CT), magnetic resonance imaging (MRI) and ultrasound (US) provided an acquisition source that produces images in digital form. Images from digital modalities can be entered much more easily into the PACS than images obtained from conventional projection X-rays, since the latter must be digitized before they can be entered. Currently about 15% of examinations are performed using digital modalities, and this ratio is steadily increasing. The ratio of digital data produced by digital techniques to that produced by traditional techniques (after digitization) is lower than 15%, because the images obtained by digital techniques contain less data than traditional X-ray studies. Traditional projection X-ray images can be entered into the PACS without producing films if the new computed radiography (CR) technique is used.

Secondly, the PACS concept is supported by the general implementation of integrated hospital information systems (HIS). The HIS provides access to all alphanumerical medical data for authorized users. Since images form such an essential part of the patient record, it is very attractive to make them accessible through a computer system together with the HIS data.

Thirdly, the PACS concept has been greatly aided by the rapid developments in information technology, e.g., electro-optics, very large scale integration, fiber optics, high-speed central processing unit (CPU), fast magnetic disk memory, magneto-optical storage, complex data base management, and information systems.

The potential benefits of PACS include the following:

- When back-up procedures are performed, the digital storage of images guarantees the continuous presence of the images. Since images will in fact consist of digital files, they can be copied at almost no cost and as often as required. This means that a set of images can be used simultaneously for various procedures at different locations, for example, for primary reporting, for therapy to decide whether new images are needed, as reference for the acquisition of new images in the same patient, and for research and education. This also implies that the images obtained during new examinations can be made available to the clinician much faster than is possible in the film-based situation, where images are first needed for performing primary diagnosis. This could lead to a faster therapy, and thus to a reduction in the length of patient stay.
- The storage of images in a PACS will avoid the potentially lengthy searches for films that occur so often now.
- If digital images can be obtained without generating film first, then large savings could be made in materials and manpower. If film storage were avoided, savings would also be made in floor space and archive personnel.
- If the images and alphanumerical data from a patient can be presented in a coherent way, the radiologist and the clinician may be able to correlate them. This might lead to better diagnosis and therapy, and thus to better patient care.
- If images are in digital form, digital imaging techniques can be utilized to support the diagnostic process. Quantitative parameters might then be calculated which can be used as search keys in data base queries. Certain features of abnormalities could be enhanced to increase their visual detectability. Another advantage of image processing is the possibility of three-dimensional representation of anatomic structures based on adjacent cross-sectional images (e.g., MRI or CT slices). The utilization of the three-dimensional display in diagnosis is currently still very limited, but this could change in the future.
- Once images are available in digital form, they may be transmitted, even over a great distance, via digital communication links, for examples, from a basic medical facility to a more advanced hospital for consultation.

1.2 Description

To actually enjoy these potential benefits, a hospital-wide PACS needs to be realized. The creation of such a system is a giant task, since the volume of image data involved is immense. Assuming that a single chest image contains 6 MB, the total yearly image production of a hospital represents 1–2 TB (1000–2000 GB) of digital data. To fulfill these requirements in

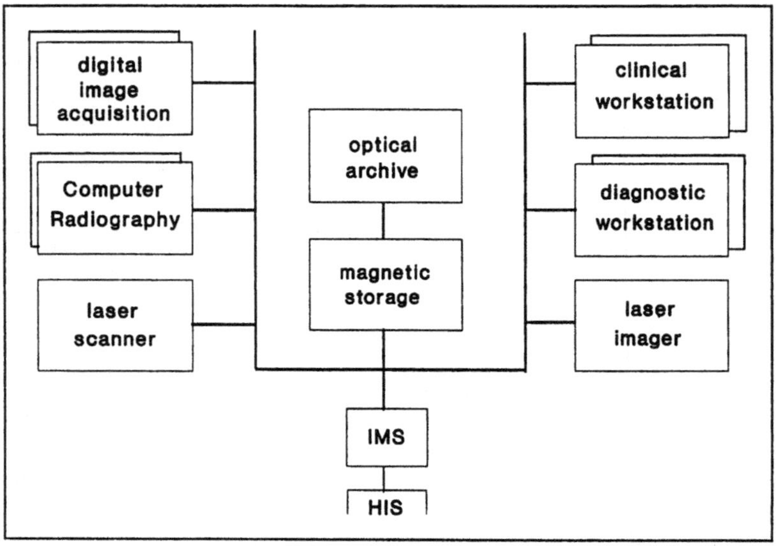

Fig. 1.1. The generic architecture of PACS consists of image entry equipment (*on the left*), image display/print devices (*on the right*), image data storage facilities (*in the center*), an image management system (*IMS*), a coupling with the hospital information system (*HIS*), and a network that interconnects all components. The number of components and the structure of the network are indicated only schematically. (From Ottes et al. 1990)

the hospital, a PACS would have to consist of various types of components (Fig. 1.1). The realization of a hospital-wide PACS requires the utmost from existing areas of information technology, and maybe more. An overview of the techniques for the digitization, compression, storage, retrieval, communication, and display of digital radiological images is given by Huang (1987).

1.2.1 Image Entry

In the very early days of PACS, it was thought that video cameras could be used to digitize films. Since it was found, however, that digital radiological images produced in this way had insufficient diagnostic quality, the technique was soon abandoned for most types of images, although it might provide sufficient image quality for US. The laser scanner technique is currently considered the best method of film digitization because of its high resolution, speed, and excellent image quality.

The new technique of CR (Kato 1990), which has been developed by Fuji on the basis of earlier research by Kodak, provides direct acquisition of digital images in conventional X-ray examinations without the expensive use of film. With CR, the film in the cassette is replaced by a light-stimulable phosphor plate. After exposure the image information on the phosphor plate is activated by means of a scanning laser beam. The light emitted, which is a measure of the incident X-ray radiation, is detected and converted to digital data. The plate can be erased and used again many times for other acquisitions. The potential medical advantages of CR are dose reduction, because of a higher sensitivity, and less under- and overexposures (and thus less retakes) because phosphor has a larger sensitivity range than film.

Currently, a new technique using large arrays of charge coupled devices (CCDs) is being developed for use in the direct digital acquisition of X-ray images. This method is very promising, because it would eliminate the handing of cassettes and the use of film and laser scanning devices. However, no prototype product has yet been created.

The early interfaces between digital imaging techniques and PACS were based on frame grabbing. With this technique, the digital signal sent to the cathode ray tube (CRT) of the modality viewing station is also fed into the interface and used to regenerate the digital file. The disadvantage is that this image contains less information than the original because it has been effected by window and level operations on the viewing station and because it is only 8 bits deep, instead of the 10–12 bits of the original image file. Nevertheless, this technique might be sufficient for US images, which have an accuracy of 8 bits or less. Currently, digital interfaces that transmit all information into the original image file are regarded as the only acceptable solution. Standards for file format and communication protocol have been developed, and some implementations have been realized.

1.2.2 Communication

The capacity of existing local area network products, for example those based on the Ethernet protocol, is insufficient to allow the distribution of the images that are acquired and viewed per day in the hospital. Transmission of a chest image (6 MB) would take about 1 min, which is an unacceptable speed for interactive image retrieval. This delay could be reduced by compressing the data. Because of the large size of the data files to be communicated, a high-speed broadband network and the integrated services digital networks (ISDN) or the fiber distributed data interface (FDDI) protocols will be required.

1.2.3 Storage

For the on-line archival of the most recent 1 or 2 years of generated images, multiple jukeboxes with optical disks have been proposed. These jukeboxes cannot, however, be used to retrieve images interactively, because it would take too much time. The retrieval speed of the optical disk is rather slow (about 30 s for 6 MB), and limited network speed would bring the response time down further. Each viewing station must be equipped with fast (parallel) magnetic disks to store the images that are expected to be utilized by the users of that viewing station. Intelligent image migration strategies have to be used to prefetch exactly those images that will be needed from the archive to the local magnetic storage buffer of each viewing station.

1.2.4 Data Compression

The required storage space and transmission time could be reduced if the digital images underwent data compression. There are two different methods of data compression: error free (reversible) or lossy (irreversible).

The error-free method does not cause any degradation of the image, but only yields a limited reduction of the file size between 2:1 and 3:1, depending on the image content. With lossy compression, much higher rates of reduction can be obtained, but as the compression factor increases, the loss of information in the image also increases. Especially in the United States, where medical malpractice leads to high legal claims, imaging equipment with built-in lossy compression is not and will not easily be accepted by the market. Another disadvantage is that data compression and reconstruction (needed before the image can be displayed) involve complex and elaborate calculations, requiring much computer power, which partly offsets the reduction in response time. Data compression could lead to artifacts in the image, especially when it is combined with image processing.

1.2.5 Presentation

In the film-based system, films are displayed on light boxes. In the hospital the type of light box used depends on the task of the medical user, Radiologists use an automatic alternator for primary diagnosis; this is a light box with a large viewing surface (for 12 or more chest films). The automatic alternator has a set of panels which can be moved in front of the light box one at a time. Multiple sets of films can be put on the panels before the reporting session, so that during these sessions changing from one set to the other is performed by means of pushing a button and is completed within 1 or 2 s.

Referring physicians, Radiology technicians and other medical professionals use light boxes of various sizes with a single fixed window; these light boxes are installed at many sites in the hospital.

Each of the functional features of PACS viewing workstations is determined by a number of parameters. The number of images that can be displayed simultaneously is primarily determined by the number of screens. The quality of the displayed images depends on many paramenters, such as the information contained in the image file itself, e.g., the matrix size of that file. Image quality is further determined by the screen size, the matrix size of the screen, the frame repetition rate, and the phosphor (color, decay time, layer thickness, and brilliance). Furthermore, image quality could be improved by image processing facilities.

The application software should provide tools to search and retrieve images and related patient information. It should allow image manipulation, e.g., adjustment of brightness and contrast (often called level and window) and position, orientation, and magnification of the image on the screen. Furthermore, because radiological studies often consist of many images (MRI studies consist of up to 50 slices) and reporting often requires comparison with previous studies, it is essential to have good tools for navigation through such a series of images. Depending on the technique used to generate the image and the medical specialty, specific analysis tools (e.g., anatomic geometrical measurements, densitometric measurement) should be available. The response times for all actions should be acceptably low.

Viewing stations are usually subdivided in different classes depending on the task they are used for. The most advanced viewing station is that for primary diagnosis, with four or more screens, 2000 × 2000 viewing capacity, and extended application software capabilities. Viewing stations with 2–4 screens and less software functionality (no processing, less navigation) might be sufficient for the referring physician. At other locations such as the operating theater, so-called output-only stations with just one screen and virtually no manipulation capability will be sufficient. A special class of viewing stations is that used for conferences. Here the size of the monitors should be sufficiently large to allow viewing from a distance by many spectators, a large number of screens (eight) is needed for comparison of the images from the patient with textbook images, and full software functionality is required.

Facilities for printing images on film must remain available, even in the still imaginary hospitals where all internal image handling is performed by means of PACS. In some cases, images will be requested by other hospitals or small medical practices which do not have PACS. Film imagers which produce films with sufficient image quality are all based on the laser scanner principle, where rows of image pixels are transferred to the film one by one by means of an intensity-modulated scanning laser beam.

1.2.6 Data Base Management

Integration of the HIS (and radiology information systems, RIS) data base into the PACS data base is required for various reasons:

- Data from the HIS (e.g., patient demographics) are needed for the identification of the images in the PACS.
- Images should be displayed on the PACS viewing station together with the related alphanumerical patient information (e.g., previous reports, medical history, anamnesis, and laboratory test results) from the HIS.
- HIS functionality, such as report editing and queries into the patient's medical history, should be available on the PACS viewing station.

- To obtain acceptable response times, intelligent image migration strategies based on data from the HIS, e.g., patient location and appointment, will be required (Bakker 1986).

The alphanumerical data required for PACS are largely the same as the data already available in the HIS data base. For performance reasons, it could be attractive to duplicate part of the HIS data base into the PACS data base. Duplicating too much data will lead to unnecessary operations to maintain the consistency between the two data bases (Bakker et al. 1990).

1.2.7 Organization and Procedures

To obtain all of the above potential benefits, the organization of the hospital must be adapted including the involved clinical procedures. For example, the advantage of images being available more quickly is limited if the reports on the images have not been completed. Thus to provide the complete results of the examination faster than with the film-based system, it is necessary to perform immediate reporting.

1.3 Genesis

Various external developments have – as indicated above – triggered the start of PACS, e.g., the development of mass-storage technology and the increased use of digital modalities. The first conference dedicated to PACS was held in the United States in 1982 (Duerinckx 1982). The first special PACS occasion in Europe was the NATO workshop in Braunlage in 1984 (Hoehne 1984). The first sign of PACS activities in Japan was the establishment of the Japan Association of PACS (J-PACS) in 1982.

Most of the participants of the first conference on PACS had a technical background, and came from universities. The implementation groups at the hospitals had not been formed at this time. Looking at the proceedings of the first PACS conference (Duerinckx 1982), early PACS research focused mainly on the potential opportunities of developing technology for archiving, communication, and the presentation of medical images. The general belief was that these technologies would soon be able to fulfill the hospital requirements, for example, that the optical disk technology would be able to supply the required capacity for image archiving, and that the PACS requirements for communication and presentation of the images could be provided soon with the fast developing fiber-optic network and CRT display technology, respectively. The possibilities of teleradiology were already discussed at that time. It was recognized at an early stage that standardization of file formats and interfaces would be crucial for the implementation of PACS. This led to the foundation of the American College of Radiologists/National Electrical Manufacturers Association (ACR/NEMA) standardization committee. The mutual relationship between PACS and image processing was clearly identified.

Early PACS research focused mainly on the technical development and clinical application of isolated components, primarily workstations and archive devices. Most of the first scientists involved in PACS had backgrounds in the development of those information technologies which were expected to be used in PACS such as network, display, storage, and image processing technology. Other scientists were psychophysicists and radiologists involved in diagnostic image quality research, and financial managers and health economists interested in cost analysis.

Current research focuses on the implementation of PACS with limited functionality in part of the hospital. These partial implementations are supported by dedicated technical developments. In addition, evaluation research is being performed on a number of issues such as diagnostic image quality evaluation, PACS performance analysis, adaptation of the hospital organization and procedures, and technology assessment. Some groups are also studying system integration aspects of PACS, such as PACS–HIS–RIS integration, network architecture and protocols, and system availability.

In future the development and implementation of full and hospital-wide PACS should be taken in hand.

Surprisingly many of the concepts which are still viable today were already presented at the very first conference dedicated to PACS. However, a few of the early ideas in PACS were abandoned at a later stage.

At some moment in time, a new type of mass-storage technology, i.e., vertical magnetization, was expected to become of use in PACS, however, this plan never matured. The same seems to hold for the optical tape which potentially could provide mass storage for very low cost. Until now no usable product has appeared on the market.

Two other examples are related to the problem of the limited intensity range of a CRT compared with the light box. One early idea was to solve this by using color, but this idea was rejected as soon as it became clear that color in X-ray images was not acceptable to radiologists. Another potential solution was to increase the perceived contrast by applying contrast enhancemen (adaptive histogram equalization). This was studied thoroughly, but because of apparent and unavoidable artifacts, it was not accepted either.

Another early expectation in PACS was that digital image processing to support the diagnostic process would be developed and implemented soon. The development of a clinically usable technique appeared, however, to be much more complicated than expected, and up to now there are very few examples of the actual clinical use of such software.

1.4 PACS Research

Past and current research topics on PACS will be treated individually and for a number of evaluation issues (Greinacher et al. 1985).

1.4.1 Workstations

The research on workstations has many aspects: first of all, insight must be obtained into the clinical requirements, then the required software and hardware should be developed, and finally the realized viewing station must be evaluated in the clinical environment (Arenson et al. 1990).

The spatial resolution required of the workstation monitors depends on the modality used to obtain the images. Nuclear medicine images have a very small matrix size (some have a matrix size of 64 × 64) compared with most radiological images. This does however not imply that nuclear medicine can use common PACS viewing stations with only one screen, because in contrast to other radiological images, most nuclear medicine images are presented in color. In fact, special mini-PACS systems have been developed and implemented in nuclear medicine departments. These can be based on general purpose hardware because of the limited image file size and the relatively small number of images produced per year.

Another modality with a limited matrix size is US, where a video image (512 × 512 and 8 bits deep) provides sufficient image quality. Because of the smaller image matrix, many requirements are less severe than for other image modalities. This is the reason why a large portion of the few (partial) PACS systems that are actually applied in clinical routine are used exclusively for US images.

The digital imaging modalities such as CT, MRI, and digital subtraction angiography (DSA) have a smaller matrix size (512 × 512 or 256 × 256), but still require a higher contrast range (10–12 bits per matrix element). However, because digital modality studies comprise many images (up to 50 for an MRI examination), the display surface of a viewing station for digital modality studies must be at least as large as that for traditional X-ray examinations. Furthermore, the software facilities for navigation through a digital modality study consisting of 20–50 images must be much more complex than those required for traditional X-ray procedures, which usually consist of 2–3 images.

The conventional projection X-ray techniques (e.g., chest, bone, and abdomen), which still account for over 80% of all radiological examinations, require a large image file (2048 × 2048 and 10–12 bits per pixel). The issue of whether these images have to be displayed on a monitor with a 2000 × 2000 matrix must still be investigated. The alternative is to use a 1000 × 1000 monitor, on which part of the image can be enlarged up to its true resolution. Mammography images will probably form a separate group, requiring an image matrix of more than 2000 × 2000 and a display of at least 2000 × 2000, since the reporting of mammography films (searching for extremely small microcalcifications) is often done with a magnifying glass.

The requirements for image dimensions mentioned above are those needed for primary diagnosis. It has been suggested that for other tasks the image requirements may be less severe. Some PACS manufacturers have adapted this idea in their PACS configuration. In the radiological department, the images are distributed and displayed with their full resolution and accuracy, but the image file size, and thus the resolution and/or accuracy, is reduced before the images are distributed to and displayed in the referring departments. This brings savings in the costs of the network and the viewing stations, but it is yet unclear whether the reduced image quality is really acceptable for referring physicians.

A lot of work has been carried out in the development of the various image query, display, manipulation, processing, and analysis software modules. The hardware on which viewing stations are based can be subdivided into general purpose platforms and dedicated devices. The diagnostic stations, meant for primary diagnosis, are always based on dedicated hardware and include special graphics boards to control the monitors. Most of the referring stations are created around general purpose (e.g., reduced instruction set computer, RISC based) workstations.

In addition to the hardware components and the software modules, it is important to provide a viewing station with a good human interface. Decisions must be made which operations are performed automatically depending on the image, and which must be explicitly evoked by the user. Many physical tools are available for the human–machine interaction, e.g., key board, function keys, dials, track ball, mouse, and touch screen. It is clear that a selection must be made. Important developments have been made at the University of Arizona, for example, where an advanced touch screen workstation has been realized in cooperation with Toshiba.

The clinical application of these multimodality viewing stations has been limited until now. The evaluation of viewing stations requires them to be used for realistic tasks in the clinical environment. This is only possible when they are incorporated into a working PACS environment, to provide the images required for the tasks.

1.4.2 Storage Devices

Research has been performed into the development of file management software for jukeboxes with optical disks to be used for long-term image archiving. Alternative strategies have been devised for the distribution of the newly acquired images across the optical disks. Chronological storage leads to a maximum filling of the storage space: the oldest disk must be removed when all disks are completely filled. The allocation of sets of disks to groups of patients will reduce the number of disks containing images of one patient, and thus fewer disks need to be moved around in the jukebox to read the images of one patient. This strategy will, however, lead to a lesser degree of filling.

Other studies have been carried out into the applicability of sets of magnetic disks for the temporal storage of those images which will be needed for viewing in the short term. Parallel retrieval from multiple disks provides faster access. The issue of prefetching attracts more and more attention, because many developers recognize that PACS is only viable if some kind of prefetching is used.

1.4.3 Network

Originally the PACS network was devised as one homogeneous structure, where all nodes were connected by one and the same kind of technique. The topology could either be a single line, a closed ring, or a star, possibly a multistar. If one single network structure could not transmit as much data as required, then the network could be divided into two or more segments by introducing bridges.

Recently, more precise schemes for the network structure have been proposed. The load of the network should be reduced by dividing it into separate areas so that most traffic remains within each of the areas and a relatively small fraction of the traffic passes from one area to another. Depending on the organizational structure of the hospital, areas which are combinations of modalities and medical specialities could be found, for example, in neurology, chest, and pediatrics.

The fastest connections are required between the workstations and the image archive. It is here that images are retrieved interactively. The requirements for the link between acquisition devices and archive facilities are less severe. Speed is not critical, but sufficient capacity for the transmission of all acquired images is needed. For reasons of performance and for reasons of availability (fault tolerance), it would be useful to establish some connections with multiple network paths. A network such as this with more than one possible route between two nodes, will require a much more complex traffic control system than a network with only one possible route.

1.4.4 Teleradiology

A special development related to PACS is that of teleradiology, a term used to indicate the transmission and display of radiological images, including the relevant patient information, with the objective that the reporting of the images may take place at a location remote from where the images were acquired. The technical requirements for a teleradiology system are easier to fulfill than those for a complete PACS. Teleradiology comprises image entry, communication (not within a hospital, but between hospitals, and at a lower speed than PACS), and display. It was expected early in the 1980s that teleradiology would be a good stepping stone towards PACS. Various teleradiology systems were developed, and the United States army, which is often confronted in combat situations as well as in peace time with the need for teleradiology, performed two extensive teleradiology field trials. The results showed that equipment reliability, image quality, ease of use, and performance speed were insufficient to allow professional acceptance of the system (Harrington 1985).

1.4.5 System Integration

Implementation of PACS requires a tight coupling with the information systems relevant for PACS, i.e., HIS and RIS, in the hospital. PACS requires demographic patient data from the HIS for the identification of the acquired images. PACS also needs alphanumerical medical data to be displayed in coherence with the images. PACS users need access to HIS functions, e.g., facilities to perform queries into the medical history. PACS image management strategies need HIS information as parameters for the related algorithms.

Much preparatory work in this area has been done by work group VIII "RIS/HIS/PACS" of the ACR/NEMA committee. A dozen actual PACS–HIS or PACS–RIS couplings have been realized in clinical sites over three continents. Up to now most couplings are unidirectional and connect the existing RIS with the PACS. An example of the development and the clinical evaluation of a coupling with an integrated HIS, including a RIS, has been performed within the scope of the Dutch PACS project (Lodder et al. 1989).

When computer systems comprise so many components, they become vulnerable. Failures in one component may lead to total system breakdown unless special measures have been taken. The usage integrity of large information systems such as PACS, and even more so HIS is also at risk, unless special precautions are taken.

The availability of images in the archives is positively influenced because optical disk storage media are less vulnerable than magnetic tape or magnetic disk. Magnetic interference cannot damage the data, and mechanical contacts with the read/write head do not occur in optical disks. The latest system architecture developments suggest that some critical components are duplicated (e.g., the image data base management system). Magnetic disks for the temporal storage of unique copies of newly acquired images are duplicated (mirrored disks). Of course, such measures will lead to extra costs.

The existing access authorization rules from the HIS should be used for access to the PACS, since the HIS data is accessible through the PACS. For the PACS, user identification passwords or magnetic/smart cards can be used.

Since performance is an important factor in the acceptance of a PACS by its users, it is of great importance to make an estimation of the expected performance before the PACS is actually implemented. The attempt to implement a PACS that demonstrates insufficient performance will lead to aversion to PACS, which will in turn hinder future implementations. A useful tool for performance analysis is computer simulation. Various studies in this area have been performed based on stochastic processes (Martinez et al. 1990) and on semantic data models and parallel decision processes (Stut et al. 1990).

1.4.6 Standardization

In the area of file formats and communication protocols for digital radiological images, various standards have been published. The earliest and most important one is the ACR/NEMA standard. The medical imaging processing standard (MIPS) standard has been derived from the ACR/NEMA standard, but it is adapted to the Japanese characters. The standard product interface (SPI) standard, developed by Siemens and Philips together, is an extension of ACR/NEMA. SPI supports the grouping of images, which is unknown in ACR/NEMA. The Papyrus standard, developed in the Geneva University Hospital, allows multiple images to be stored in a single file.

Various hardware interface boards have been realized both by university groups and by the industry. An extensive evaluation, including actual tests of the communication between two types of such boards (from different vendors), have led to the suggestion to split the standard. The idea is to choose an existing protocol such as transmission control protocol/internet protocol (TCP/IP) and Ethernet for the lower layers (of the open standard interconnect, OSI, communication frame work) and to keep the ACR/NEMA standard only for the upper layers (McNeill et al. 1990).

1.4.7 Diagnostic Image Quality

Much research has been done in an attempt to demonstrate that the diagnostic quality of digital images displayed on a monitor is not inferior to that of the same images on film viewed on a light box. These investigations give an indication of the specifications of PACS components which are required to assure diagnostic quality. Many studies have been done to measure the effect of data compression and other processing techniques on diagnostic quality, and various methods have been used. Radiologists have been asked to give their subjective idea of the quality of the images, but the subjective idea of a radiologist about the image quality of a certain image does not correspond with his ability to make the correct diagnosis based on that image. The method which is commonly accepted is the receiver operating characteristics technique (Swets and Pickett 1982).

1.4.8 Technology Assessment

Before a PACS system is implemented purely as a tool for the daily routine, rather than a research experiment, the economic and health care implications of such an introduction must be evaluated. Important elements in a technology assessment (TA) of PACS are the costs of the system components, of its introduction and of its operation, and of the changes it will bring in the hospital. On the other hand, direct savings are made because films are no longer produced, archived, or handled. Furthermore, PACS is expected to improve the efficiency of the image logistics, and thus save time for the medical professionals and improve health care for the patients. A thorough study, which takes the effects of the decreasing prices of information technology products into account, indicates that the costs of PACS might be compensated by its savings at the turn of the century (Van Gennip et al. 1991). This outcome depends heavily on the assumptions about the necessary functionality, especially of the workstations, on the number of workstations, and on the cost figures.

1.4.9 PACS Manufacturers

The major PACS manufacturers (and some of their main evaluation sites) are AT&T/Philips (Georgetown/USA, Bologna/Italy), Hitachi (Kyoto, Japan), NEC (Hokkaido, Japan), Siemens (Graz, Austria, Iowa, USA) and Toshiba (Kochi, Japan). Other companies offer PACS components. Various film manufacturers such as Agfa, Fuji, Kodak, Konica and 3M sell film digitizers, film imagers, and image cameras. CR systems are sold by Fuji, Philips, and Siemens (and soon Agfa). The development activities of these manufacturers are concentrated in North America and Japan. Only a small amount of development is taking place in Europe.

1.5 Clinical Implementation and Evaluation

Considering that most concepts of PACS have been present from the very beginning, the actual realization and implementation of PACS is proceeding surprisingly slowly. There are many reasons for this. First of all, PACS is a multidisciplinary problem, which has many technical aspects in various areas such as communication hardware and software, mass storage techniques, display devices, and data base and information systems. It is not possible for most single vendors to assimilate such a mixture of hardware and software knowledge. With time, it became clear that the clinical requirements had been underestimated. The acceptance of PACS by medical professionals has been slowed down because of their doubts about image quality and the performance of the PACS until now. Implementation has also been hampered by the fact that the equipment is very expensive, while tangible savings are not sufficiently large, and potential health care and organizational benefits as yet difficult to demonstrate.

From the experience gained in some of the recent PACS implementation projects, one might conclude that much has been learned from these studies (BAZIS 1990, Elliott 1990), for example, that the reliability and the performance of the equipment is very important for its acceptation by the medical professionals, and that it is essential for PACS to be integrated with HIS (and RIS). It has also become clear that the performance of PACS based on the current information technologies depends critically on the implementation of intelligent image management software, and that the potential benefits are mainly in the improvement of the logistic procedures.

On the basis of the first 10 years of PACS, it is realistic to say that the clinical application of full and hospital-wide PACS is probably another 10 years away. However, it appears technically feasible to implement a partial PACS now, and this is an attractive and necessary stepping stone towards full-blown PACS. Currently about up to 30 hospitals have implemented a limited scale PACS which is used to some extent in clinical routine. The archiving of digital images has not yet replaced the production of films. In all implementations, at least for legal reasons and in some cases also to obtain reimbursement, all images are still also made on film.

A PACS implementation is mostly carried out by a larger (university) hospital, and is preferably not only supported by the radiology department, but also by the central administration, because PACS provides more benefits when it is also installed at the referring departments and when it is connected to the central HIS. There are various types of implementations. One possibility is to install a PACS from one single PACS vendor. In fact, the full system is always obtained from multiple vendors because of the interfaces between the PACS, the acquisition modalities, and the HIS. If all PACS components come from one vendor, there is currently not much choice; about five manufacturers offer a complete set of PACS components. In this case, many responsibilities can be delegated to the manufacturer, although this is not without costs. Besides, the hospital will strongly be at the mercy of that manufacturer. If specifications are not meeting the actual clinical need, and that is very well possible since the clinical procedures will change with the implementation of a PACS, changing the equipment beyond the original specifications will be difficult and costly. Adaptations to local requirements, which are certainly needed, will be very hard. Still, the hospital remains responsible for the integration of PACS into the other information systems. PACS–RIS–HIS interfacing between systems from different vendors will not be easy, even if all systems use the same communication protocol; the allocation of user functions and systems tasks is not yet standardized. Future extensions are difficult because the size of the implementation is limited by the capacity of the components that the selected manufacturer sells.

Another choice is that of the multivendor PACS solution. In this case it will not be easy to get connecting components, even on the communication level, since although standards exist, they are either not implemented or might be interpreted differently, in which case the hospital will have to do the interfacing by itself.

The third, most challenging, option is that the hospital buys general purpose components from many different manufacturers and creates the

PACS system itself. One advantage is that the individual components will be much cheaper, but the method will require a lot of effort to adapt the components to fit the PACS requirements. The network architecture and capacity of individual storage components can be chosen to fit the local structure of the hospital. Products based on the latest technological developments can be used in this option. The great disadvantage is that the hospital's commitments are much larger: it needs to buy the components, but also needs to pay the salaries of an experienced development team, and the software development costs have to be provided by one institute. These sizable expenses make this option only feasible for hospitals that are large and that can obtain considerable funding, from either the government or the industry. Furthermore, hardware and software maintenance will be much more complicated in this case since the products come from many manufacturers, and have been changed in one-of-a-kind specials.

Funding for implementations comes from different sources. In North America from the industry, from the military, and from the central government (e.g., National Institutes of Health). In Europe, it comes mainly from the government (e.g., the European Community or at national or state level). In Japan, the implementation is more nationally guided, while funds are obtained from the industry and from the government (Akisada 1990).

1.6 Organizations and Conferences

1.6.1 Organizations

Various organizations are active in the PACS field. The ACR/NEMA standardization committee was formed at the beginning of 1983 under the auspices of the American College of Radiologists, representing the users, and the National Electrical Manufacturers Association, representing the manufacturers. The early target of this committee was to develop a standard interface for the exchange of images and related data between medical imaging devices and PACS components. Various working groups were formed to treat issues such as hardware and protocols, data format, RIS–HIS–PACS, and data compression. As a result of these activities, the first version of the ACR/NEMA 300 standard was published in 1985. The second version of the 300 standard was published in 1988 (ACR/NEMA 1988). This and standards on other aspects (PACS–HIS–RIS interface) are continually being developed further (Horii 1991).

The European Committee for Recommendation – Standards in Computer aspects of Diagnostic Imaging (ECR-SCDI) was founded on December 10, 1990. The objective of this committee is – as its name already indicates – to devise recommendations and standards for computer applications within the field of diagnostic imaging. It is sponsored by the European Association in Radiology (EAR) and EuroPACS. EuroPACS is the European association of research, development, and user groups in the field of PACS. The objective of EuroPACS is to promote the exchange of information in the field. EuroPACS was founded during the NATO workshop in Braunlage, September 1984. The main activities of EuroPACS are the organization of the annual international conference and the publication of its newsletter. The newsletter contains information about forthcoming conferences, current PACS projects in Europe, and a list of the members and other PACS interested scientists that receive the newsletter.

The J-PACS committee was founded in 1982 and is composed of representatives from the industry. Its aim is to promote, coordinate, and cooperate in developing and implementing PACS technology. The JRS-PACS committee, which is composed of members of the Japan Radiological Society, is working to bring scientists and industry closer together in PACS activities.

In Japan, the MIPS standardization committee has been brought together by the Ministry of Industry and Trade (MITI) to study the standardization of medical image processing systems. In 1987 the draft MIPS digital interface standard, based primarily on the ACR/NEMA standard, was published.

The Society for Computer Applications in Radiology (SCAR) was founded in 1988. It organizes the biannual SCAR meeting in the USA and sponsors the CAR conference in Europe. SCAR publishes the quarterly *Journal of digital imaging*, which started in February 1989. Recently, in November 1990, SCAR started to distribute its own newsletter *SCAR news*.

1.6.2 Conferences

The earliest conference on PACS was held as the First International Conference and Workshop on Picture Archiving and Communication Systems (PACS) in Newport Beach, California, January 18–21, 1982 (Duerinckx 1982). This meeting has proven to be the first of still continuing series of meetings all organized by the International Society for Optical Engineering (SPIE). During the more recent SPIE meetings, PACS design and evaluation was treated during one of the four tracks. Short presentations on individual research activities were contributed.

The first meeting on PACS in Japan was the First International Symposium on PACS and Personal Health Data (PHD) held in July, 1984. This meeting has been repeated each year in combination with the Medical Imaging Technology meeting. The combination has been sponsored by the Japan Association of Medical Imaging Technology (JAMIT).

Two NATO Advanced Study Institute workshops in the PACS field were held. Both workshops lasted for 2 weeks. Scientists from all NATO countries presented their research and discussed their opinions. The audience came from very different disciplines such as computer hardware and software scientists, medical doctors, physicists, and administrators.

The first PACS-related NATO workshop entitled Pictorial Information Systems in Medicine was held in 1984, in Braunlage, FRG (Höhne 1986). This workshop, which was held in the early days of PACS, was primarily oriented around the technologies that were expected to create the various building blocks for a PACS such as information system technology, image processing technology, and display technology. The current situation in the film-based radiology department was illustrated. Some PACS research results and the very first clinical experiences with small-scale PACS were presented. The audience of this workshop appeared to be quite dominated by the technical scientists.

The second PACS-related NATO workshop, titled Picture Archiving and Communication Systems in Medicine, was held in Evian, France (Huang et al. 1991). The invited presentations from this workshop can be subdivided into three groups. Firstly, lectures on the technical specifications of PACS components and system integration were given. Secondly, the current PACS and related research in each of various countries were presented. Thirdly, results of clinical evaluations and PACS research projects were demonstrated. Finally, many short papers about current work were presented. During this workshop there was a good balance between the potential users (medical doctors), the developers of PACS (hardware and software engineers), and others involved (scientists, administrators) which certainly contributed to the fruitful multifaceted discussions.

The first EuroPACS meeting took place in September 1984. Since then an international meeting of EuroPACS has been organized each year. The EuroPACS meetings are of an informal character, and each of them is hosted by a different group. The presentations are generally concise and concern actual research work. Over the years, the meeting has been held in various European countries, namely, FRG, France, Sweden, The Netherlands, Belgium, and Italy. The proceedings of the meeting are not produced as such, but a collection of papers from some of the meetings has been published (Newell and de Valk 1988).

Every 2 years since 1985, a computer-assisted radiology (CAR) meeting has been organized in Berlin, Germany (Lemke et al. 1985). The topics at the conference are digital image acquisition (MRI, CT, CR, DSA, US), image management and communication, medical workstations, and HIS–RIS–PACS integration. Further topics include application systems for computer-assisted radiodiagnosis, radiotherapy, neuroradiology, and orthopedics. The CAR conference is combined with an extended technical exhibit. In June 1990, the first S/CAR meeting was organized under the auspices of the SCAR society (Arenson and Friedenberg 1990). In the future the location of the CAR and SCAR meeting will alternate between Europe and the United States.

The first international conference on Image Management and Communication in Patient Care (IMAC) was held in Washington DC, USA, June 4–8, 1989 (Mun et al. 1990). The second IMAC conference was held in Kyoto, Japan, April 10–13, 1991. IMAC meetings are truly international meetings that do not so much focus on technical research, but rather explore the role of PACS in health care, the current technical and organizational barriers for implementation, quality of care issues, technology assessment, and evaluation methodology.

Many other conferences, although not purely devoted to PACS, include papers on PACS and PACS-related topics. Such meetings are, for example, the Radiological Society of North America (RSNA) and the European International Conference on Radiology (ICR) in the field of radiology and the MEDINFO (organized by the IMIA-International Medical Informatics Association), and Medical Informatics Europe (MIE) conferences, in the field of computer science.

References

ACR/NEMA (1988) ACR/NEMA 300–1988. Standard for digital imaging and communications. National Electrical Manufacturers Association, 2101 L Street, Washington, DC 20037, USA

Akisada M (1990) Present status and perspective of PACS activities in Japan, (1990) In: Muu SK, Grebermann M, Hendee WR, Shannon R (eds) Proceedings of the First International Conference on Image Management and Communication in Patient Care: implementation and impact. June 4–8, 1989, Washington, DC, USA. IEEE Computer Society, Los Alamitos, CA, USA

Arenson RL, Friedenberg RM (eds) (1990) Computer applications to assist radiology. S/CAR90. June 13–16, 1990, Anaheim, California, USA. Symposia Foundation, Carlsbad, CA, USA

Arenson RL, Chakrabarty DP, Seshadri SB, Kundel HL (1990) The digital imaging workstation. Radiology 176: 303–315

Bakker AR, Didden H, de Valk JPJ, Massar ADA (1986) Considerations on an algorithm for activation of images in a multi-layered storage system within a PACS. In: Schneider RH, Dwyer SJ III (eds) Proceedings of Application of Optical Instrumentation in Medicine XIV and Picture Archiving and Communication Systems (PACSIV) for Medical Applications. Proc SPIE 626: 637–640

Bakker AR, Lodder H, Kouwenberg JML (1990) Traffic between PACS and HIS/RIS: data or information? In: Dwyer SJ III, Jost RG (eds) Proceedings of Medical Imaging IV: PACS System Design and Evaluation. Proc SPIE 1234: 495–500

BAZIS, Utrecht University Hospital, Philips (1990) Concluding report: Dutch PACS project picture archiving and communication system, phase I (1986–1989). Available from BAZIS, Leiden, The Netherlands

Duerinckx AJ (ed) (1982) First international conference and workshop on picture archiving and communication systems (PACS) for medical applications. SPIE 318

Elliott LP, Mun SK, Horii SC, Benson H (1990) Digital imaging network system (DINS) evaluation report, March 1990. Available from Department of Radiology, Georgetown University Medical Center, Dept. of Radiology, 3800 Reservoir Road NW, Washington, DC 20007, USA

Greinacher CFC, Fuchs D, Müller K (1985) PACS – A topic of the future becomes reality. Electromedica 53: 96–103

Harrington MB, Miller KD, Kerlin BD (1985) The 1984–85 teleradiology field trial executive summary, December 1985. Available from MITRE, 7525 Colshire Drive, Mc Lean, Virginia 22102–3481, USA

Höhne KH (ed) (1986) Pictorial information systems in medicine. Springer, Berlin Heidelberg New York (NATO ASI series, vol 19)

Horii SC (1991) An introduction to the ACR/NEMA standards. In: Huang HK (ed) Elements of digital radiology. Prentice-Hall, Englewood Cliffs, NJ, USA

Huang HK, Ratib O, Bakker AR, Witte G (eds) (1991) Picture archiving and communication systems in medicine. Proceedings of the NATO ASI workshop, Evian, France, October 14–26, 1990. Springer, Berlin Heidelberg New York (in press)

Kato H (1990) Computed radiography. In: Proceedings of the First International Conference on Image Management and Communication in Patient care: implementation and impact. June 4–8, 1989, Washington, DC. IEEE Computer Society, Los Alamitos, CA, USA, pp 108–116

Lemke HU, Rhodes ML, Jaffee CC, Felix R (1985) Proceedings of the international symptosium CAR'85 computer assisted radiology. Springer, Berlin Heidelberg New York

Lodder H, Van Poppel BM, De Valk JPJ, Wilmink HBM, Ising C, Bakker AR (1989) HIS-PACS coupling in practice. In: Schneider RH, Dwyer SJ III, Jort RG (eds) Proceedings of Medical Imaging III: PACS System Design and Evaluation. Proc SPIE 1093: 301–306

Martinez R, Sanders WH, Alsafadi Y, Nam J, Ozeki T, Komatsu K (1990) Performance evaluation of a picture archiving and communication system using stochastic activity networks. In: Dwyer SJ III, Jost RG (eds) Proceeds of Medical Imaging IV: PACS system design and evaluation. Proc SPIE 1234: 167–178

McNeill KM, Osada M, Martinez R, Tawara K, Maloney K, Vercillo R, Ozeki T, Komatsu K, Dallas WJ, Fukushima Y, Toshimitsu A (1990) Evaluation of the ACR/NEMA standard for communications in digital radiology. IEEE Transactions on medical imaging, 9–13 September 1990

Mun SK, Greberman M, Hendee WR, Shannon R (eds) (1990) Proceedings of the first international conference on image management and communication in patient care: implementation and impact. June 4–8, 1989, Washington, DC, IEEE Computer Society, Los Alamitos, CA, USA

Newell JA, de Valk JPJ (eds) Med Informa 13(4)

Ottes FP, Bakker AR, Kouwenberg JML (1990) Implementation of picture archiving and communication systems in hospitals guided by dedicated software. In: O'Moore R, Bengtsson S, Bryant JR, Bryden JS (eds) Proceedings of the 9th international congress on medical informatics in europe (MIE 90), Glasgow, 20–23 August 1990. Springer, Berlin Heidelberg New York Tokyo (Lecture Notes in Medical Informatics, vol 40), pp 521–526

Stut WJJ, Van Steen MR, Groenewegen LPJ, Bakker AR (1990) Picture archiving and communication system design issues: the importance of modelling and simulation. J Digital Imaging 3/4: 246–253

Swets JA, Pickett RM (1982) Evaluation of diagnostic systems: methods from signal detection theory. Academic, New York

Van Gennip EMSJ, Van Poppel BM, Bakker AR, Ottes FP, Kouwenberg JML, Wilmink JBM (1991) An analysis of the costs of a hospital wide picture and archiving communication system with the software package CAPACITY. Eur J Radiol 12: 69–78

2 Medical Requirements for Clinical Integration

M. Osteaux, R. Van den Broeck, Y. Temmerman, and B. Wein

2.1 Introduction

2.1.1 The Clinical Advantages of PACS Technology

Picture archiving and communication systems (PACS) technology has – at least potentially – substantial advantages over the conventional technique, and there is no doubt that PACS will gain acceptance if the necessary research and development is permitted. With this in mind, it is, however, necessary to understand the functional medical needs and the nontechnical obstacles that hamper its implementation in the hospital environment. It must be remembered that the medical community has been accustomed to handling conventional (film-based) radiology for almost a century. This tradition is embedded deeply in the organization of the health care system, and this is true not only for the department of radiology, but also for the hospital community as a whole and for communication with extramural specialists and general practitioners.

The "good old film" also has a number of advantages which must be considered. The spatial resolution of film is high – up to 10 pairs of lines per millimeter – and its handling is quite easy. For viewing, a simple light box or even the light from a window is sufficient. Conventional films can be sampled and sorted in folders, which then physically accompany a patient on his or her way through a hospital. The production of conventional films is straightforward and not as expensive in terms of logistics as the digital method of sampling and distributing images. We can state that in order to outperform the conventional method, PACS must bring major advantages in clinical use and must be integrated into the whole chain of medical events, inside and outside the department of radiology and even the hospital. The clinical advantages of PACS (see Chaps. 1 and 9) are discussed in the following.

PACS leads to better (easier, faster) access to archived images. Using the conventional system, primary reporting can be performed efficiently. The radiologist reports on films placed on a specialized light box directly after the study or within a maximum of 1 day, since the films are kept in the department until needed for reporting. Access to films from preliminary examinations is, however, more difficult, since these must be fetched from archives. Problems may occur if earlier images cannot be retrieved within a period of 1 h or half a day or if indeed they are lost totally. Depending on the medical indication for X-ray examinations, i.e., whether emergency, follow-up, or routine, this might also have adverse effects on treatment. Comparison with preliminary examination is a key issue in medicine in several situations. In oncology, for example, comparisons with earlier documents are the basic tool for evaluating the efficacy of treatment, in orthopedics comparisons are made for medicolegal reasons, and in emergency they are made to find out any acute changes in patients.

One important factor is the period between the time when the patient consults or is hospitalized and the time when, after a correct diagnosis has been made, an efficient treatment is instituted. Shortening that interval is at least a factor of psychological comfort to the patient; in some situations, it can even be medically important or even life-saving. It is also a cost-saving factor for the health care system, especially for inpatients. Therefore, everything that can shorten the delays in the diagnostic chain represents a substantial qualitative advance. PACS technology can be a major clinical improvement here.

Image manipulation capabilities are also an important factor. If the information is kept on a digital basis, the possibility of using the image as input for different types of specialized diagnostic exploitations is retained (e.g., multiplanar reconstruction from magnetic resonance imaging (MRI), three-dimensional data sets, three-dimensional reconstruction, automated image analysis) or for computer-aided therapeutic procedures (e.g., radiotherapeutic treatment planning, stereotaxy, and surgical simulation).

Sharing of infrastructure is more an organizational than a medical advantage. The link between different systems allows the use of a common infrastructure (typically image storage, laser printer, and digitizer) and allows a module of equipment to be bypassed during maintenance without bringing all medical activities to a standstill.

The implementation of PACS may be advantageous for scientific and educational purposes. Digital archiving constitutes an ideal basis for scientific and educational retrieval and collection, especially if a dedicated indexing technique is used. PACS technology also lends itself very well to coupling with decision-support systems.

In order to reproduce the described advantages in clinical practice, however PACS must be integrated well into the hospital system. In order to achieve that goal, it is necessary to analyze correctly the functional activities connected with imaging within the hospital.

2.2 The Structure of Imaging Activities Within the Hospital

2.2.1 Some Definitions: Radiology, Diagnostic Imaging, Medical Imaging, Microscopy, Endoscopy

Radiology or diagnostic radiology has evolved in several directions since Roentgen's discovery at the end of the nineteenth century. Conventional radiology encompasses bone and joint radiography, chest and breast imaging, and various specialized applications of contrast media such as in digestive radiology, intravenous pyelography, angiography, and lymphography. In the 1970s, some digital imaging techniques appeared in radiology such as computed tomography (CT) and digital substraction angiography (DSA), which make use of secondary digitization of fluoroscopy. There is also a more recent trend towards replacing film as primary support for information in conventional radiology by electronic reading and digitization (phosphor storage systems, for example).

The two last decades have also seen a tremendous development of techniques that use physical methods other than the transmission of X-rays such as ultrasonography and MRI. These two modalities have been incorporated into the functional cluster of radiology. A new generic name has been created to cover the whole field, i.e., X-ray and non-X-ray, namely, diagnostic imaging. Diagnostic imaging also encompasses nuclear medicine. Nuclear medicine, which makes use of the internal administration of isotope tracers is (partly) incorporated into the radiological concept in the United States and the FRG. In the rest of Europe, the place of nuclear medicine varies according to country, but it is generally considered as a separate specialty. Finally, the word "radiology" designates a cluster of imaging modalities, including nuclear medicine in the United States, which would be better labeled "diagnostic imaging".

Diagnostic imaging encompasses conventional radiology, angiography, DSA, CT, digital radiology, echography, MRI, and nuclear medicine. Diagnostic imaging must be regarded as a functional entity within the hospital and outside, too, since it also involves groups of specialists, specific scientific societies, specialized journals, and a specific cluster of industries manufacturing equipment.

Medical imaging is a generic term, designating every medical procedure where the diagnosis is based upon the technical realization and interpretation of images. It includes not only diagnostic imaging, but also other methods such as microscopy, endoscopy, and specific techniques for plastic surgery and dermatology. Regrettably, several European languages such as French, German, Dutch and Spanish have translated diagnostic imaging as medical imaging. This terminology is confusing and impedes correct understanding and planning of PACS technology in hospitals. PACS technology has been developed to deal with diagnostic imaging only.

The specific problems of microscopy, endoscopy, or other medical imaging sources are not within the scope of this book. However, in order to be able to define a correct strategy for PACS as an overall information system in the hospital, a short description of these fields is necessary. Microscopy in clinical use refers mostly to conventional light transmission microscopy, while electron microscopy remains mainly a research tool. Microscopy is widely used in diverse specialties such as anatomopathology (histology), cytology, genetics, and hematology. Within the hospital, the number of images generated by anatomopathology and hematology is already quite considerable, but mass screening by cytology (for detection of cancer of the cervix uteri or differentiation of fine needle aspiration material) produces an enormous amount of additional material. The objective requirements of microscopy, i.e., spatial and color resolution, differ widely from those of diagnostic imaging. Automated diagnosis by means of form recognition and expert systems have been developed, especially in the fields of hematology and genetics, and the industry dealing with these fields is totally different from the one dealing with diagnostic imaging.

Endoscopy refers to direct visualization of internal human cavities by the introduction of specific endoscopes, using the technique of light transmission by optical fiber, or, more recently, miniaturized camera and digital capabilities. Endoscopy is used in a large number of medical specialties including gastroenterology, urology, pneumology, orthopedics, and surgery, just to mention a few. For each cavity examined, specialized apparatus and manufacturers exist. Physically, the spatial resolution and restitution of the color are of tremendous diagnostic importance. It must be observed that endoscopy is moving relatively rapidly towards digitalization. Various works are presently being undertaken to incorporate endoscopy in a PACS-like system, but these are still in an early phase.

Finally, the specific functional requirements and optimal architecture systems for microscopy and endoscopy, must be described and experienced by specialists in these fields, and the authors of this book definitely do not come into this category. However, by analogy with the necessary concept of decentralization within PACS (see Chap. 9), we can suggest:

1. The development of a dedicated decentralized system tailored to suit the specific needs of user clusters. This should have a dedicated local area network and specific standards.
2. The need for integration with the common monitor of specialized information systems, e.g., a hospital information system (HIS) with the same motivation as for PACS (see Chap. 5).

The idea of centralization of all image data of multiple origins can only create enormous difficulties for access and contradictory specifications for workstation and user interfaces, and jeopardize the process of standardization. There is no real medical need for this, since only the relevant groups of experts need direct access to these different classes of images.

2.2.2 The Relationship Between Hospital Structure and Its Diagnostic Imaging Activity: The AZ-Vrije Universiteit Brussels as a Case Study

In order to understand the flow of image production and the medical uses of these images, it is first necessary to describe the structure of a hospital, indicating where images might be needed. We will analyze the situation using the example of an existing hospital, namely the AZ-Vrije Universiteit Brussels (AZ-VUB). Table 2.1 presents the most important general data for the AZ-VUB.

Table 2.1. General data on the case study hospital (AZ-VUB)

Beds (n)	700
Mean occupancy (%)	80
Average length of stay (days)	7.5
Number of clinics (n)	47
One-day patient visits (per year)	340 000
Radiological examinations (per year)	150 000
Nuclear medicine examinations (per year)	10 000
Total film surface produced per year (m^2)	30 000
Total amount of film sheets (per year)	270 000
Surface of image archive (m^2)	435

This hospital can be divided into five large parts:

1. Hospitalization block
2. Emergency department
3. Medicotechnical block, including radiology, medical imaging, and radiotherapy
4. Polyclinic, including the function measurement department
5. Pediatric and technical blocks, including administration

Description of Medical Image Production Units

In a hospital, various types of medical images are produced in different locations, as shown in Table 2.2.

The department of radiology and medical imaging produces the largest number of pictures, nearly 1 million per year in the AZ-VUB (Table 2.3). These images form an important part of examinations, as description of them results in a report. It is, therefore, important to keep the images available for several reasons, e.g., exact localization of lesions, follow-up, and comparison. In most cases the requesting physician needs to view the pictures along with the report, whereby sometimes the images are of paramount importance, e.g., in the treatment of fractured limbs. This results in important flows of image folders (IFs) and in certain cases in a demand for the fast availability of images and reports.

The department of nuclear medicine carries out about 10 000 digital examinations a year, 50% of which are morphological studies, e.g., bone and thyroidal scintigraphy. From these morphological studies, a hard copy on film and a report are produced, and both of these are kept in the patient's alphanumerical record. The other half of the examinations consist of function-related images, e.g., angiography and single photon emission computed tomography (SPECT), which are computed into numbers to give a picture of the functionality of the organ. One color Polaroid print containing approximately ten images accompanies the report to illustrate the examination. Both are also filed in the patient's alphanumerical report. The

Table 2.2. Survey of the different kinds of images used in different hospital departments

Department	Type of image	Medium
Radiology and medical imaging	Conventional X-ray	Film
	Digital X-ray	
	CT	Film hard copy/digital storage
	MR	Film hard copy/digital storage
	DSA	Film hard copy
	US	Film hard copy
Nuclear imaging	Morphological studies (Bone scintigraphy)	Film hard copy/digital storage
	Functional studies (SPECT or angiography)	Polaroid color print
Radiotherapy	Simulation X-ray	Video paper color print Film
	Dose and field calculation images	Paper print/digital storage
Surgery quarters	Conventional X-ray	Film
	Digital fluoroscopy	Film hard copy
Stomatology	Conventional X-ray	Film
Endoscopy department	Endoscopic images	Colour video tape Video paper color print Polaroid Photographic color prints
Plastic surgery	Morphological studies	Polaroid and photographic color prints
Dermatology	Skin images	Polaroid and photographic color prints
Pathology	Microscopic images	Photographic color prints
	Conventional X-ray	Film
	Morphological studies	Photographic color prints
Ophthalmology	Retina angiography	Polaroid prints and slides
	US	Polaroid

department stores all the images produced in digital form (raw data). This is possible because of the low resolution of the images and their small number (16 angiography studies, resolution 64 × 64; 64 SPECT studies, resolution 64 × 64; 2 bone scintigraphy studies, resolution 1024 × 256).

In the radiotherapy department, field simulation is necessary before irradiation, and approximately 12000 patients a year undergo this type of simulation. Field simulation images are produced by positioning the patient as if he were going to be treated by radiation, but only normal energy X-rays are actually used. The images produced are only relevant for the radiotherapist carrying out treatment and are mostly kept at the department in special folders, during treatment and follow-up of the patient.

In some cases CT images are used to calculate the radiation field and the dose of the isometric curves. Here, then, CT is used first (only a small number of images are needed), and the images obtained are digitally trans-

Table 2.3. Number of different types of images produced per year using different imaging techniques in the AZ-VUB (data from 1990)

Technique	Type of image	Amount/year (n)
Conventional X-ray	Skeleton	100 000
	Chest	75 000
	Urology/digestive system/gynecology	80 000
	Blood vessels	40 000
	Special Exam	5 000
	Total	300 000
CT	Brain	120 000
	Skeleton/joints	70 000
	Chest/abdomen	100 000
	Total	290 000
MRI	Brain/spine	85 000
	Chest/abdomen	15 000
	Joints	60 000
	Total	160 000
DSA		13 000
US		150 000
Nuclear medicine	Morphological	10 000
	Functional	20 000
	Total	30 000
Total		943 000

ferred to the dose-planning device, which then draws the dose–isometric curves around the determined target. The images obtained are also only relevant to the radiotherapist carrying out treatment and are kept in digital form, while a hard copy of the dose calculation is made on paper.

X-ray examinations are performed during and just after surgery. Recently it has become possible to obtain hard copies of images from digital fluoroscopic devices. These pictures are of importance on site, since they determine, for example, if a fractured bone has been correctly repositioned.

The department of stomatology produces three kinds of images, all using conventional X-ray techniques, i.e., small dental views, Orthopantomographs (overview of the total jaw), and teleradiographs of the skull. These images are kept in separate folders with the orthodental patient files, which are kept in the department.

The endoscopic department, e.g., for broncho-, duodeno-, recto-, or arthrofibroscopy, registers several examinations by means of color videotape or photography. The video images can be printed in color on paper, as can the photographs. These images are, for example, relevant to the follow-up endoscopic treatment. They are temporarily kept in the department.

The departments of plastic surgery and dematology sometimes require photographic color prints, and these are kept in the patient's alphanumerical record.

The department of anatomopathology identifies tissues by microscope. Microscopic images are only recorded for scientific purposes, and the report is of primary importance. However, the prepared tissue slices are archived in the department. The images themselves have no real value for the requesting physician, the prepared slices are archived in case further reviewing or consultation is necessary. Sometimes color print photographs are made.

2.2.3 Flow of Images Produced by the Radiology Department

The radiology department consists of a central unit with five clusters (angiography, ultrasound (US) urological and gastrointestinal radiology, CT, and skeleton, chest, and special radiology) and three satellites (pediatric radiology, MRI, and emergency).

The angiography unit consists of two DSA units, one coronarography unit with a 35-mm camera, one lithotriptic unit, a central reporting space with an alternator, and two image evaluation spaces, both with CRT and Lbs. All examinations (digital and conventional) are reported within 1 day. Patients sent by other hospitals take a brief report with the images along with them back to the physician treating them. Later, a full report is sent by mail. Hospitalized patients are transported back to the nursing wards. The images are sent with them in urgent cases, otherwise the images follow later via the routine twice daily distribution. Reports are dictated on tape and typed on a word procesor into the HIS central patient data base, and a hard copy of the report is also distributed via the routine system twice a day.

For US, three units are available, one with Doppler and one central reporting space with a small Lb. All US examinations are reported immediately. The images are given to the outpatients with a brief report. Images of examinations from hospitalized patients are sent with the alphanumerical report to the nursing wards. A brief report is written into the alphanumerical report, and a hard copy of the dictated report follows by distribution.

The urological and gastrointestinal radiography unit consists of three screening rooms, all with a 10 × 10 camera, and one central reporting space with two alternators. In urgent cases the patient receives a brief report immediately after the examination. For hospitalized patients, a short note is written after the examination into the alphanumerical record. The reported IFs are collected several times a day and distributed twice a day by messengers of the department to all nursing wards. If outpatients are consulting the same day they are given the IF to return to the requesting physician. Otherwise, IFs are collected several times a day and brought to the dispatch room of the radiology department, from where they are distributed to the image archive or the requesting department. For the patients of general practitioners, the IF is kept in the dispatch room until a hard copy of the report is available. The hard copy and the IF are then sent together to the general practitioner by mail.

There are two CT units, each of which has a small reporting space with an Lb, two remote reporting sites with alternators, and a remote digital reporting station with three high-resolution CRT. Since the radiologist takes part in the examinations and performs most of them himself, the examinations are reported after his active CT work is finished (mostly half a day). He then has several possibilities.

He may take the IFs with him and produce a hard copy of his report in one of the remote reporting sites or on alternator immediately after finishing his active work.

Alternatively, he may put the images in a central collector and report them later. The IFs are then available in case something urgent happens and they are needed immediately. All IFs without a report and those returned by the responsible physicians also arrive in this collector. The radiologist may also choose to write his report on the PACS digital reporting console; the hard copy is then made after reporting is completed. All IFs are distributed to the nursing wards or to the dispatch room to be sent to the image archive or requesting departments, or they are sent by mail to other hospitals or general practitioners.

The skeleton, chest and special radiography unit consists of one specialized chest X-ray device, five conventional X-ray devices, one central reporting site with two large Lbs and one alternator, three quality control Lbs, a distribution center for the nursing wards, and a dispatch room for X-rays from the emergency department. Skeleton and chest X-rays are reported immediately.

Patients referred from other clinics or by general practitioners are given the IF to take back with them to the consultant if they are returning there the same day; if not, the IFs are collected several times a day and brought to the dispatch room to be sent to the image archive or requesting clinic. Reports are dictated on tape and typed into the HIS. Hard copies are sent later.

Outpatients also take their IF with them, and a brief written report accompanies it. Later a full report is sent by mail.

For hospitalized patients, examination films and reports are distributed twice a day to the nursing wards. If needed, they can be collected earlier. Intensive care units receive their IFs immediately, and a hard copy of the report usually follows half a day later. If necessary, the radiologist contacts his colleague by telephone to advise him about urgent or unexpected cases.

A satellite of the radiology department situated in the center of the pediatric department, which consists of two conventional X-ray devices, one US unit, and two reporting sites with large Lbs. Image flow is mostly similar to that in the central department. The distribution and mailing is carried out locally from the reception desk. IFs are brought to the nursing wards for hospitalized patients, to the pediatric image archive, or are given to the patient if he is returning to the consultant. The pediatric radiologist brings the results of CT and MRI examinations with him back from the central department or the MRI building, where the examinations were performed.

He reports them at the local reporting site and distributes them from the reception desk.

The second satellite of radiology and medical imaging is situated outside the hospital and connected by a tunnel, and consists of two MRI units, a remote evaluation station, a remote image processing station, and a reporting site with an alternator.

It is possible for the radiologist to use the PACS reporting facilities at the central department, because the images can be transferred to the PACS environment. MRI images are often sent into PACS to relieve the local storage, because some examinations require a large amount of images, for example, to be processed into three-dimensional constructions. They can easily be returned via the network to the image processing station on request. The IFs are collected and distributed locally from the reception desk of the MRI satellite.

The emergency department constitutes the third satellite and is on duty 24 h a day. It consists of two conventional rooms, a reporting site with a small Lb and a reporting station (a personal computer, PC, connected to the HIS network), and one US unit during the night and at weekends. Due to the nature of the emergency department, several examinations are required with a minimum delay. The radiologist types his report into a word processor connected with the HIS for patient information (demographic information). A hard copy is produced directly, and the report is sent into the HIS after supervision.

All examinations from the radiology satellite emergency are checked each day, for example, as to whether they have been reported, whether they have been sent to the archive or nursing ward, whether they have been sent out with the patient, and whether the examination was supervised. These checks are carried out in the central department of the dispatch for emergency radiology examinations. A dedicated person takes care of the distribution of the IFs to the image archive, nursing wards, or polyclinic, or into the cases in the collector of the radiologists who were on duty the day the examinations were performed, so that they can report them. The same thing happens with the IFs without a report which come from the nursing wards.

Digital Versus Analogue Images

It is also interesting to split the images into digital and analogue. In 1990, the AZ-VUB was not equipped with phosphor plate radiology, so the relevant digital modalities are CT, MRI, US, DSA, and some secondary digitization of film. The digital modalities account for 30% of the total number of examinations (Fig. 2.1). However, since the digital modalities generate more images per examination, the proportion is inverted for the number of images: 70% are digitally generated (Fig. 2.2).

If we then translate this into bytes, then conventional radiology represents more than 90% (Fig. 2.3)!

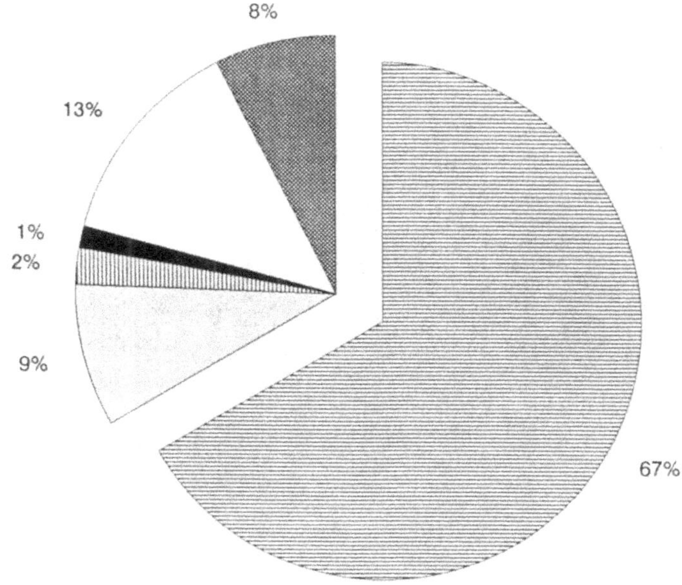

Fig. 2.1. A comparison of the number of examinations performed using digital and film-based techniques for 1990 in the AZ-VUB (*horizontal lines*, conventional X-ray; *gray shading*, CT; *vertical lines*, MRI: *black shading*, DSA; *white shading*, US; *cross hatching*, nuclear medicine)

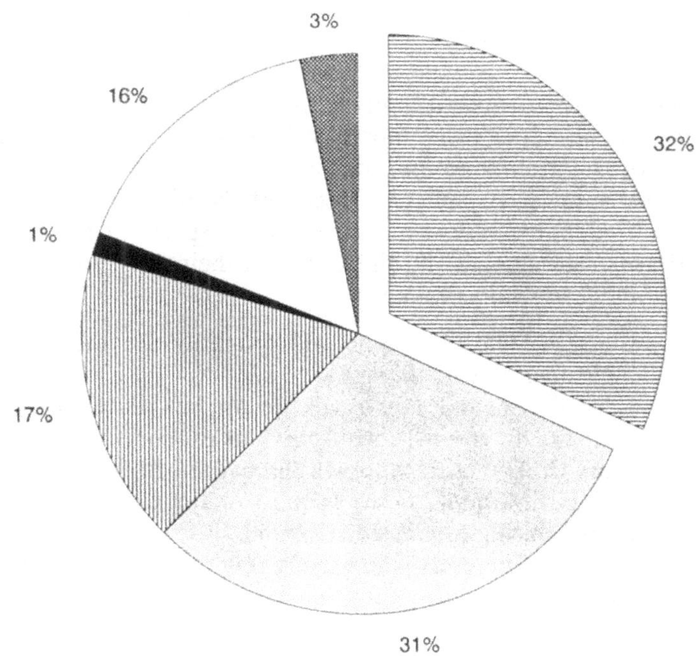

Fig. 2.2. A comparison of the number of images produced using digital and film-based techniques for 1990 in the AZ-VUB (*Horizontal lines*, conventional X-ray; *gray shading*, CT; *vertical lines*, MRI; *black shading*, DSA; *white shading*, US; *cross hatching*, nuclear medicine)

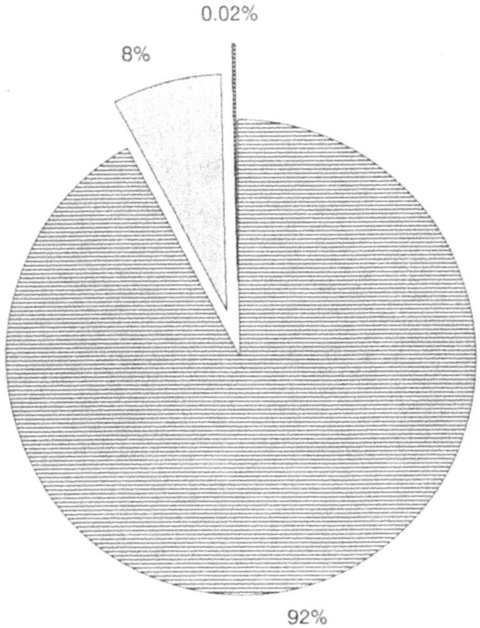

Fig. 2.3. A comparison of the number of images produced using digital and film-based techniques (cf. Fig. 2) calculated in bytes for 1990 in the AZ-VUB. Each conventional image is considered for a matrix of 2000 × 2000 (*horizontal lines*, conventional X-ray; *gray shading*, CT–MRI–US–DSA; *cross hatching*, nuclear medicine)

2.2.4 The Different User Clusters of Diagnostic Imaging and Their Specific Needs

PACS has to cope with an overall distribution to several locations and the functional demands of those working in the hospital. This means a variety of workstation concepts, and necessary image retrieval speeds and image transfer rates. A global hierarchy of the diagnostic image users can be set up by defining different classes with respect to the frequency with which they consult images and the nature of their consultation. Schematically, this can be described as follows:

- Class A. The users who will primarily use the images themselves for their diagnosis or therapy.
- Class B. The users who will use the images to check the validity of the report or to compare with previous examinations ("reviewing").
- Class C. The users who will discuss selected cases with colleagues. This may be informal, at the request of the clinician for a specific case, or formal during organized seminars.
- Class D. The users who usually rely on the report, and only occasionally consult the images.

Class A: Primary Use of Images – (Primary) Reporting by Radiologists. The images are the interpretation tool for radiologists, who will use them "on the spot" (the typical example being the emergency department) or within 24 h for making a report. The report is usually dictated by the radiologist and then typed into the radiological information system or the HIS by a secretary. Alternatively, the report can be entered directly by the radiologist, using, for example, some dedicated form of text processing or perhaps, in the future, voice recognition.

Primary reporting requires a large set of images to be immediately available. Conventionally, this is achieved with the folders of the series of the patients to be reported arranged upon a large automatic light box. Reporting in a PACS environment is performed using a multimodality workstation (dedicated PACS workstation). The folders to be reported are preliminarily loaded and stored locally at the console, or can be retrieved for comparison via high-speed image networks. For a number of cases, reporting also involves the necessity of comparing different examinations or a development over time.

Class A: Primary Diagnostic Use by Nonradiologists. For certain classes of specific examinations related to medical specialties, nonradiologists will use the images for diognosis. Examples of this are bone radiology for orthopedists, chest X-rays for pneumologists, angiocardiography for cardiologists intravenous pyelography for urologists, CT and MRI for neurologists and neurosurgeons, and intensive care unit imaging for anesthesists.

The requirements of these subclasses of users can be tailored to the specific examinations that they will use in routine. For example, in neurological examinations mainly CT and MRI are required, modalities which produce images with a relatively small spatial resolution, but in which the examinations are composed of a large set of images. The user interface must be very different in this sort of environment from that required, for example, in angiocardiography. This concept is illustrated in Fig. 2.4, which summarizes the amount of diagnostic imaging used for outpatients. The pattern is not only quite different for each specialty, but also in comparison with inpatients for the same specialty. Note the predominant consumption of CT and MRI for the neurological cluster, US for gynecology and obstetrics, and conventional X-rays for orthopedics (represented here as bone and joints).

Class A: Primary Use of Images As a Guide or Tool for Therapeutic Purposes. Images typically serve as a guide or tool for therapy for orthopedists during fracture reduction, for example, for surgeons in preoperative planning, and for radiotherapeutic planning. These applications will mostly presuppose specialized workstations fed by the digital input of the PACS environment.

Class B: Reviewing. Reviewing must be possible within every hospitalization unit and for every subdiscipline of internal medicine and surgery when consultations take place. For reviewing, only unsophisticated image manipulation capability is required, the emphasis being on speed and user friendliness.

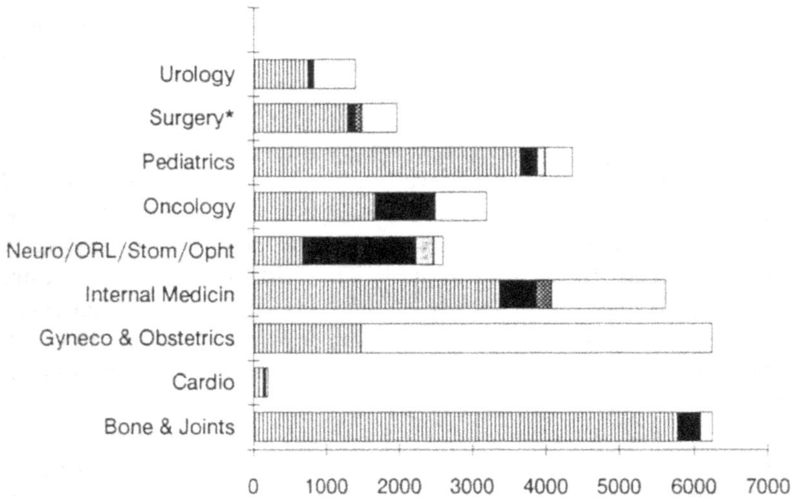

Fig. 2.4. Number of examinations according to imaging technique used by individual departments of the AZ-VUB in 1989 (*asterisk*, surgery does not include orthopedics, which is classified under bones and joints; *white shading*, US; *cross hatching*, DSA; *gray shading*, MRI; *black shading*, CT; *vertical lines*, conventional X-ray)

Class C: Discussion and Consultation. Informal discussion and consultation with the radiologists must take place at a PACS reporting console (multimodality console). For formal seminars or conferences, dedicated equipment must be available, for example, a remote control and screen connected to a PACS workstation.

Class D: Occasional Consultation. Occasional consultation of images does not justify direct access to a specialized workstation. Access to the reports via the HIS is sufficient for routine work.

This applies to specialities which do not routinely use radiology, for example, a dermatologist may occasionally require some radiological examination for his patient. It may also apply to classes of examinations which are not routinely used by the specialist, for example, the gastroenterologist will be placed in class A for examinations of the digestive tract or CT of the abdomen, but in class D for neurological examinations.

2.3 Medical Requirements in Terms of Access to Images

For primary reporting, as already mentioned, the radiologist needs instant access to the image set (IF) of the unreported examinations. Real-time access means that the time of access must be almost unnoticeable (a fraction of a second). This means that the unreported examination must be stored locally at the place where it will be reported. The topology and organization of the PACS system must also serve the needs of the other class A users with a very short access time.

For reviewing, organized facilities must be provided, namely, image acquired from intensive care examinations or examinations of inpatients must be stored locally while the relevant patients are hospitalized. Examinations of patients foreseen for consultations must also be stored locally (see Chap. 5, Sect. 5.3). This can be organized for medically relevant classes of patients, for example, oncology.

For reviewing unforeseen cases, a longer waiting time must be accepted by the clinician, but PACS will in any case be faster than conventional archiving.

Comparisons with previous examinations can also be organized in certain recognized situations, for example, in oncology and orthopedics.

Meeting these requirements for access time to the images is fundamental for the clinical acceptance of PACS. They were not met by the first generation systems, which used central archiving, a star network configuration, and nonhierarchized structure. This is one of the reasons why these systems were never used for primary reporting.

2.4 Medical Needs in Terms of Spatial Resolution

A very important and much researched question, which concerns not only the field of PACS itself, but also the whole concept of digital radiology, is the question of the spatial resolution required. A correct evaluation is more complex than it may appear, as it is not a theoretical, physical, spatial resolution that is of importance, but its performance in diagnosis, which requires a combined appreciation of the spatial and the density resolutions. The problem also varies according to the intrinsic resolution of each modality, the magnitude of the field of view (the portion of the space relevant to the examination), and the type of clinical question addressed. Therefore, the problem must be considered for each combination of these three factors and examined using the receiver-operating characteristic (ROC) method.

Research has also shown that resolution is only one of the factors which plays a role in image quality. The requirements of spatial resolution vary according to different factors including the signal-to-noise ratio of the system, sharpness, and the physical size and contrast of the object being examined. Changing one of more of the above-mentioned features could influence the required spatial resolution. The weight of opinion today would like the display resolution to be a 2048 × 2048 pixel matrix, in some critical applications at least.

A clear idea of the signification of the different matrices in terms of the spatial resolution for a chest film (40 × 40 cm film) is provided by the following list:

- 512 × 512 = 0.625 lines/mm (equivalent to 0.8 mm pixel size)
- 1024 × 1024 = 1.25 lines/mm (equivalent to 0.4 mm pixel size)
- 2048 × 2048 = 2.5 lines/mm (equivalent to 0.2 mm pixel size)
- 4096 × 4096 = 5.0 lines/mm (equivalent to 0.1 mm pixel size)

2.4.1 Spatial Resolution Required for Digital Thorax Radiology

The golden standard for spatial resolution is the resolution of conventional X-ray film. This resolution is comparable to a 4096 × 4096 pixel matrix, but the actual digitized X-ray film and interactive video display cannot cope with this very high spatial resolution demand.

However, it is possible with the available laser digitizers to scan a conventional X-ray film with this high resolution, so that the image data are available with a 4096 × 4096 matrix in the computer memory. Zoom functions on an interactive video display offer the possibility of imaging only a part of the image at full resolution. One wonders whether there is really a need for this very high spatial resolution? Recent studies have rejected this necessity.

The weight of opinion has settled for a 2048 × 2048 pixel matrix. As already mentioned, spatial resolution is only one of the properties of image quality, so it seems that the performance of a given pixel matrix of 2048 × 2048 is not equal for both digital hardcopy and interactive video display. Hayrapetian et al. (1989) concluded that a pixel matrix of 2048 × 2048 is sufficient to replace the conventional screen–light box combination by an interactive video display at least for examinations of the septal lines and lung nodules. Seeley (1987) also agrees that 2048 × 2048 would be sufficient for an entire digital radiology department. Cox et al. (1990) disagree with this statement. Cox states it is premature to say that the currently available 2048 × 2048 interactive video displays can generate images equivalent to conventional X-ray images. He also refers, however, to the advantages of using interactive video displays. For instance, a great improvement in the accuracy of diagnosing noduli situated in the lung parenchyma can be achieved using the video display. Cox's research indicated that there is a significant difference in image quality and diagnostic accuracy between interactive video display and digitized hard copy if both have the same spatial resolution. The performance of digitized hard copy is much higher as far as interstitial and obstructive lung disease are concerned. For interstitial pathology, the performance of digitized hard copy and conventional X-ray are equal.

There is an important difference in diagnostic accuracy between conventional X-ray film and interactive video display as far as interstitial pathology is concerned. By contrast, the performance of digitized hard copy and conventional X-ray are equal for interstitial pathology. This proves that the lower image quality on the video display is not due to the digitalization process itself. One of the causes could be the fact that the users were not familiar with the computer displays. When making their diagnosis, they were using the same standards as for conventional X-rays. With the window-center adjustment function, they created an interstitial intensification themselves, which led to a false-positive diagnosis in many cases.

There was also a difference in performance for the diagnosis of obstructive lung disease, which was caused by a lower sensitivity for small differences in contrast. Finally, a lower sensitivity was noted for the diagnosis of pneumothorax. This was due to the inherent loss of edge definition (the raster scanning operation of the monitor), an effect which could be at least partially eliminated by the use of image magnification and edge-enhancement algorithms. Other features which diminish image quality are the lower image luminance, the higher signal-to-noise ratio, and the image flutter.

According to Kundel (1986), very good quality images can be obtained using a digital system with a lower signal-to-noise ratio or an image receptor with a greater dynamic range than a conventional light box–film combination.

Conclusions

The majority of researchers agree that a 2048 × 2048 pixel matrix image could replace conventional X-rays of the thorax without a significant loss of information and diagnostic accuracy.

2.4.2 Digital Skeletal Radiography

Murphey (1989) used subperiosteal bone resorption to test the spatial resolution required for bone imaging, because this is one of the most demanding tests in terms of resolution in skeletal imaging. In this research program, very high resolutions were used, equivalent to a pixel matrix of 1024 × 1024, 2048 × 2048, 4096 × 4096, and 8192 × 8192. There was a significant loss of diagnostic accuracy in detecting subperiosteal bone resorption with a pixel matrix of 8192 × 8192, as well as for lower spatial resolution values. The technology currently available cannot provide these high spatial resolution images, therefore magnification techniques should be used, as they were in this research program. At present displays of 2048 × 2048 are available. On these screens a fourfold magnification would be necessary, and they would provide the examiner with only one-quarter of the total image.

2.4.3 Digital Gastrointestinal Imaging

Only a few radiologists have examined the spatial resolution requirements for digital gastrointestinal imaging. One of these was Kastan (Kastan et al. 1987), who studied subtle mucosal changes of inflammatory bowel disease and normal colonic mucosa. One of the conclusions of this study was that there were no significant differences for mean sensitivities between the original image and those with pixel size 0.1 mm, 0.2 mm, and 0.4 mm. A pixel size of 0.4 mm is comparable to a pixel matrix of 1024 × 1024. Of course there was a slightly better performance for the highest resolution of 0.1 mm.

2.4.4 CT and MRI

The intrinsic spatial resolution of CT and MRI is typically expressed in a matrix of 256 or 512. There is (naturally) no problem in the full exploitation of these images on available workstations. However, contrast resolution is very high (12 bits), and image protocols have to address this problem.

2.4.5 Ultrasound

The intrinsic spatial resolution of most (digital) US systems is less than 512. Existing PACS systems, therefore, already exceed the necessary specifications in terms of spatial resolution.

2.4.6 Conclusion

In a PACS environment, there are no limitations on the spatial resolution of the results of digital imaging techniques such as CT, MRI, and US. For specific applications (e.g., digital radiology and secondary digitization of films) and especially when dealing with large field of view (e.g., chest films), a spatial resolution of 2048 × 2048 seems to be the minimum acceptable for viewing stations. Below this, a loss of diagnostic accuracy would occur. For some imaging techniques, a resolution of 2048 × 2048 would even not be sufficient (e.g., skeletal radiography, radiography of the breast). In these cases, higher spatial resolution can be obtained by using the image magnification technique.

Different studies have clearly shown that spatial resolution is not the only important feature in image quality. This was demonstrated by the difference in image quality for images with a given spatial resolution displayed on digitized hard copies or interactive video displays. Important problems for an interactive video display are image flutter, signal-to-noise ratio, physical dimensions of the screen, and lower luminance.

2.5 Medical Needs in Terms of User Friendliness

Complex manipulation of images belongs to the world of imaging techniques. Within the multimodality environment of PACS, emphasis must be put on speed, simplicity, and good presentation of the documents. In most hospitals, the system will be used by a large number of different people, e.g., physicians with no or only superficial knowledge of computer science. Extensive use of the keyboard and dialogues must be avoided. The systems must also be safeguarded against erroneous erasing or changes within the data base.

2.6 Medical Needs in Terms of Patient Data Consistency

Patient data (identity and other alphanumerical information) must naturally be identical in every information system in the hospital, otherwise the information could be erroneously interpreted, or even totally lost. Also, experience shows that the need to reintroduce manually and repetitively, via the keyboard, the identity of a patient is incompatible with many clinical situations and constitutes a factor of nonacceptance of PACS. It is, therefore, mandatory for these functions to be automatized by the system (see Chap. 4.1).

2.7 Medical Need for Image Manipulation: Image Compression

As already mentioned, complex image reconstruction or manipulation is an intrinsic part of the use of imaging techniques and, therefore, by definition, not of the PACS environment. Most of these operations are specific to each modality and are performed by the relevant software of the acquisition system. The typical "basic" set of functions of a PACS multimodality workstation must include: image arrangement, flip-rotation, zooming, windowing–centering (with programmable preset values), and possibly some tools for measuring distances, angles, areas, or volumes.

Image arrangement simulates the disposition of the films on the light box by the radiologist, who sequentially "composes" the examination from separate pictures, in order to gain a global idea of the examination. The system must also provide a facility for comparing the images with former studies.

Flip-rotation is necessary to present correctly pictures that have been introduced in the wrong orientation in the system (typically, this is frequent when conventional images have been digitized).

Zooming, or the capability to one isolated image enlarged to the full screen, is necessary for the study of small details on one picture.

Windowing–centering is a classical function, present in every digital modality. In the PACS world, the multimodality environment makes the free choice of these values somewhat awkward, since the rationale and values vary considerably depending on the type of examination.

The images must, therefore, be presented automatically in a preset, programmed value of center and window, according to the modality, region investigated, and clinical problem. Secondary changes must also be possible.

Measurement tools can be useful in different modalities (e.g., distances, angulations, surfaces, and radiological densities), however, these functions will always be more efficiently applied on the specialized console of the relevant technique.

Image data compression is on the one hand highly desirable (if not necessary!) for PACS technology, and on the other hand potentially dangerous for diagnostic efficacy and medicolegal implications. The first reason for its desirability stems from the need for enormous amounts of storage space to archive the huge amounts of data generated by the different acquisition nodes on a PACS network. As memory on optical disks is not yet inexpensive, data compression is required to make the archiving cheaper and at the same time more practical, since it means faster retrieval of images from the optical disk. A second important reason why image compression is needed is for the flow of data over the PACS network, since compressed images may be transported faster over the network. This leads to fewer collisions on the network and a faster retrieval of images.

As far as retrieving images is concerned, one should ensure that the act of compression and decompression does not take up significantly more time than sending the uncompressed image through the network; this necessitates specialized hardware. Different methods of image compression are available, for instance, run-length coder/decoder (Cookson and Thoma 1988) and discrete cosine transform (DCT) (Chan et al. 1989). In general, one could say that the compression methods with a high compression ratio are irreversible. The methods with low performance, such as run-length encoding, are reversible.

Over the last few years, several studies on image compression have been published in the international literature. Most observers used DCT to compress their images and used the ROC method to study the diagnostic accuracy which could be obtained using a certain compression ratio. Bramble et al. (1989) reported no significant difference in diagnostic accuracy up to a compression ratio of 28:1, but Ishigaki et al. (1990) reported a significant difference in diagnostic accuracy for an image compression ratio higher than 20:1. Chan finds no difference in image quality for image compression ratios lower than 10:1. Most authors agree that image compression ratios lower than 10:1 are not detrimental to image quality, so it seems acceptable from the technical point of view to use an image compression ratio of 10:1 for daily clinical use. By using the run-length encoding method, loss of original data can be avoided. One major disadvantage of this technique, however, is that compression ratios can be as low as 3:1 and 4:1.

Further fundamental research should be carried out to develop faster and more powerful algorithms, which should then be implemented via dedicated hardware. On the other hand, extensive clinical evaluation is still necessary in order to prove the medical acceptability of this technologically important technique.

References

Bramble JM, Cook LT, Murphey MD, Martin NL, Anderson WH, Hensley KS (1989) Image data compression in magnification hand radiographs. Radiology 170: 133–136
Chakraborty DP, Breatnach ES, Yester MV, Soto B, Barnes GT, Fraser RG (1986) Digital and conventional chest imaging: a modified ROC study of observer performance using simulated nodules. Radiology 158: 35–39
Chan KK, Lou SL, Huang HK (1989) Radiological image compression using full-frame cosine transform with adaptive bit-allocation. Comput Med Imaging Graph 13(2): 153–159
Cookson JP, Thoma GR (1988) X-ray image compression using run length coding. J Med Syst 12(4): 201–209
Cox GG, Cook LT, McMillan JH, Rosenthal SJ, Dwyer SJ (1990) Chest radiography: comparison of high-resolution digital displays with conventional and digital film. Radiology 176: 771–776
Fraser RG, Sanders C, Barnes GT, MacMahon H, Giger ML, Doi K, Templeton AW, Cox GG, Dwyer SJ, Merritt CR, Jones JP (1989) Digital imaging of the chest. Radiology 171: 297–307
Goodman LR, Foley WD, Wilson CR, Rimm AA, Lawson TL (1986) Digital and conventional chest images: observer performance with film digital radiography system. Radiology 158: 27–33
Goodman LR, Foley WD, Wilson CR, Tikofsky RS, HOffmann RG (1988) Pneumothorax and other lung disease: effect of altered resolution and edge enhancement on diagnosis with digitised radiographs. Radiology 167: 83–88
Hayrapetian A, Aberie DR, Huang HK, Fiske R, Morioka C, Valentino D, Boechat MI (1989) Comparison of 2048-line digital display formats and conventional radiographs: an ROC study. AJR 152: 1113–1118
Huang HK, Mankovich NJ, Taira RK, Cho PS, Stewart BK, Ho BK, Chan KK, Ishimitsu Y (1988) Picture archiving and communication systems for radiological images: state of the art. CRC Crit Rev Diagn Imaging 28(4): 383–427
Ishigaki T, Sakuma S, Ikeda M, Itoh Y, Suzuki M, Iwai S (1990) Clinical evaluation of irreversible image compresion: analysis of chest imaging with computed radiography. Radiology 175: 739–743
Kastan DJ, Ackerman LV, Feczko PJ (1987) Digital gastrointestinal imaging: the effect of pixel size on detection of subtle mucosal abnormalities. Radiology 162: 853–856
Kundel HL (1986) Digital projection radiography of the chest. Radiology 158: 274–276
Lams PM, Cocklin ML (1986) Spatial resolution requirements for digital chest radiographs: an ROC study of observer performance in selected cases. Radiology 158: 11–19
MacMahon H, Vyborny CJ, Metz CE, Doi K, Sabeti V, Solomon SL (1986) Digital radiography of subtle pulmonary abnormalities: an ROC study of the effect of pixel size on observer performance. Radiology 158: 21–26
Metz CE (1986) ROC methodology in radiologic imaging. Invest Radiol 21: 720–733
Murphey DM (1989) Digital skeletal radiography: spatial resolution requirements for detection of subperiosteal resorption. AJR 152: 541–546
Schaefer CM, Greene R, Oestmann JW, Hall DA, Llewellyn HJ, McCarthyn KA, Pile-Spellman ER, Rubens JR (1990) Digital storage phosphor imaging versus conventional film radiography in CT-documented chest disease. Radiology 174: 207–210
Seeley GW, Fisher HD, Stempski MO, Borgstrom M, Bjelland J, Capp MP (1987) Total digital radiology department: spatial resolution requirements. AJR 148: 421–426

3 Looking for Indicators of a Reference Hospital

H. LODDER, B.M. VAN POPPEL, and A.R. BAKKER

3.1 Introduction

As with hospital information systems (HIS) and radiology information systems (RIS), picture archiving and communication systems (PACS) have been (and are still being further) developed for use in hospitals. Since each hospital has its own characteristics, it is not sufficient to buy and implement a standard HIS, RIS, and/or PACS; adjustments to the local dimensions and working methods, for example, will be necessary. Nevertheless, for both the hospital management and the vendors, a reference hospital is evidently needed. PACS vendors, for example, need a reference hospital to serve as the basis for the definition of their standard product. Within the context of this study, the concept of a reference hospital is limited to those aspects related to PACS.

We have collected data on the situation in the Netherlands to investigate whether so-called indicators can be found for what we have called a Dutch reference hospital. As the next step, data from other European hospitals were added to the Dutch figures in order to see whether indicators exist for a European reference hospital or – if there is too much diversity – whether a set of indicators can be found for each country or group of countries. The information from the European hospitals was obtained using a questionnaire, which is described in Sect. 3.2. In Sect. 3.3, a number of possible indicators are introduced along with their mutual relations. In Sect. 3.4 we present some results for the Dutch situation and then some preliminary results for the European case. Possible explanations are given for the variability observed. In Sect. 3.5, we conclude with some suggestions for the next step(s) to take in continuing this study.

3.2 Questionnaire

In order to obtain a general view of the main characteristics of those European hospitals which showed interest in PACS, a questionnaire was developed and sent to over 30 hospitals throughout Europe. One of the selection criteria was the affinity for PACS, because in our experience, hospitals keen to introduce PACS had often already conducted an in-house inquiry to get reliable data on aspects important for (future) PACS imple-

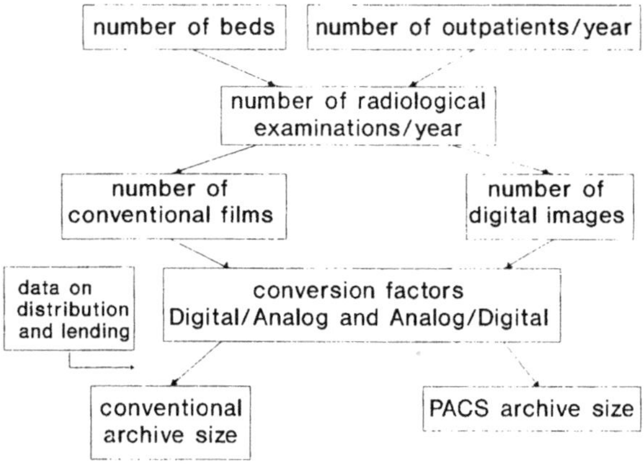

Fig. 3.1. Schema of indicators which might characterize a European reference hospital and from which archive size may be derived

mentation. Such aspects include the total number of radiological examinations per year, their distribution over different imaging modalities (both conventional and digital), and the net film usage per year, as well as data on the functionality of the available information systems (e.g., HIS and RIS) and on logistics and archiving procedures, which are of great value. As an indicator for "PACS affinity", we used EuroPACS membership and personal contacts during PACS conferences.

The questionnaire was divided into 5 parts:

- General hospital data
- HIS/RIS functionality
- Radiology department
- (Radiodiagnostic) procedures
- (Film) archiving

3.3 Basic Schema of Possible Indicators

We started this investigation to obtain indicators which might characterize a reference hospital, as indicated in Fig. 3.1.

By successively plotting the data values of the entities on both sides of each arrow in Fig. 3.1, an estimation of the relationship between those entities is obtained. We expect, for example, the number of radiological examinations per year to be a function of the number of beds and the number of outpatients per year. However, we have to find out whether the number of radiological examinations per year can be derived from these two data entities alone, or whether other dependencies also exist. If we suppose that the schema of Fig. 3.1 holds true, then an indication of the PACS archive size can, for example, be obtained from the number of beds, the number of outpatients per year, the ratio of digital to conventional images, and the necessary period of archiving.

We are, therefore, interested in searching for indicators such as:

- Number of radiological examinations per year per bed and/or number of radiological examinations per outpatient per visit
- Number of conventional films per radiological examination
- Number of digital images per radiological examination
- Number of square meters of conventional film used
- Number of megabytes (MB) required per digital image
- Ratio of digital to conventional images
- Ratio of digital to conventional radiological examinations

and conversion factors such as:

- Number of MB per square meter for conventional films
- Number of square meters per MB for digital images

3.4 Preliminary Results

3.4.1 Some Results for the Dutch Situation

In order to get some feeling for indicators, we will first look at the data gathered from 36 Dutch hospitals (both university and nonuniversity hospitals) within the framework of a study on PACS design. The first results of this study were presented at the MIC'89 conference in Belgium (van Poppel 1989). First we will try to ascertain whether the productivity of the radiology department is proportional to the dimensions of the hospital, measured in number of beds and/or number of outpatient visits/year. In Figs. 3.2 and 3.3, the number of radiological examinations is plotted against the number of beds and the number of outpatient visits/year, respectively. Although the number of university hospitals is relatively small compared with the number of general hospitals, the differences appear to be relatively few.

Without distinguishing between university and nonuniversity hospitals, the approximate relationships for Dutch hospitals shown in Table 3.1 are found. These relationships imply that the production of the radiology department for one bed corresponds to the production for about 320 outpatient visits.

The next step (see Fig. 3.1) is to determine the relationship between the production of the radiology department, measured in the number of radiological examinations, and the number of conventional films produced on the one hand and the number of digital images on the other. Rather than taking the *number* of conventional films into account, we can look at the

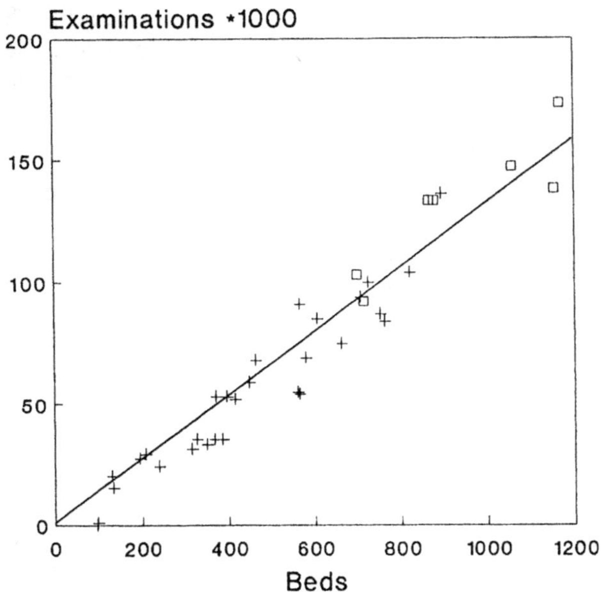

Fig. 3.2. Correlation of number of beds to number of radiological examinations performed in Dutch hospitals. Data were obtained from 36 hospitals with a total of 19000 beds (*square*, university hospital; *plus sign*, nonuniversity hospital)

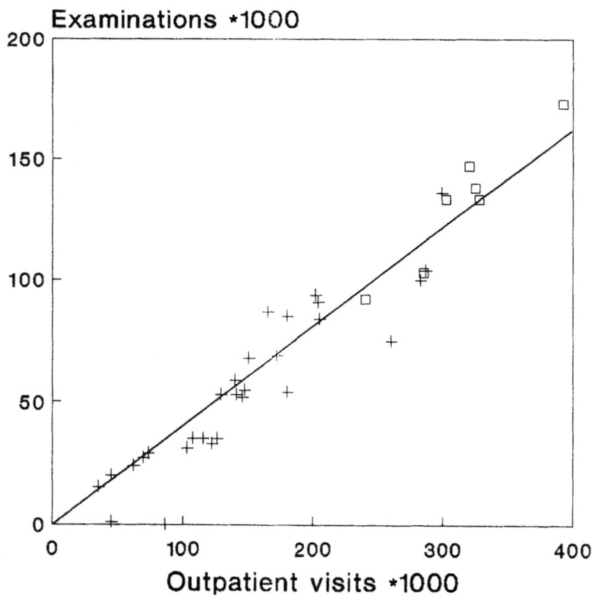

Fig. 3.3. Correlation of number of outpatient visits to number of radiological examinations performed in Dutch hospitals. Data were obtained from 36 hospitals with a total of 19000 beds (*square*, university hospital; *plus sign*, nonuniversity hospital)

amount of film used in square meters, and for digitally acquired images the number of MB needed for storage can be investigated.

Although this seems quite straightforward, it appeared in our investigations that most hospitals do not have reliable figures available on these matters, some do not even have any figures at all. Fortunately, we had

Table 3.1. Indicators for Dutch hospitals

Examinations/bed per year (*n*)	145
Examinations/outpatient visit (*n*)	0.45
Conventional films/radiological examination (*n*)	2.5
Digital images/radiological examination (*n*)	5.4
Square meters/conventional film (m^2)	0.1
MB/digital image (MB)	0.07
Ratio digital/conventional images (%)	30
Ratio digital/conventional examinations (%)	15

Table 3.2. Relationship between radiology production, number of pictures, net film used, and storage requirements for conventional and digital imaging techniques (1987 data from two Dutch University Hospitals)

Imaging technique	Hospital	
	AZL (Leiden)	AZU (Utrecht)
Conventional		
Number of examinations/year	116000	115000
Amount of film used (m^2)	30000	30740
Number of pictures/year	296000	292000
in gigabyte (GB)	1220	1250
Number of pictures/examination	2.6	2.5
Number of MB/examination	10.5	10.8
Amount of film used/picture (cm^2)	1010	1050
Amount of film used/examination (cm^2)	2580	2670
Digital		
Number of examinations/year	17000	18000
Number of images/year	88000	103000
in GB	6.2	7.1
in m^2 film	4770	5480
Number of images/examination	5.2	5.6
Number of MB/examination	0.4	0.4
film used/image (cm^2)	540	530
film used/examination (cm^2)	2810	2990

carried out a rather detailed investigation into these matters in two Dutch academic hospitals (AZL in Leiden and AZU in Utrecht) in 1988.

The main results of this investigation (1987 figures) are shown in Table 3.2.

For conversion from m^2 to MB for both conventional and digital images (van Poppel 1989a) it was assumed that a conventional standard thorax image with format 14×17 inch (about $0.15\,m^2$) is represented on average by 6 MB. This results in a mean information density of $6/0.15 = 40\,MB/m^2$.

An estimate for the information density of digital modality images shows that the information density is considerably lower than for the con-

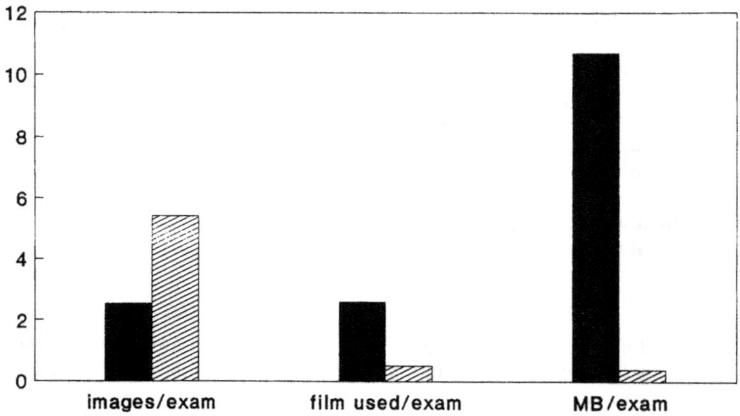

Fig. 3.4. Comparison of conventional and digital imaging techniques in two Dutch university hospitals. Film used per examination is measured in $m^2 \times 0.1$ (*black shading*, conventional technique; *diagonal stripes*, digital techniques)

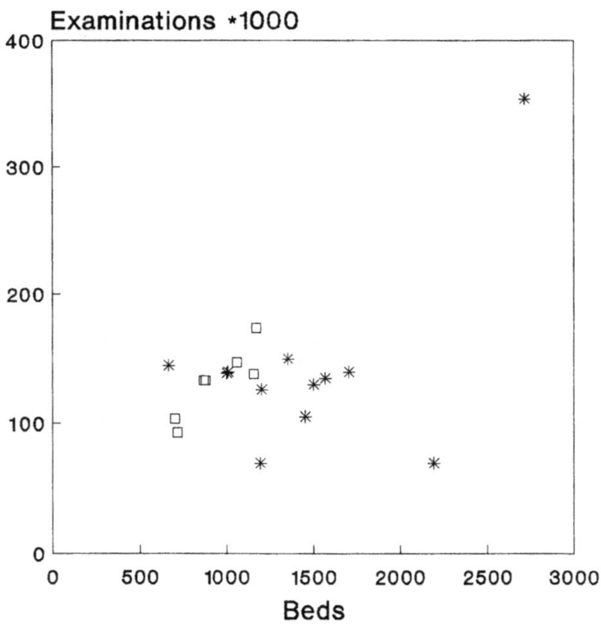

Fig. 3.5. Correlation of number of beds to number of radiological examinations performed in Dutch and non-Dutch academic hospitals (*square*, Dutch; *asterisk*, non-Dutch)

ventional images, e.g., a computed tomography (CT) image, shown on $500\,cm^2$ (normally seven CT images on $3500\,cm^2$) has an average pixel matrix of 256×256 with a depth of 8 bits. The mean information density for CTs is, therefore, $1.3\,MB/m^2$.

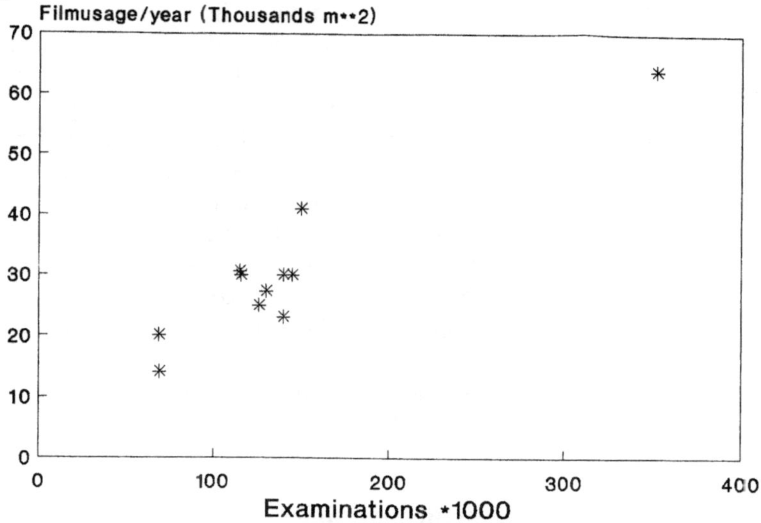

Fig. 3.6. Correlation of number of radiological examinations performed to amount of film used per year (in thousands m^2)

When all the images acquired are expressed in net film used (m^2), the net amount of film used per examination is about the same for both the digital and conventional modalities, because the higher number of images per examination for digital examinations is compensated by the lower net amount of film used per image.

3.4.2 First Steps Outside the Netherlands

Using the results from 3.4.1, it may be interesting to find out whether the data gathered from other European countries confirm the relationships found in the Dutch situation, or whether they disagree with them. It must be noted that care should be taken in interpreting the data because the number of responses as yet received (15) is limited. The data in Fig. 3.5 (beds versus examinations) indicate that for European university hospitals the relationship between hospital size and annual radiology production is not as straightforward as it is for Dutch university hospitals alone. Also, the cluster of points in Fig. 3.6 does not really support the existence of a simple ratio between the two entities.

There may be several explanations for the observed noncorrelation of Dutch and non-Dutch hospital data:

1. The differences between countries (e.g., in the way hospitals are organized) are too large to make the search for a European reference hospital useful. As an alternative, perhaps a set of indicators can be found for each country or group of countries.

2. Comparing these two sets of data is like comparing two objects as different from each other as apples and oranges, because there are, as yet, no standard definitions for parameters such as radiology production, number of beds, outpatient visit, film usage, or image. For example, ultrasound is not always included in the total radiology production, and the number of beds does not always include incubators, childrens' beds, nursing home beds, and intensive care beds. Furthermore, for many hospitals it is a problem to ascertain annual film usage; the most reliable method, e.g., to compensate for film drop-out, seems to be to observe both sides of the process, i.e., how many films were purchased by the hospital, and how many films have been passed on to the physicians.
3. The number of hospitals studied is still too small to form a sound statistical basis from which to draw conclusions.

3.5 Indications for Further Inquiries

The preliminary results described in Sect. 3.4 encourage us to carry out further research in order to get answers to the following questions:

To what extent are the semantics of the relevant parameters (and their relation to each other) comparable in all European countries? This question refers to the need for standardization of definitions, as was also clearly expressed during the workshop on standards in Europe, held on Crete (Institute of Computer Science 1990).

A question closely related to the relation between the parameters is which data model is used (Koens et al. 1988)?

In Sect. 3.3 we started with a set of indicators which seemed relevant to PACS. How far does this set meet our needs, or is an extension of the number of indicators necessary?

When may we, or how many hospital data must be collected and processed before we may, dispense with the idea of a European reference hospital?

To what extent do we have to distinguish between university hospitals and nonuniversity hospitals? For the time being it looks as if the only category with PACS affinity is the university hospital.

Thus far we have only looked at a very limited set of data from the questionnaire. We have not yet worked out the data received to questions of HIS/RIS functionality, working procedures, and archiving. Do we have to develop indicators for these parameters too?

What is still missing at the moment is an adequate error analysis, e.g., the straight lines in some of the diagrams have to be regarded as rough indication, not as statistically reliable linear relations.

The only conclusion we can draw at this moment, based on the (preliminary) results thus far, is that the indicators found for Dutch hospitals are not automatically applicable to other countries. Although answers first have to be found to the questions above, it seems that all the steps mentioned in the basic schema of indicators have to be taken for each country or group of countries.

References

Institute of Computer Science (1990) Proceedings of the working group on PACS standards in Europe, Heraklion, Crete, May 1990

Koens ML, Lodder H, Bijl K, de Valk JPJ, Bakker AR (1988) Dutch team merges HIS/RIS with PACS; next step: improve, coordinate data model. Radiology Today 5 (11)

van Poppel BM (1989) Manual of the software package CAPACITY. BAZIS internal report June 1989

van Poppel BM, Bakker AR, Mattheus R, Elsakkers PH, Wilmink JBM (1989) Cost evaluation of PACS using the software package CAPACITY (in Dutch). In: de Moor GJE (ed) Proceedings Medical Informatics Conference MIC'89, Antwerp, Belgium, September 1989

4 Communication Between Hospital and Radiology Information Systems and Picture Archiving and Communication Systems

4.1 Integrated Information Systems in the Hospital

A.R. Bakker

4.1.1 Background

Appropriate medical care is determined by data on the patient's condition on the one hand, and the knowledge and experience of the physician on the other. In the early days of health care, a patient had to deal with only one physician, who collected the observations himself and had the knowledge and experience stored in his own brain. With the advancement of medicine, increasing amounts of data had to be recorded, and these were no longer stored only in the brain of the physician, but gradually also recorded on paper: the medical record was born.

Due to the growing complexity of medicine, the field was divided into specialist areas which together supply care to the patient. The medical support functions were assigned to special departments such as clinical laboratories, radiology, and pharmacy. This process of further specialization is still going on. As a consequence, we are confronted within the hospital with an ever increasing volume of data, which must be collected and recorded. Since (parts of) these data are needed by the many health care workers who play a part in the care process and also by the support departments, the volume of information exchange is increasing rapidly.

A substantial percentage of the man-hours available in a hospital is spent on handling information and communication. In nursing, this percentage is estimated at 20%–30% (Heemskerk van Holtz 1988). Nevertheless, the situation is far from ideal.

4.1.2 Computers in the Hospital: The Concept of HIS

In view of the intensive use of information and communication, it is not surprising that the potential benefits of computer application were recognized at an early stage. In the early 1960s, attempts were already being made to use computers to register diagnoses, to support the clinical chemistry laboratory, to analyze physiological signals (e.g., electrocardiography, ECG), and to manage the financial administration. It was soon recognized that such isolated applications were only of limited value, since the information handling process in a hospital cannot easily be separated into independent categories; integration is a keyword in hospitals. This observation and the rather disappointing experiences led at the end of the 1960s to the concept of a integrated hospital information system (HIS), initially also termed a total hospital information system. According to Collen (1988):

"the goal of a hospital information system is to use computers and communications equipment to collect, store, process, retrieve, and communicate patient care and administrative information for all hospital affiliated activities, and satisfy the functional requirements of all authorized users".

Bakker et al. 1989 mention the following characteristics of such systems:

"– coherent storage of data (both medical and administrative) in a central database
- access to data, for authorized users, from the work location, whenever needed, in a presentation adapted to the needs of the individual user
- the system takes care of some coordinating tasks".

At the time the concept emerged, only alphanumerical data was being considered. The concept is not, however, restricted to this and by nature also covers images, curves, scanned documents, speech recording, and other data recording methods (Kaihara and Watanabe 1988).

4.1.3 Potential Benefits of HIS: Some Examples

A few examples may illustrate the attractiveness of the concept. If all medical and administrative patient data were stored in a computer and were retrievable from workstations available throughout the hospital, the health care workers in the hospital would have direct access to up-to-date patient data of this sort, not only those collected by themselves, but also those collected by others. This would improve the quality of the diagnostic and therapeutic process significantly.

The foregoing holds even more true for patients being treated by more than one specialist department. Activities could be coordinated and duplication of tests could be avoided. In emergency situations data on current diagnoses, recent operations, and current medication can be of great value and sometimes even life saving.

The possible interactions of various medications issued by different physicians could be detected, and complications could be avoided. In nursing, the direct recording of data at the bedside could prevent the occurrence of errors and omissions. Orders for medical examinations could be entered directly, and their effect on diet and treatment could be derived and entered automatically into the patient's "work schedule". When viewing images, radiologists would have access to both previous images and other medical data. The consumption of drugs and supplies could be fed directly into a stock control system that would generate orders to suppliers when the stock level fell below a certain limit. Medical activities such as operations, laboratory tests, radiology examinations, and drug supply would directly feed the financial administration and billing.

4.1.4 Objectives of an HIS

The goals of an HIS are to improve the quality and efficiency of the health care provided. This translates into the following objectives (Collen 1988):

1. Establish a database capable of providing an integrated, continuing, computer-stored medical record for all patient care data and make it directly accessible to all authorized health care providers 100% of the time.
2. Communicate patient data to and from all hospital clinical and administrative services, within all affiliated medical facilities.
3. Support all health care provider functions, including order entry and results reporting, patient history and examination findings, consultation and procedure reports; and communicate individual patient data to and from all authorized health care professionals by user friendly terminals.
4. Provide clinical and administrative decision support.
5. Establish and maintain files for hospital administrative and business functions, including patient eligibility, registration, scheduling, personnel and resources.
6. Assist with quality assurance, accreditation, and regulatory requirements.
7. Support research and education requirements.

4.1.5 Short History of HIS

The HIS concept described in the previous section promises so many advantages that it is not surprising to find that many persons and institutions were motivated to try to translate it into a real system. In doing so, they expected to be able to apply information technology to the improvement of both the quality and the efficiency of hospital care. The history of HIS development and the experiences gained may be of help when preparing for the realization of PACS in a hospital.

In the 1970s, many projects were already being initiated to try to translate the HIS concept into operational systems and applications. The vast majority of these initial projects led to complete failures, only a few were a partial success.

Although the use of HIS is now widely accepted in hospitals (at least in Europe and the United States), we are still far from realizing the ideal, complete HIS. Only a limited number of the objectives as described above have been realized, and one might wonder why this is so. A rough estimate indicates that until now, a total of 100000 man-years have been invested in HIS development, mainly in the USA and Europe. The realization of HIS has turned out to be substantially more difficult and time-consuming than expected. When contemplating the implementation of picture archiving and communication systems (PACS), it is good to bear this in mind.

4.1.6 Problems Encountered in HIS Realization

It is often rather easy to identify reasons for failures and disappointments in retrospect. Nevertheless, it seems worthwhile to have a look at these reasons since some of them may still hamper the development of HIS and perhaps of PACS as well. Limitations in the technology available have been one of the major reasons for problems. Initial HIS projects were confronted with serious hardware limitations in central processing unit (CPU) power, storage capacity, and transmission speed. This led to poor response times which resulted in problems with user acceptance. The system software turned out not to be adequate for the volume of transactions generated, and the data base software was another serious bottleneck.

With respect to the application software, it turned out that the information handling in a hospital was significantly more complex than anticipated. This, combined with limited experience in designing conversational software for a wide user population, also often led to rejection of the solutions proposed. Because of the costs of hardware in most systems, no duplication of equipment was applied. As a consequence, the reliability of the services supplied was found to be too low to be able to rely on the system as a commodity for daily hospital care; again a reason for nonacceptance.

Over the years some of the problems have been solved or at least reduced in size. It is well accepted now that a modern hospital should have some sort of HIS. However, several problems still exist, and their solution is not yet within reach. Later in this chapter, the further development of HIS and the major obstacles will be considered, but first we will discuss the current situation.

4.1.7 Approaches to HIS Realization

4.1.7.1 Different Approaches Possible

Although the concept of HIS outlined above is widely accepted as the ideal situation to be strived for, the approximations to this ideal as realized by the different groups who are active in HIS development show a wide degree of variation. Evidently, the summit is being approached from different directions, and since the summit is still a long way off, the various groups may, theoretically, still be far apart; this turns out to be indeed the case. First of all, the choice will have to be made as to which operational functions should be supported by the HIS and what priority should be given to each of them. This determines to a large extent the way the HIS will present itself to the users in the hospital. To make this more clear, we will consider a few examples.

4.1.7.2 The Administrative Approach

Some HIS projects started with the emphasis on billing and accounting. These applications are reasonably well defined, the number of terminals is limited, and the dependency of the hospital on the functioning of the HIS is not critical (billing can wait for a day if there is a technical problem). Especially in the USA, several systems are offered on a commercial basis that emphasize this aspect of the hospital. This approach has quite a low risk level, however, it can hardly demonstrate to those directly involved in providing care what the attractiveness of the HIS concept is.

4.1.7.3 HIS from the Medical Support Departments

Some other HIS projects placed the emphasis on medical support departments such as clinical laboratories, radiology department, and pharmacy to improve the communication process in the hospital and gradually fill a central data bank with useful medical data. The systems provide valuable support for the routine process within the support departments and contribute to timely and more accurate reporting. From the data recorded, billing data can be derived directly.

This approach leads to more demands on technology. A considerable number of terminals is required, otherwise on-line reporting cannot function adequately and demonstrate its benefits. The medical support departments cannot stand still for half a day, as the billing process can, so a high degree of availability is required. The processes to be supported are reasonably well known, nevertheless, specifying the functionality is more complex than in the administrative approach. The on-line transactions are manifold and not always easy.

4.1.7.4 Clinical Support Departmental Approach

Some projects have a more limited scope and do not aim to realize an information system for the whole hospital, but rather concentrate on one department, e.g., the radiology department or the pharmacy. The advantage of this approach is that the user group is not too broad, and can thus be more easily addressed. From the point of view of hospital management, the cooperation of the different departmental systems is a point of concern.

Other projects try to serve directly the primary process of the hospital by supporting doctors and nurses. Examples of applications are conversational anamnesis, patient monitoring, recording of vital signs, supporting protocols, progress notes, duty rosters, and expert systems to support the diagnosic process. For nursing, it has turned out that support of the communication with other departments is a crucial aspect. Most nursing applications can flourish only when other departments have an information system that is accessible from the nursing application.

4.1.7.5 The Logistics Approach

Starting with support of the logistics of the hospital might be another approach. The flow of materials, drugs, meals, and patients through the hospital could, for example, well be supported by an information system that schedules appointments, supplies meals in time (taking account of the current diet and examinations scheduled), and generates orders when stock runs below a given threshold.

4.1.8 Realising HIS: Choosing an Approach

The present incarnations of HIS differ widely. Some give in-depth support of a limited number of functions (e.g., within one department), while others try to offer services throughout the hospital with limited functionality. The choice depends on the climate in the hospital and on the resources available. One should not think only of the available budget, but primarily of the availability of motivated and capable people, both from the user and the data processing (DP) sides.

The choice of approach in realization is also heavily influenced by the target group of users. If the institution management is the main target group, the system will have to grasp what is going on in the institution; a broad but sheer coverage is needed, often with an emphasis on financial data and on resource utilization. If the department managers are the main target group, achieving efficiency and quality in the department will be the main aim of the development. If doctors or nurses are the main target group, the support of the direct process of diagnosis and care will be the main issue.

Attitudes to and the status of DP will differ from institution to institution, so it is not surprising to find quite different approaches being used. In view of the huge amount of manpower required to realize (parts of) an HIS, the development groups have to make choices, and it is interesting to note that, even for the groups that survived, the approaches are quite diverse.

There is also a wide variety of technical solutions. The first attempts to realize an HIS were based on mainframe computers. This approach still exists. With the advent of minicomputers, some groups embraced this new technology; and this approach also still exists. Furthermore, the introduction of personal computer (PC) networks inspired other groups to try to use this technology to realize HIS. Within the minicomputer approach, we find systems of both a centralized and a distributed structure, i.e., a network of departmental systems.

4.1.9 Common Characteristics of HIS

Because of the different approaches adopted in the realization of HIS, as indicated in the previous section, and owing to the lack of a widely accepted terminology, users might easily get confused. In this section, the common principles in the vast majority of HIS incarnations will be presented.

A focal point in an HIS is a common data bank where both medical and administrative patient data are stored. Typical types of medical data are results of laboratory tests, radiology examinations, diagnoses, medication orders, ECG findings, reports on operations, and discharge letters. Typical examples in the administrative domain are admission/discharge data, insurance data, care provided, invoices, and appointments. Many data within a hospital are primarily of a medical nature, but have an administrative meaning as well. One task of an HIS is to take advantage of this duality, by collecting data to support the primary process and feed the administrative part of the HIS with these medical data.

The backbone in any HIS is the patient identification file or patient master index, holding patient identification and some demographic data. In most systems, the patients are given a unique number that gives technically direct access to that patient's data. If the number is unknown, the patient identification file allows a quick search for the patient to be made by means of index keys, based on, for example, the patient's birthdate and some characters of the name, although searching for the name only will often lead to ambiguity. In some countries there is a national identification number that can be used within the HIS as well; special provisions have to be made in this case for foreigners and newborn babies.

Another common characteristic of most HIS is interactivity, which results in a widespread use of terminals. Display/keyboard combinations are predominant, and these are sometimes equipped with printing facilities, or there are separate printing terminals. Besides keyboard input, in some systems light pen input and touch screens are being used. The use of PCs as terminals/workstations is increasing, but not at the pace initially expected. The conversational workload of a fully developed HIS is substantial and, despite technological advances, often at the limits of the available capacity; problems with response times are not uncommon.

4.1.10 Structure of HIS

The application domain of an HIS is tremendous, even when the ambition level is relatively low. To be able to manage the application software, the HIS must be structured by being separated into subsystems. Such subsystems are then meant to supply a more or less coherent set of functions, e.g., for one department or one function of the hospital. Typical examples of this are the radiology information system, the clinical laboratory information system, the personnel information system, the order entry system, the invoicing system, and the pharmacy system. Such systems are logically grouped around the common data bank and supply users with access to the data.

Since the various functions of the HIS are not isolated, the subsystems should be able to benefit from each other. Communication between the different subsystems is essential, since this will the HIS give its integrated character.

Unfortunately no standard exists to define the decomposition of HIS into subsystems. As a consequence, subsystems developed by different groups do not fit together. Trying to build an integrated HIS from the best subsystems available is at present an illusion. For PACS, it might be possible to arrive at such a standard, since the PACS community is more aware of the need for standardization, and, moreover, the application domain is much narrower than that of HIS. Such a standard is essential for an open PACS, but will not create itself since it requires resources and commitment.

4.1.11 IMIA Working Group 10 "Hospital Information Systems"

The International Medical Informatics Association (IMIA) is the organization behind the MEDINFO world congresses which have taken place every 3 years since 1974; the next congress will take place in Geneva in 1992. Members of the association are the national societies for medical informations. IMIA has a number of working groups that pay attention to specific topics, and working group 10 is currently dealing with HIS. The working group organizes working conferences and special sessions or workshops during major international conferences. In 1988, a working conference was organized on the future of HIS called "Towards New Hospital Information Systems" (Bakker et al. 1988). In 1991, the next working conference "Trends in Modern HIS" will take place at Göttingen, Germany.

4.1.12 Main Obstacles for the Further Development of HIS

At the 1988 working conference of the IMIA working group 10, the main obstacle blocking the further, fruitful development of HIS was identified as the lack of standardization, which creates several problems. Since there is no blueprint for the separation of an HIS into subsystems, it is impossible to compose an integrated HIS from modules supplied by different producers. Even for the subsystems that are presented under the same generic name, the functions supported may be quite different. This can be illustrated for the example of clinical laboratory systems:

- In some laboratory systems, the invoicing function is included, while in other systems it is supposed to be taken care of by the invoicing subsystem of the HIS.
- Reporting is often considered as a function of the laboratory system, however, in some approaches reporting is supposed to be included in a

separate subsystem that also takes care of the reporting of other results and integrate this service.

- In some laboratory systems, we find an order entry facility, in other systems, however, order entry is considered to be a subsystem in its own right, or is considered to be a function of the nursing system.

In this example, we have considered only the top level functions; at the lower levels, the lack of uniformity is even worse. If we ever hope to achieve a more or less open HIS, we need a common reference structure that describes which functions are assigned to which module. With increasing integration this need will increase.

Another standardization problem is the lack of a standard data definition. This not only hampers the exchange of data between systems in different institutions (a common language being required to be able to communicate), it is also a requirement if systems from different origins are expected to communicate within an institution. Furthermore, standard record layouts are required for data interchange, and standard protocols if the data are to be transmitted. With the gradual introduction of electronic data interchange (EDI) in health care, this issue is gaining importance. Standardization is also an issue at the user interface, even if the software modules of the HIS are supplied by the same vendor. Fortunately, the issue of standardization is now receiving considerable attention in Europe too. Recently, the European Committee for Standardization (CEN) set up its Technical Committee 251 to deal with standards in medical informatics (Mattheus 1991).

Although the concept of HIS is well accepted, no widely accepted definition of an HIS exists. Some groups keep HIS restricted to information handling within an institution, while others conceive HIS as going beyond the limits of institutions (for them HIS stands for health information system). Working group 10 was asked during the 1988 working conference to devise a definition proposal; hopefully this will be presented soon.

Another important issue is the meaning and materialization of the label "integrated"; undoubtedly it means something like "the whole is more than the summation of the parts". Within the HIS, the different applications or subsystems must benefit from each other. The following types of integration at least can be distinguished (Leguit 1989):

1. Functional integration, meaning that, within the domain of one application or subsystem, functions of other applications can be used. All patient-related subsystems should use patient identification functions of the patient registration subsystem. It should be possible to compose user task packages using functions from different subsystems, e.g., so that secretaries in the wards may handle retrieval of medical data, ordering tests, ordering meals, discharge letters, and appointments.
2. Data integration, meaning that subsystems can use data registered by other subsystems; for example, when routing reports, meals, drugs, or materials, the location of the patient should be available from the

admission/discharge/transfer (ADT) subsystem, and recording of the tests and examinations performed should be input into the invoicing subsystem.
3. Hardware integration, meaning that the system should present itself to the user as a unity, or at least permit access to all functions by means of the same terminal/workstation.

The requirements listed above look quite simple, however, in practice it turns out that even these "simple" requirements are difficult to meet. When subsystems come from different suppliers, the best one can hope for nowadays is proper interfacing and no integration. More attention should be paid to the nature of integration and the method of realizing it, since with the evolution of applications the need for integration will grow. In the laboratory subsystem, for example, the current medication of the patient is not yet checked when a test is ordered; this requirement, however, can be expected in the near future, since current medication may affect the test result, making it useless or even misleading.

4.1.13 HIS and Data Protection

4.1.13.1 Three Data Protection Issues

Although the opportunities for easy and remote access to the data stored in the HIS databank can be of great value to the quality of care and the efficiency of the institution, easy access may also be or become a threat to the privacy of the patients. In addition to that, the integrity of the data and programs deserves attention, as corrupted or lost data might harm the patient and the hospital. A third issue is the availability of the services of the HIS. Users will rely on HIS facilities to be able to work efficiently and for the proper functioning of their departments. If the system's service were interrupted, this might harm the patient and the functioning of the hospital.

The IMIA set up working group 4 to investigate data protection in Health Information Systems. The working group has published three books on the subject (Griesser 1977; Griesser et al. 1980, 1983) and organizes workshops during major international medical informatics conferences.

The threats to data protection may be related to hardware, environment, software, or organization. Sometime the threat will arise from an intended action from someone who wants to get hold of confidential data or wants to corrupt data, but often the threats will be unintentional. To reduce the risks or the expected damage related to the various threats, measures will have to be implemented in relation to hardware, software, and organization. In the literature, many proposals can be found for measures which should be implemented (Griesser 1980) and some case descriptions (Louwerse and Kouwenberg 1984). Measures will reduce the risks, although it will not be possible to reduce the risk to zero; the proposed measures and their costs will always have to be balanced against the effects they will have on the risk level.

4.1.13.2 HIS and Usage Integrity

With the introduction of HIS, many users in the hospital have access to data that are often rather sensitive. This is not principally new, but the use of remote terminals and the storage of data in a central data bank give the problem another dimension, which make the usual measures taken to protect paper registrations no longer adequate. On the other hand, a well-organized HIS may offer the patients better protection than they have in the paper system, since here the specific access rights of each user can be defined, and the user will only be allowed to see those categories of data he is authorized for and only for those patients that he has to deal with.

Interest in the protection of privacy led in 1981 to the recommendation on automated medical data banks by the Council of Europe, which was followed in many countries by national legislation. It is well accepted nowadays that a medical information system should have a regulation describing the goal of the registration, its organization, the rights of the patients (information, inspection, correction, and deletion), the user access rights, and the supply of information outside the institution (e.g., for research purposes). The effective protection of privacy is heavily dependent on the attitude of the users. They should be (made) aware of the threats to privacy of the patients that may arise from careless use of the system. The upper management echelons of the institution itself and professional organizations both have the responsibility of stimulating the awareness and the implementation of adequate measures, such as user identification control, specific user access rights ("need to know" principle), and restrictions to query facilities.

4.1.13.3 HIS and Data/Program Integrity

The data and programs stored in an HIS are of great, sometimes even vital value. One should be aware of threats to the integrity of these data, which might, for example, get lost or corrupted due to malfunctioning of the equipment, environmental conditions (e.g., fire, smoke), software errors, or errors in operating. Typical measures to prevent this are making back-up copies of the data bank, implementing software to log mutations and recover the data bank, testing software acceptance, and setting up a professional computer center.

4.1.13.4 HIS and Availability of Data

In the previous section we considered the safeguarding of the quality of the data, another important aspect of an HIS is the availability of the data to the user. The data bank may be correct and consistent and nevertheless be unavailable to the user because the hardware or software is not operational.

In a situation when all appointments are made by means of the system, when all reporting is performed by the system, when the supply of meals and drugs is scheduled by the system, and when nurses and doctors depend on the system for their direct patient care, an interruption of service will cause significant problems.

It should be realized that the services of the HIS will have to be available 24 h a day, 7 days a week. An availability of 100% will of course never be reached, but to realize an acceptable level of availability, certain measures have to be taken such as:

- Duplication of the central computer configuration
- Duplication of air-conditioning
- Back-up power supply
- Automatic fire extinguishers
- Mirrored disks
- Back-up computer center

4.1.14 His Workload: A Case Description

The volume of data to be recorded in an HIS, the number of terminals needed, and the number of transactions were all seriously underestimated initially. It has turned out that the workload is considerable, often leading to problems with performance. It is not just the volume of transactions that causes the problems, the situation is complicated by the large variation in transaction type and the wide variety of data to be handled.

Some workload data for the HIS at Leiden University Hospital, The Netherlands (875 beds and over 300 000 outpatient visits/year) can serve as an illustration (Bakker 1990). The HIS here is of an integrated nature and covers many functions of the hospital, ranging from patient registration to general ledger, from clinical chemistry to stock control, from meal supply to infection statistics, from operation registration to payroll, and from appointment scheduling to invoicing. The system is organized around a central data bank containing the data of over 800 000 patients. Terminals are installed throughout the hospital, and their total number exceeds 1000, so there are more terminals than beds. The heart of the system is a fully duplicated configuration, The system is operational 24 h a day, 7 days a week, and the realized availability is 99.8%, round the clock. The number of user interactions (carriage return symbols to which the HIS has to react) in the day shift exceeds 800 000; the number of user numbers issued exceeds 4000.

Although the HIS at Leiden already supports many functions of the hospital it can be expected to expand further. The main developments will involve:

- Support of direct medical care (nurses and doctors)
- Support of the logistic aspects of the hospital

- Communication beyond the limits of the hospital
- Support of management at both institutional and departmental levels.

It is expected that the workload will grow by about 20% per year, (therefore doubling in 4 years).

4.2 Radiology Information Systems

R. VAN DE VELDE

4.2.1 Introduction

In medicine there is a clear trend towards the increasing use of noninvasive imaging techniques to determine the optimal diagnostic and therapeutic procedures for patients. Radiology departments have grown in importance and have become huge organizations in terms of personnel, technologically advanced medical equipment for medical specialties, and the imaging procedures performed daily. The costs and revenues of this department have to be monitored very carefully.

It is obvious that radiology departments nowadays are also seeking methods to provide efficient, qualitative, medical and administrative services to patients, physicians, and technologists. In this chapter, the general concepts of radiology information systems (RIS) are emphasized as well as the aspects of integration between hospital information systems (HIS) and RIS with their alphanumerical data on the one hand, and picture archiving and communication systems (PACS) with their huge amount of image data, including the management of image data bases and traffic, on the other hand. The realization of so-called PACS is still in its starting phase, which makes the situation more or less comparable to that for HIS in the 1970s. The main difference is the tremendous volume of data to be stored and transported by PACS which follows from the large volume of data contained in images, although the number of tables in the image data base of PACS is much lower than in an HIS. As PACS are becoming increasingly important, it is interesting to compare the differences and similarities of both systems (Table 4.1). It is obvious that the alphanumerical data available in the HIS is a prerequisite and will be indispensable for managing the image data base.

We are moving towards a diagnostic imaging environment that will provide all medical patient images, but it must be clear that images do not stand alone, and the need for information derived from various clinical information systems is obvious. To maximize the value of a specific examination, physicians need information from many sources other than past and present images. The integration of information is necessary for any system to survive, but this will become increasingly difficult due to the continuing changes in technology and practice patterns. The definition of integration deserves extra attention (Fig. 4.1). This might be clarified by keeping in mind that a clinical user needs an integrated overview of all relevant patient

Table 4.1. A comparison of HIS and PACS

Feature	HIS	PACS
Size of data base (GB)	1–20	1000–20 000
Number of tables (n)	400	20
Length of tables	10–100 B	1–6 MB
Response time (S)	<3	>3
Number of WS (n)	100	10
Types of WS	cheap; numerical	expensive; bit-mapped

GB, gigabyle; *MB*, megabyte; *WS*, workstation

data, namely, image data from PACS and alphanumerical data from HIS and RIS at the right time and in the right place. The physician acquires images through the PACS from patients identified by the HIS, coupled with numerical and text data in medical reports about examinations from the RIS at the relevant time and place.

Both users at the image acquisition end and users at the hospital clinic end should, thus, be involved in setting up PACS. It is also obvious that the coupling of PACS and HIS – so-called integration – should be realized as early as possible, where the information in the HIS data base may serve to manage large image data bases, probably many terabytes.

4.2.2 PACS, HIS, and RIS: Natural Couples

PACS is not viable when it is not integrated both with the RIS and with the HIS. The RIS has to be integrated with the HIS to make use of the single central hospital (alphanumerical) data base. A PACS can be connected with the HIS (possibly integrated) and have a common part with the RIS, which is in fact included in the HIS if the RIS is an integrated part of the HIS. Of course there will be a part of the HIS with no relation to PACS and RIS, and vice versa (Fig. 4.2). The end user or clinician has to perceive all these subsystems as one logically related system.

4.2.3 Radiology Information Systems

The RIS has to be considered as the front end of each PACS. The current goal of an RIS should be to use the computer for registration, scheduling, reporting, and communication of all relevant patient data and for all activities and functions within the imaging department. Furthermore, it should be horizontally integrated with the nursing communication system in order to provide order scheduling. Let us consider the individual parts of an RIS in some more detail. In Fig. 4.3 a data flow diagram of an RIS is presented and

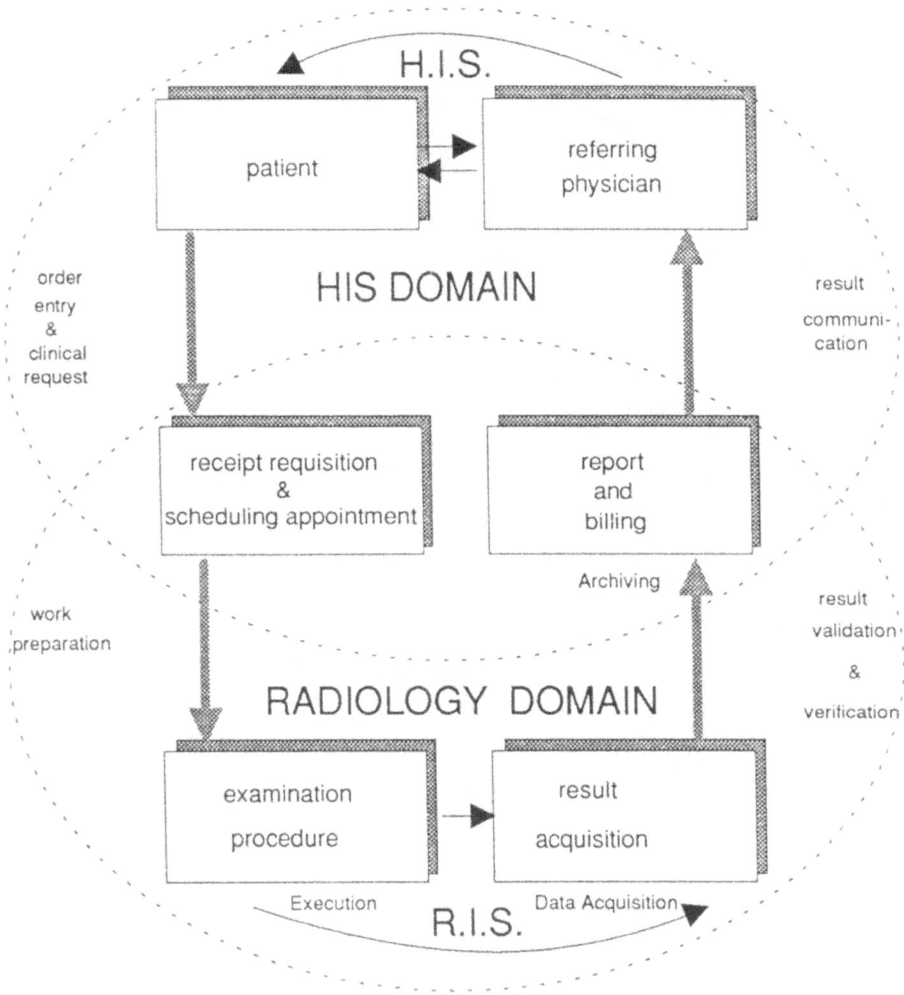

Fig. 4.1. The key elements of a radiology information system representing the main flows and relationships

Table 4.2 gives an overview of the main activities in an RIS from requisition to reporting activity.

4.2.3.1 Examination Requisition

The radiology process starts with the creation of the examination requisition by the referring physician, for future diagnosis and treatment therapy. The patient identification and demographic data have to be retrieved, if registered previously in the admission/discharge/transfer (ADT) system from the

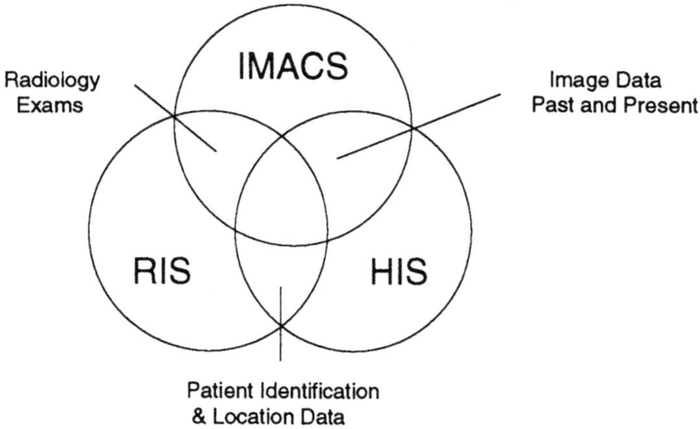

Fig. 4.2. Optimal integration will be achieved in the management of images (PACS) if those stored in the image archive are coupled with examination data from the RIS and with patient data from the HIS

Table 4.2. Overview of the main activities and related subsystems in an RIS/HIS/PACS environment

Action	Subsystem	Computer peripheral
1. Clinical request	HIS	Terminal
2. Appointment and scheduling	HIS–RIS	Bit-mapped workstation
3. Image acquisition	RIS–PACS	PACS workstation (local CPU)
4. Data processing	PACS	PACS workstation (local CPU)
5. Interpretation and reporting and approval	RIS–PACS	PACS workstation
6. Communication to referring physician	PACS–HIS	Simple viewing station
7. Archiving	PACS–HIS	Long-storage archive
8. Retrieval history	HIS–PACS	Simple viewing station

CPU, central processing unit

HIS in a transparent user environment via several access pathways such as phonetic search and medical record number and coupled to the requisition. If the patient is not registered, the admission function has to be included in the RIS and fed to the HIS. This requisition requires:

- Patient selection
- Identification of the patient's clinical problem
- Identification of the imaging studies that have to be carried out for the patient

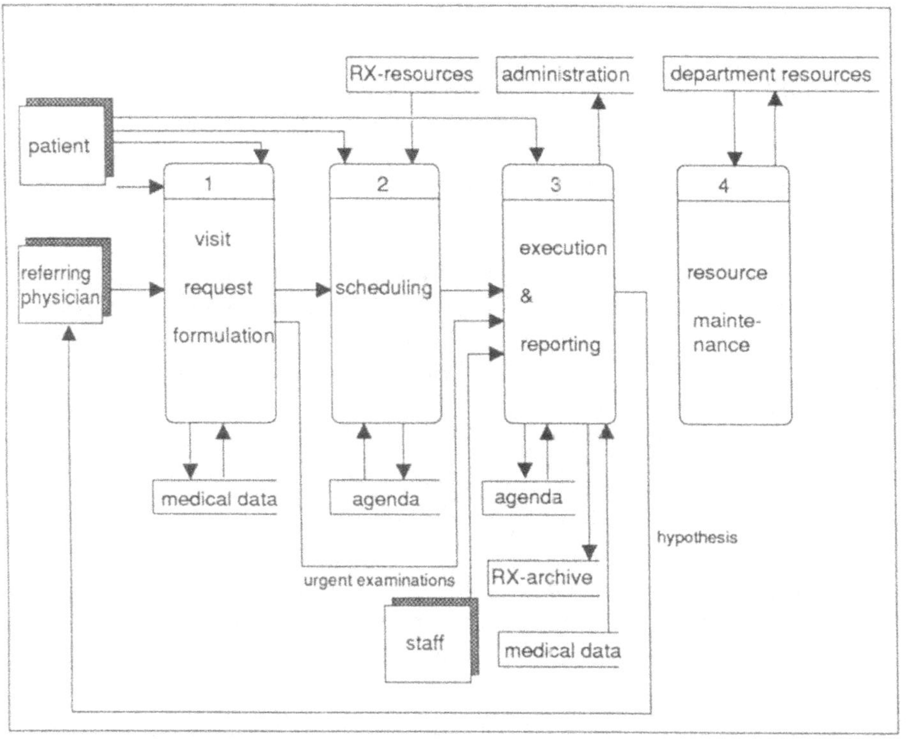

Fig. 4.3. Data flow diagram of an RIS (*RX*, radiology department). (From Gane and Sarsen 1979)

- Possible prefetching previous radiology examination results
- The automatic control of the request with previous or future, similar or duplicate examinations, which have to be flagged
- The indication of conflicts between examinations

Various documents have to be printed for preparing and streamlining the work. These documents include transportation sheets, indicating where transporters have to move the patient; flash cards to identify the patient's imaging study; and examination preparation cards (work lists) to be used by the radiologists at the time of examination to assemble information on, e.g., drugs used and patient's time of arrival and departure. Some institutions use bar code labels to assist them in fast retrieval and registration of patient data.

4.2.3.2 Scheduling

After the requisition has been entered into the system, the examination has to be scheduled at a certain examination room and time. Scheduling criteria are defined according to the specific needs of the department. It is obvious that the basic scheduling mechanism in an appointment system forms the basis of this for the radiology department, i.e., length of examination, scheduling templates, slot length, available resources, agenda, and graphic user interface (GUI) (Van de Velde 1987). Scheduling systems in radiology vary substantially, but all have the common feature of booking appointments in advance for various examinations. The scheduling procedure involves the following activities:

1. Transmission of orders entered by nursing stations or referring services directly into the department schedule prior to receiving the paperwork from the floors.
2. Maintaining the daily patient schedule by room, providing a better distribution of workload.
3. Preventing, permitting, or highlighting overbooking.
4. Preventing duplicate, conflicting, or incompatible examination scheduling with previous or future examinations, if not already detected at a previous stage.
5. Indicating the sequence of examination checking.
6. Retrieving active cases by any one of a wide range of selection criterial such as patient, room number, radiologist, or referring physician.
7. Supporting automatic label printing for flash cards and film tracking.
8. Calculating the workload of each section in real time.
9. Supporting automatic transportation notes.
10. Pringing the daily schedule by appointment time, resource (i.e., examination room), or inpatient location.
11. Requisition of the radiologist approval before certain examinations can be scheduled.

4.2.3.3 Acquisition

The acquisition phase includes the creation of images and their registration in the PACS. The examination preparation cards (or work lists) indicate to the technician which examinations have to be performed. Before starting the examinations, patient identification data have to be coupled with the images, either by using the flash cards (labels) for conventional films, or electronically for digital imaging modalities such as computed tomography (CT) scans or magnetic resonance imaging (MRI). Each image has further to be identified by a unique identifier coupled with the examination. Historical images are sometimes also needed during the execution of the examination.

The patient-tracking module registers the time each examination performed for that patient started and ended. A registration of time intervals allows the hospital to look for trends and to strive for an improvement in patient flow. It can also form the basis for generating productivity and utilization reports. An alternative method is the use of bar codes. Before the patient arrives, requisition orders or the work list can be printed using bar codes. The requisitions are bar-coded with the patient identification number and other instructions such as examination code and patient's medical record number. When the technician is carrying out the procedure, he may read the data at a glance, adding his confirmation and charge.

4.2.3.4 Diagnostic Reporting

After completion of the examination, the next stage is the interpretation, generation, and communication of the results to the referring physician. During reporting, the previous reports included in the patient's medical record are often consulted. This report generation process is the least developed component of every RIS system (Greenes and Brinkley 1990). Nowadays, transcription by secretaries of dictated reports in combination with text processing facilities and stored radiological tests is by far the most common and preferred system used for report genertation by radiologists. Report generation systems using structured (coded) reports are only successful in domains where the content and organization of reports are well structured. Up to now, several other experiments and methods of report generation have been tried over the years, not always with success. One of these methods is based on a dialogue between the computer and radiologist (e.g., in the Missouri automated radiology system, MARS). The report is built up by making iterative selections from a standard thesaurus (library) of terms, which are subdivided into examination type, anatomy, and diagnosis (Lehr et al. 1973). Another technique has emerged through the development of touch-sensitive terminals on which diagnostic possibilities are indicated. The physician may prepare his report by touching the appropriate items on a touch-sensitive screen. These systems have not been well accepted in Europe. Commercial systems were produced by CGR and Siemens (e.g., Sirep) (Wheeler 1979). Another approach utilizes mark-sense sheets (Mani and Jones 1973) or some form of coded or mnemonic input by the radiologist (Raport system).

Some experiments are being carried out nowadays using more sophisticated voice-recognition methods for data entry in report generation. A speech-recognition system produces machine-readable reports from dictated phrases using (for the moment) a lexicon of 1000–7000 words (Kurzweill Company, USA). It is clear that – although very promising – this technology does not seem to be ready yet for general use in report generation, since surrounding noise and pronounciation are still obstacles.

Every procedure can be coded according to the diagnosis, using, for example, the American College of Radiology (ACR) classification. This can be an integral part of the diagnostic reporting subsystem and is highly desirable for retrieving cases according to medical diagnosis. Radiologists may use system terminals to apply approval codes (electronic signature) and do final editing of the reports themselves, even from remote locations. Reports remain online for any designated period.

4.2.3.5 Teaching File

For teaching and research purposes, a number of cases are indicated as valuable and stored in a data base of diagnostic information, i.e., a teaching file. Afterwards, it is possible to retrieve all desired information for teaching and research purposes by specifying certain criteria.

4.2.3.6 Results Reporting: Mailing Facility

After the results have been created and verified (if necessary), they will be sent to the referring physicians or to the patient's location (inpatient or outpatient department). It is most desirable to do this with mailing facilities.

4.2.3.7 Film and Patient Tracking

To reduce the loss incurred by unreturned film loans, a film management and leading system is still necessary.

The main objectives of a film-tracking system are:

- To support the operational functions of archive management.
- To keep track of X-rays.
- To provide for check-out of a film jacket (via bar-coding) to any temporary location or referring physician outside or inside the department.
- To provide for check-in from any temporary location.
- To provide an on-line film location inquiry in order to locate the film quickly, as the films for a patient can be scattered over different locations. Some hospitals use bar-code readers as automatic data entry for this purpose.

For future PACS, it is worthwhile to compare the transactions within a film library and a PACS (Table 4.3). Nevertheless, (Matheus 1989), since digital images are not "returned", there is no transaction similar to returning films to the film room. Occasionally, however, the radiologist may wish to store a newly made transformed image or annotated overlay. Furthermore, images copied from archival to intermediate storage do not have to be copied back to archive storage after being used. Here again, bar-code labels with patient number can be used for conventional film tracking.

4.2.3.8 Management Reports and Billing

Finally, the system has to provide billing data to be processed by a general billing module. The effective management of a radiology department requires tools which are adequate to understand the operation of the department thoroughly, to have enough accurate data to suggest changes in its

Table 4.3. Comparison of PACS and film library transactions

Film library transaction	PACS transaction
Inactive file room to active file room	Archival to intermediate storage
New films to active file room	Image generators to PACS viewing station
Active file room to light box	Intermediate storage to PACS viewing station
Light box to active file room	None
Active file room to inactive file room	Movement of new images from intermediate to archival (storage)
Active file room to borrowers	Intermediate storage to remote display
Borrowers to active file room	None

operation, and to monitor the effectiveness of these decisions once new actions have been taken. So, the system has to provide comprehensive statistical information.

The framework for management reporting can be divided into three categories:

1. Daily management.
   - The daily log lists patients in chronological order and by department section.
   - The new patient report lists all new patients by origin.
   - The incomplete activity report lists incomplete exams that have been performed, or not transcribed and approved. It helps determine the efficiency of the department.
   - The system maintains teaching files according to physician and ACR code.
2. Operation management.
   - The room productivity reports provide valuable utilization data for workflow monitoring.
   - The facility and equipment utilization reports provide information for equipment usage.
   - The revenue report summarizes clinical fees by cost center.
   - The activity report lists all departmental activities by type of examination and by patient type.
3. Personnel management.
   - Technologist productivity reports.
   - Physician productivity reports.

4.2.3.9 Inventory Tracking

A departmental inventory tracking module is necessary to provide the user with the ability to notify the system of changes in inventory and to monitor the on-hand value of the inventory. This capability can be used to identify consumption trends as well as measure the costs of maintaining inventory levels. Economic order quantities are determined for all products in the system.

4.2.3.10 Equipment Maintenance

Information about preventive and unscheduled maintenance is maintained for a user-defined set of equipment. The information recorded includes equipment identifier, manufacturer, services, dates of all maintenance, type of maintenance, problems, cost of repair, part replaced, and time down. Query reports may be run to summarized or select maintenance records using any of the data recorded as a sort or selection criteria.

4.2.4 The Relationship of PACS to HIS

4.2.4.1 Image Acquisition Nodes

As part of the examination identification, a unique identification of the patient is required. Such a unique identification will be present in the HIS and must be copied into the equipment for the acquisition of digital images coupled to the PACS. The best moment to couple the examination identification to the image is when the image is created. Because a visit can consist of one or more examinations, the RIS has to be extended with the notions of folder and subfolder for image storage.

Rough overall calculations indicate that the total digital image storage capacity will be measured in terabytes. Even with a reduction factor of 10,

Table 4.4. Advantages of an RIS

Improvement	Cause
For the patient	Reduced waiting time
Patient result reporting	Flexible report formats Decrease in turnaround time Decrease in lost results
Resource managment	Appropriate workload in advance by theatre Inventory control record
Administration	Accurate billing input Accurate workload Optimalization of workflow
Personnel performance	Increased efficiency
Film management	Increased film control Loan lists Automatic link with PACS

this is still a tremendous amount of data. It is more or less accepted that the physical storage structure should be layered into three parts:

1. A relatively slow but huge archive containing all the images in the hospital.
2. A faster but smaller intermediate buffer with images that are needed in the very near future.
3. A small but very fast working memory for daily routine.

The HIS can play an important role in deciding the place and the moment to store the images. Besides hardware solutions, software and algorithms that manage the correct and in-time allocation of images to a specific layer will be required. Without a close coupling of HIS and PACS, this strategy is impossible.

4.2.4.2 Image Communication Network

A standardized network must be the PACS backbone and must include a link to the HIS for control and management purposes, although this link could be physically isolated from the image transport link.

4.2.4.3 Image Viewing Stations

Since there are many different types of image users in a hospital, it may be expected that there will be different types of stations for the display of images. The HIS has also an important role in the proper presentation of both alphanumerical and image data in an integrated way.

4.2.5 Distributed Radiology Systems: A Possible Architecture

Early RIS ran mainly on separate, independent minicomputer systems, or sometimes on the central computer facility. Compared with other departments, radiology departments are characterized by the need for more computational and especially more communicative needs. The advantages of an RIS are presented in Table 4.4. In a real computer network environment a configuration hierarchy could contain the following components (see also Fig. 4.4).

- A centralized cluster of one or more hospital information computer systems, utilized by other departmental feeder systems for demographic patient data and the long-term archiving of longitudinal medical records.
- A centralized radiology application server to collect intermediate radiology data and functions as an interradiology communication vehicle.

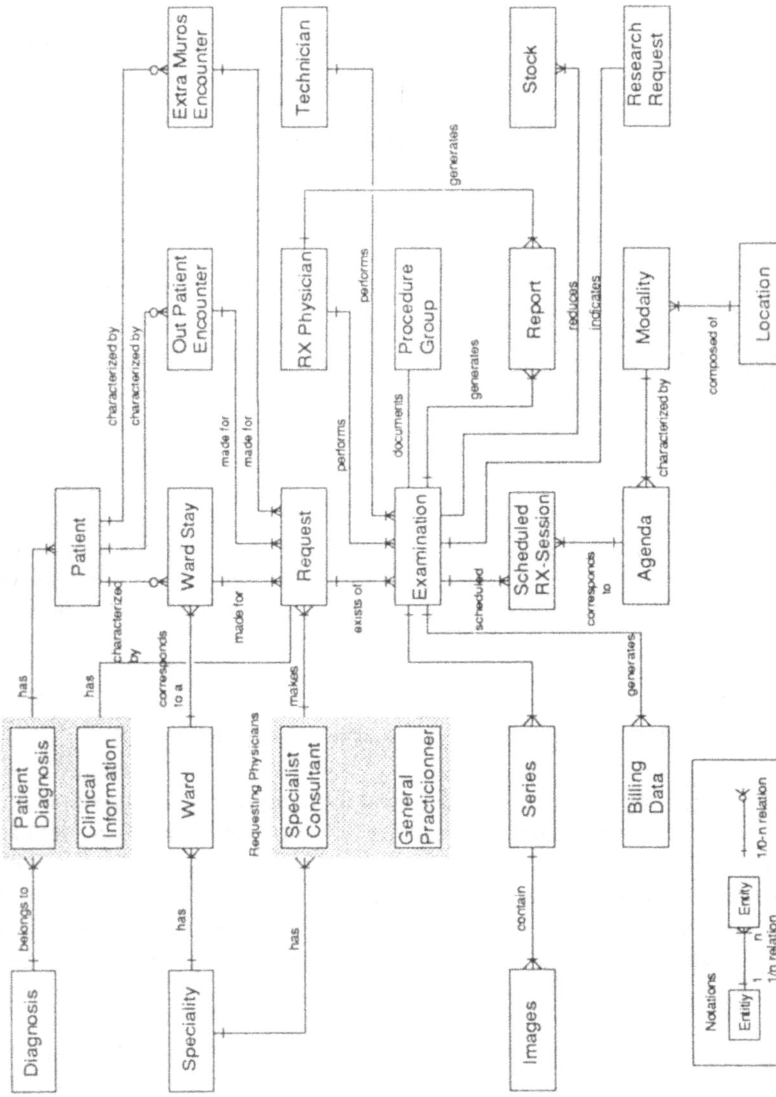

Fig. 4.4. General representation of an RIS (*RX*, radiology department)

- Microcomputers and workstations with high quality bit-mapped screens in different imaging areas for communication with the rest, to collect data, to generate reports, and to perform medical functions such as viewing or image manipulation.

Indeed, the RIS is the front end of the PACS system and of other hospital data sources.

4.3 Integration of PACS, RIS, and HIS

H. Lodder, B.M. Van Poppel, and A.R. Bakker

4.3.1 Introduction

4.3.1.1 Starting Points and Approach

From earlier chapters it should have become clear that the concept of integration plays a key role, not only if we look at clinical integration (Chap. 2), but also if we consider the way in which those information systems that have already been in existence for some time such as hospital information systems (HIS; cf. Sect. 4.1) and radiological information systems (RIS; cf. Sect. 4.2) have been designed and implemented. Within the framework of the Advanced Information in Medicine/Hospital Integrated Picture Archiving and Communication Systems (AIM/HIPACS) project, research is carried out to identify and – whenever possible – eliminate the bottlenecks that hamper implementation of a fully integrated picture archiving and communication system (PACS). In order to be able to realize a PACS which works on a hospital-wide scale, integration with other information systems such as HIS and RIS is seen as a must (Bijl 1987; Lodder 1990).

Following a top-down approach, this chapter will treat successively:

1. The concept of integration. By using a number of examples, we discuss the advantages of implementing a PACS which is integrated with an HIS and/or an RIS over implementing a PACS which stands alone. We will also remark on the different opinions that exist on the relation between HIS and RIS and between PACS and HIS and RIS. In addition, attention is paid to the differences between integration, interfacing, and coupling. We will also discuss the specifications of an (unpartitioned) HIS-RIS-PACS, which will be called HIPACS for the sake of convenience. The starting point in drafting the specifications is naturally the user. Besides the user or functional requirements, the specifications must contain performance requirements and a data model.
2. A method which can be used to bridge the gap between the HIPACS specifications and the characteristics of existing and separately developed systems such as HIS and RIS. This will prove necessary to make choices in the assignment of both functions and data to the systems. Three aspects that play an important part in HIPACS data base design will also be indicated briefly.

3. A number of conclusions that can be drawn from the experience gained thus far and some recommendations with respect to the development of a second generation PACS. The key words will in any case be integration, standardization, and partial PACS.

4.3.1.2 Reasons for PACS–HIS–RIS Integration

Because an exact definition of the concept of integration is lacking, we will here discuss the necessity of a PACS being integrated with an HIS and/or an RIS using several examples.

Example 1. For reporting on new examinations, the radiologist needs information from previous radiological examinations, i.e., both images and related reports, and other medical data from the patient. Moreover, it is preferable for all data to be presented in a coherent way on the (HI)PACS workstation. If a PACS is integrated with an HIS and an RIS, textual information from the HIS and RIS is directly accessible.

The advantage of an integrated PACS is that the radiologist only has to deal with one user interface rather than two or three. It should preferably not be necessary for him to know the origin of the data (i.e., PACS, HIS, or RIS), since this should be obvious.

Example 2. The radiologist mentioned in example 1 is used to reporting on new examinations at a great pace, and this will only be possible if all the relevant previous images and related data are easily and quickly accessible. In a PACS environment, this implies that all the necessary information should be available in the local memory of the radiologist's workstation. This is really a big problem when we have to deal with a patient's history which consists of many images. If the PACS is integrated, the HIS and/or the RIS can – as a result of an admission registered or a radiological appointment made, for example – trigger the transport of previous images within the PACS from the large, but slow optical archive to the smaller, but much faster local buffer of the workstation. Depending on the amount of intelligence applied in the software, it can be determined for each examination which historical information is relevant and must be activated, and which is not.

The strategy which may be used to optimize PACS image management using information generated by the HIS and/or RIS is called "prefetching" (cf. Sect. 5.3 for an in-depth discussion). The advantage of an integrated PACS seen here is that the response time of the system can be shortened considerably by using prefetching.

Example 3. The technician responsible for the actual acquisition of digital images must combine the images and corresponding patient data to identify the images. It is desirable for the necessary data from the HIS and/or the RIS to be available at the acquisition unit in advance so that correct identification can be made by means of simple selection from a list of data. If the PACS used is not integrated, the identification data have to be typed in (again) or entered into the PACS using a plastic card produced by the HIS or RIS.

The advantage of an integrated PACS is that identification data only has to be entered once (i.e., into the HIS or RIS). As a result, the risk of making typing errors will be eliminated.

Example 4. A radiologist or referring physician working at a PACS workstation sometimes needs functions that are only available on the HIS or the RIS. In other words, this user requires access to RIS-related information such as radiological reports (for updating and authorization), administrative data, information on previous radiological examinations and reports, and patient scheduling for radiology, as well as other HIS information such as admission discharge transfer (ADT) data, diagnoses, surgery data, pathology data, laboratory reports, and other diagnostic and therapeutic data.

The advantage of an integrated PACS is that both PACS functions and HIS/RIS functions are available from the workstation, provided that the user is authorized to use those functions. In fact, one can say that this so-called function integration is a prerequisite for offering the user a one-user interface instead of two or three.

The examples given above are concerned with the advantages of an integrated PACS from the user's point of view. A number of arguments can also be put forward from the view point of system management for integrating a PACS with an HIS and/or an RIS. The main reasons of PACS–HIS–RIS integration from the user's point of view are the need for patientinformation which is not stored in the PACS data base; the need for HIS functions which are not available on the PACS; an acceptable response time of the system; the advantage of only having to enter identification data once (i.e., in HIS or RIS, not in aquisition device); and the possibility of selecting images according to criteria from HIS information (e.g., teaching files).

From a system management point of view an integrated PACS–HIS–RIS has several advantages, for example, it is important to keep HIS and PACS data bases consistent in an efficient way. Furthermore, to be able to judge whether a certain updata of HIS data is allowed or not, one has to know whether this data is present in the PACS data base. Another advantage is that in the case of nonacceptance of messages by the PACS, it is much more efficient for the HIS to stop and wait until the PACS is in a ready-to-receive mode again. Moreover, integration of this sort is more efficient in handling the error situation that occurs when data sent to the PACS cannot be processed in the PACS data base.

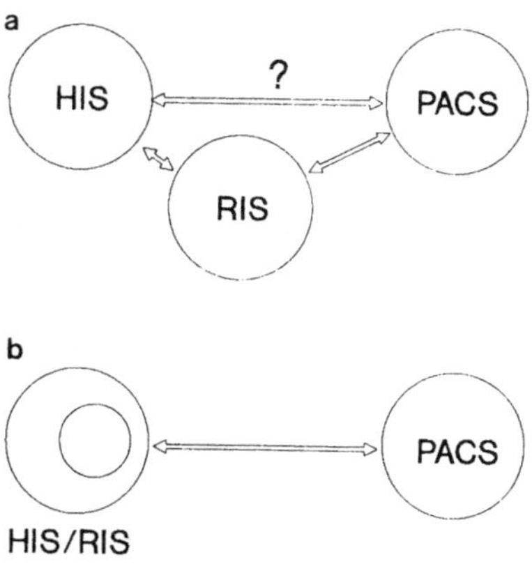

Fig. 4.5a,b. Different views on the relationship between HIS and RIS. **a** HIS and RIS as two independent systems. **b** RIS as a subsystem of HIS

4.3.1.3 Different Views on the Relationship between HIS and RIS

In this section, we will discuss the various views that exist with respect to the relation between HIS and RIS, which, of course, also has a impact on integration with PACS. In Fig. 4.5 the two alternatives are depicted. In Fig. 4.5a, HIS and RIS are regarded as two independent systems which are often linked in some way. They are not, however, integrated, which means that, for HIS-related information, the user has to use his HIS terminal and for RIS-related information, he has to consult his RIS terminal. This departmental system approach usually implies the existence of many more separate information systems, e.g., for cardiology, surgery, and neurology. In that case the HIS is actually just a general information system for administrative and financial purposes. For this approach, PACS–HIS–RIS integration implies – depending on the extent to which HIS and RIS already have been coupled – the realization of more than one interface with the PACS.

In Fig 4.5b, the RIS is seen as a subsystem of the HIS. This type of integrated HIS contains in principle all the functionality necessary to support the activities in a hospital using an automated information system (cf. Sect. 4.1 for a detailed explanation of the integrated HIS concept). From this point of view, the integration of HIS and PACS is just one logical step.

4.3.1.4 Coupling, Interfacing, and Integrating

Before describing the requirements for an ideal future HIPACS, we would like to go into some more detail about the concepts of interfacing, integrating, and coupling. Interfacing two systems means linking the two systems; the interface description involves the dependencies which exist between elements from different systems. One of the most important issues in interfacing two systems is to determine where the interface should be positioned.

If no functions are supported by both systems, the interface should simply be located between the elements of both systems that have to communicate. If there are comparable functions in both systems – such as in the currently available HIS, RIS, and PACS systems – a choice has to be made between the possibilities. In Sect. 4.3.2, we start out independently of any consideration of HIS, RIS, or PACS by specifying the user and performance requirements of an ideal HIPACS. These specifications are based on the functions performed by, for example, a radiology department together with other departments which (may) use the functions offered by HIPACS. In Sect. 4.3.3, choices are made with respect to the demarcation of functions and related data.

In general an interface between two systems is associated with the borderline between them, and a coupling between two systems refers rather to the physical link between the systems. In general one can say that by integrating two (or more) systems, a new system is created which has more intrinsic possibilities than the sum of the functionalities of each of the separate systems.

In other words interfacing can be seen as the first step towards integration. The more Open Systems Interconnect (OSI) layers are supported, the larger this step will be. If there is also agreement on the semantics of the entities to be communicated, the level of integration has been reached.

4.3.2 Specifications of a Global HIPACS

4.3.2.1 Requirements of an Ideal Global HIPACS

As already mentioned in the introduction, an unpartitioned HIPACS should offer the user all the functions needed to support his daily tasks. It should preferably not be necessary for the user to be aware that some of these functions used to be restricted to the HIS and others to the RIS, since he now only has to deal with one system, namely, HIPACS. In Fig. 4.6, this important notion is illustrated in a slightly different way with the user placed in the center.

The user in Fig. 4.6a, i.e., in the nonintegrated environment, has to cope with several different information systems, namely HIS, RIS, PACS, and maybe even more (see Sect. 4.3.1.3). The acquisition modules may also be mentioned here, because they do play a role even though they are often not regarded being part of PACS. The user in Fig. 4.6b only has to deal with one system, i.e., the HIPACS system. The tuning of functions of the different subsystems is performed by the inner shell.

Because the needs of the users should be the starting point when specifying any information system, the first thing to do is to find out which requirements the HIPACS system has to meet. In other words, what should a HIPACS offer to the user (see Sect. 4.3.2.2) and what data are we talking about (see Sect. 4.3.2.3).

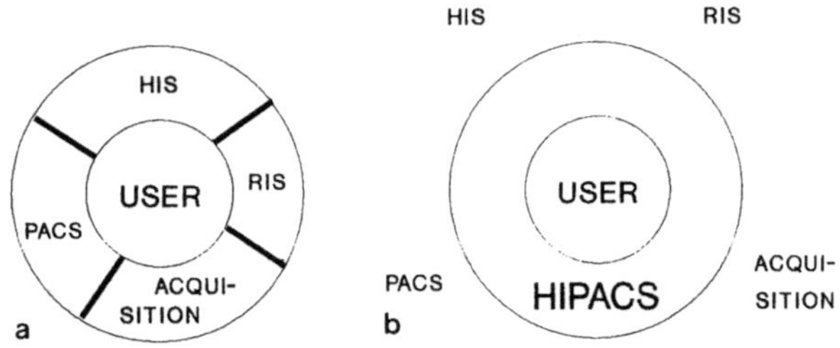

Fig. 4.6a,b. Comparison of a nonintegrated (**a**) and an integrated (**b**) system from the point of view of the user

4.3.2.2 Functional and Performance Requirements of a Global HIPACS

Before one can specify or design an information system, or in our case an interface between information systems, one has to know which requirements the information system has to meet. Requirements are often subdivided into two main categories, namely functional and performance requirements.

Functional requirements specify which data have to be processed and delivered, and these depend upon the specific information needs of the users. Performance requirements specify the quality with which the data have to be processed and delivered. These performance requirements may be regarded as the conditions which the information system has to satisfy.

If during the design of an information system too much emphasis is placed on the functional requirements only, then the development process is incomplete. It should be noted that the development of an information system is complex and costly, not just because of the realization of the functional demands, but in particular because of satisfying the performance requirements. In other words, designing an information system is largely a process of balancing the efforts, the functional requirements, and the performance requirements.

Functional Requirements

In a top-down approach, one can say that at the top level a HIPACS information system should support the following two global functions:

- Offer clinicians the possibility of retrieval of all relevant medical data, including images.
- Support the performance of new examinations, including the management of resources such as acquisition rooms, scheduling acquisitions, the administrative follow-up, and the minimization of the radiation doses applied.

A good starting point for gaining insight into the user functions of a HIPACS are the operational activities in a hospital which are somehow related to PACS and which can be described for the different classes of users. The main activities in this respect, together with relevant input and output data, are summarized in the following.

Appointment. The sequence of activities within the radiological department will be started at the request of a physician. He will request a radiological examination and add a motivation, e.g., a possible diagnosis or a description of symptoms. This request will lead to an appointment for the acquisition and to the allocation of manpower and equipment. The appointment can be adjusted to fit with other appointments. A certain strategy will be followed in order to optimize the use of the resources, e.g., optimal occupancy of the acquisition rooms. During the request process, it is possible that medical data will be discussed by the radiology department and the requesting physician. Previous images may be needed during the acquisition or during the reporting. A request for retrieval of the previous images will be sent to the film archive. In PACS, this activity is represented by prefetching the relevant images. The main activity here is, therefore, the registration of an appointment by the secretarial office of the radiology department.

Acquisition. Under the activity of acquisition we include the arrival of the patient, or, if the examination is performed at the bedside, the arrival of the X-ray equipment, the actual acquisition, and the departure of the patient or the equipment. The technician needs information on which examinations are to be performed and which patients are to be examined. This data may be put in the form of a work list for the technician. The control of the visits of patients can be supported by a module for patient tracking. After the acquisition of the images, each image has to be coupled to a unique identifier. Sometimes previous images are needed during the acquisition. The main activity here is, therefore, the acquisition of images and the identification of the image data.

Preparation for Reporting. Reporting of the examinations will be performed by the radiologists. There are various ways of assigning a stack of examinations to be reported to an individual radiologist. The historical film images needed (or expected to be needed) for reporting are added to the new examinations, and with PACS this means requesting the transmission of the needed images to the workstation. The main activity here is, therefore, the preparation of a stack of images for a radiologist.

Reporting. The radiologist makes his diagnosis on the stack of examinations prepared previously. The report is usually recorded on tape and afterwards typed into the PACS–HIS–RIS. It depends on the particular radiology department when the reports are authorized. In most teaching hospitals, reporting will be performed in two phases; first a draft report is made, then authorization follows. Images need to be kept on the local workstation until the report has been authorized. The main activity here is the creation of an authorized report.

Conference. Frequently the relevant and interesting cases are discussed by the (assistant) radiologists and the referring clinicians. This means that the new images from these patients, together with a number of previous images (and reports), if appropriate, must be available on the viewing station(s) in the conference room. In many hospitals a so-called holy hour is also scheduled each day for internal discussion between radiologists and residents. The main activity here is viewing and sometimes image manipulation.

Receiving Results. The referring clinician, who usually requests the radio-diagnostic examination, will receive the results of this examination as soon as they are available. Whether the results must contain only a written report by the radiologist or the corresponding images as well differs according to hospital. Moreover, the referring clinician needs access to other medical patient data from the HIS and/or RIS. The main activity for the referring clinician is viewing, sometimes simple image handling, and gaining access to clinical patient data from the HIS and/or RIS database.

Research/Teaching. One of the important activities in university hospitals in particular is the teaching file facility. For a given medical issue, a file of images is assembled containing cases with the medical characteristics relevant to this issue. Such queries will also be carried out for research purposes on both the image data base and the HIS and/or RIS data base.

Performance Requirements

At first sight it seems that the inventory and description of user functions is sufficient to specify an information system, but this is not true. As well as finding answers to the question of *what* a HIPACS should do, we also have investigated the question of *how* a HIPACS should do this. The latter question pertains to the performance requirements, which will be described briefly below. Because of the technical nature of this section, reference is made, where applicable, to coupling as being the physical connection between the different HIPACS components.

Specifications. It is almost unnecessary to say that the specifications on the HIS side, the RIS side, the PACS side, and the interface(s) have to be complete and up to date. This means there must be agreement about the definitions of data, the data model, the processes involved, and the manual procedures. It is not necessary to use the same definitions, but the definitions have to be described in the same terms. Standardization of the language in which specifications are drawn up will support the communication between users and system developers. It is necessary to investigate where redundant storage occurs and which considerations are involved, e.g., who manages the data, who is responsible, and which is the major application.

Adaptability of the Coupling. The coupling has to function automatically and in the background. Moreover, the coupling has to be able to react to a number of external occurrences such as the breakdown of one of the systems and disturbances in the communication. The coupling has to be able to start the communication without human action. Arrangements for monitoring software and logging follow from this requirement.

Regular Operation and Error Handling. In regular clinical operation, some technical problems with the system, e.g., a full disk, have to be solved manually, which will require qualified operators. Attention has to be given to management aspects, e.g., an operators' guide. HIS, RIS, and PACS suppliers have to participate in fulfilling these demands. The operation of the coupling should be easy to use and easy to learn.

Standards. It is advisable to make use of widely accepted standards in software, documentation, and methodology as much as possible. This is even more important because a number of activities in establishing a coupling will be undertaken by different persons from different institutions and suppliers.

Reliability/Integrity/Availability. In a clinical environment, high demands will be imposed on the reliability of data, software, and hardware. The consistency of the data itself has to be safeguarded. Besides the issues which refer to the information provision itself (e.g., completeness, correctness, timeliness, and permissibility), measures against loss, damage, and sabotage will be needed. Furthermore, arrangements have to be made to avoid human failures and unauthorized access. It is desirable that checks can be performed, e.g., a consistency check on redundantly stored data. Special attention has to be paid to a recovery procedure.

System Design. PACS will be implemented step by step. The design has to anticipate future use in terms of extensibility and flexibility. It is commonly accepted that information systems should be built as a modular structure. It may eventually involve more departments and more data and communication with other hospitals. It is advisable to define only one interface with PACS, if possible since separate communication with each PACS component should be avoided. The design must be flexible as it is impossible to predict exactly how PACS systems will be used. The specification of a coupling should be as manufacturer-independent as possible. Software and possibly hardware within the coupling should be portable. A subsequent design criterion is maintainability, especially for the specifications.

Requirements for Response Time. A short response time for image retrieval will be an important design issue. It is currently commonly accepted that prefetching is a prerequisite for PACS (see Sect. 5.3 for an extensive discussion on prefetching). It is important that the complete procedure, of which such a retrieval is only a part, be kept in mind. For example, a very fast image retrieval loses in value if there are long delays in generating accompanying reports. Depending on the output of the system, the total

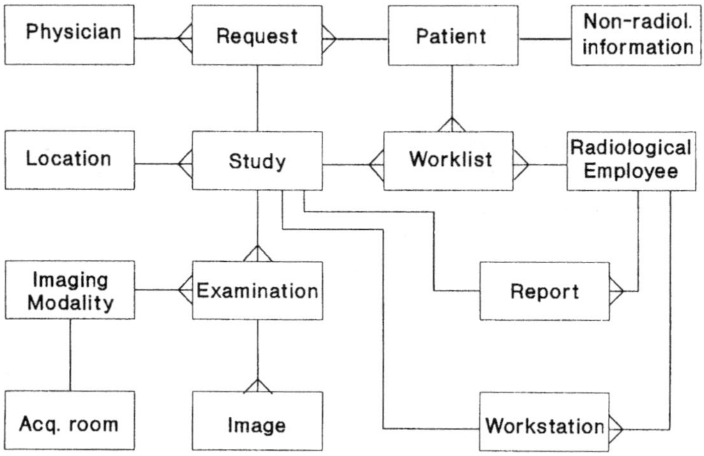

Fig. 4.7. Entity-relation diagram of the data elements that play an important role in the HIPACS system and the relations between them. The *lines* indicate the links between the entities, and the *crow's feet* indicate that the relations are one-to-many and many-to-many, rather than one-to-one

time taken to perform a task can be significantly reduced by means of the presentation of aggregated information, exception reporting, or, in the case of PACS, the presentation of images in lower resolution, for example. The demands on response time should be specified separately for every case, since response time requirements have a great influence on the design (and the costs). Another time aspect concerns the period for which data have to be stored. Longer archiving periods will mean more data must be managed and consequently management will be more difficult and only possible if more use is made of image management strategies such as prefetching.

4.3.2.3 Data Model

The data elements that play an important role in the HIPACS system are summarized and the relations between them is described in Fig. 4.7, a so-called entity-relation diagram (Lodder 1989). Each rectangle represents an entity, i.e., an item on which information is stored. The lines represent the relations between the entities, and the "crow's feet" at the end of some lines indicate that the relations are one-to-many and many-to-many relations, rather than one-to-one. For easy reference, some entities have been aggregated, while others have been omitted.

In Table 4.5, the entities used in Fig. 4.7 are summarized and provided with the most relevant attributes.

Table 4.5. Entities and the most relevant attributes used in the global data model

Entity	Attributes
Patient	Patient identification (name, birthdate, sex, address, name of physician, insurance data)
Physician	Physician identification (name, specialty, address, telephone number)
Imaging modality	Imaging modality identification (modality type, acquisition room identification)
Acquisition room	Acquisition room identification
Location	Location identification
Request	Request identification (physician identification, patient identification, medical issue, patient mobility, request date/time)
Nonradiological information	Patient identification (description, date)
Workstation	Workstation identification
Report	Report identification (study identification, radiological employee identification, typist, status)
Study	Study identification (request identification, status, radiological employee identification, location identification, study date/time)
Radiological employee	Radiological employee identification (name, function/specialty)
Image	Image identification (examination identification, resolution, pictorial index, image data)
Work list	Work list identification (patient identification, study identification, radiological employee identification, date/time)
Examination	Examination identification (study identification, examination code, radiological employee identification, imaging modality)

4.3.3 Decomposition of HIPACS into its Components HIS, RIS, and PACS

In the previous section, a global unpartitioned HIPACS was specified. The next step using the top-down approach towards a design is the demarcation into subsystems. Data and functions have to be assigned to the demarcated components in such a way that both the data traffic between the subsystems and redundant storage over the subsystems is minimized. Before trying to relate functions and data, it is convenient to distinguish a hierarchy in demarcations as well. The alternative decompositions for the first two demarcation passes can be expressed as follows. In the nonintegrated environment, HIPACS is broken down into the components HIS, RIS, and PACS at the first demarcation pass, and PACS is broken down into its subsystems at the second demarcation pass. With an integrated system, HIPACS is broken down into the components HIS and PACS at the first demarcation pass, and, at the second demarcation pass, each of these is broken down further into the respective subsystems, RIS being included in the subsystems of HIS.

In the next sections, the relation between the HIPACS functions and data will first be established using the so-called information cross technique (Sect. 4.3.3.1). Subsequently, an indication will be given as to how to find the natural (or theoretical) demarcation lins(s) (Sect. 4.3.3.2). The third step consists of the problems to be overcome in adapting theoretical findings to the real situation (Sect. 4.3.3.3). Finally some remarks will be made on the specific requirements which are important in HIPACS data base design.

4.3.3.1 Establishing the Relationship Between Functions and Data

To represent the dependencies between processes or functions and data, a so-called information cross can be used (Zachman 1982). In an information cross, the data entities and functions are plotted. Each cell of this matrix corresponds to a data entity and a function. In the cell, the data base action (create, read, update, delete) of a specific function on a specific entity is noted. It is not necessary at this stage to enter functions and data in a specific order. As soon as all relevant functions, data entities, and their relations have been entered, one can start searching for independent clusters of functions and clusters of data entities by mutually changing columns and rows respectively.

4.3.3.2 Finding the Natural/Theoretical Demarcation Line(s)

After completion of the information cross, the search begins for the clusters of functions and data which are most independent. An ideal (and merely theoretical) outcome of clustering is depicted in Table 4.6 In this example, the functions and data relating to cluster A are natural candidates for assignment to subsystem A, and the same holds for cluster B.

4.3.3.3 Adaptation to the Real Situation

Next we will apply this method to the data entities and functions of HIPACS mentioned in Sect. 4.3.2. Besides these radiology-specific functions, the functions *arrival* and *departure* have been added because of the data base actions they trigger. Table 4.7 shows the corresponding information cross for the user functions. As an example of how these data can be read, the function *patient arrival* performs two data base actions: the physician who will treat the patient (read *physician*) is linked to the patient (update *patient*).

Table 4.6. Ideal situation of demarcation of functions and data

Function / Data	f1	f2	f3	f4	f5	f6	f7	f8	f9
d1									
d2									
d3			Cluster A						
d4									
d5									
d6									
d7									
d8							Cluster B		
d9									
d10									

Occurrences of the entities examination and appointment are created by the function *appointment*, and an acquisition room will also be reserved. The functions *work list* and *acquisition* are closely related: the function *work list* gathers together all the examinations for which the appointment in an acquisition room falls within the duty roster of the technician. During *acquisition*, the image is created, and after the acquisition has been performed the patient can be deleted from the work list. Note that the data needed for the image identification are provided by the work list. *Preparation* can be seen as the first step of *reporting*. During *preparation*, a selection will be made of examinations to be reported. The pictorial index (attribute of image) will be consulted in order to select the relevant images of the patient. The stack is created, denoting the selected cases.

During *reporting*, medical data will be needed such as patient (e.g., age), examination, image, and nonradiological data (e.g., pathology reports). After the diagnosis has been recorded on tape, the case will be deleted from the stack. *Typing* here not only comprises entering the information from tape into the system – for which patient data will be needed, e.g., for the correct name and address of the patient –, but also authorization of the report by the radiologist. *Departure* is the counterpart of *arrival*, and the link between the patient and the responsible physician will be changed to not active (update *patient*). Finally, with the *review* function all possible data can be retrieved (data base action *read*).

Note that in Table 4.7 we have taken the integrated HIS approach as a starting point, so that the first demarcation pass results in two subsystems, one to be assigned to HIS and one to PACS. In a nonintegrated environment, the first demarcation pass should result in at least three subsystems, which would then be assigned to HIS, RIS, and PACS. However, in the interest of illustrating the demarcation concept this distinction has not been made here.

Table 4.7. Demarcation of functions and data using an integrated HIS approach

Function	HIS				PACS				
Data	Arrival	Departure	Appointment	Typing	Preparation	Reporting	Work list	Acquisition	Review
HIS									
Patient	U	U	R	R		R	R		R
Examination			C		R	R	R		R
Nonradiological data						R			R
Appointment			C		R		R		R
Report				U	R	C			R
Acquisition room			R				R		
Physician	R								
PACS									
Image					R	R		C	R
Work list							C	U	
Stack					C	U			

C, create; *U*, update; *R*, read

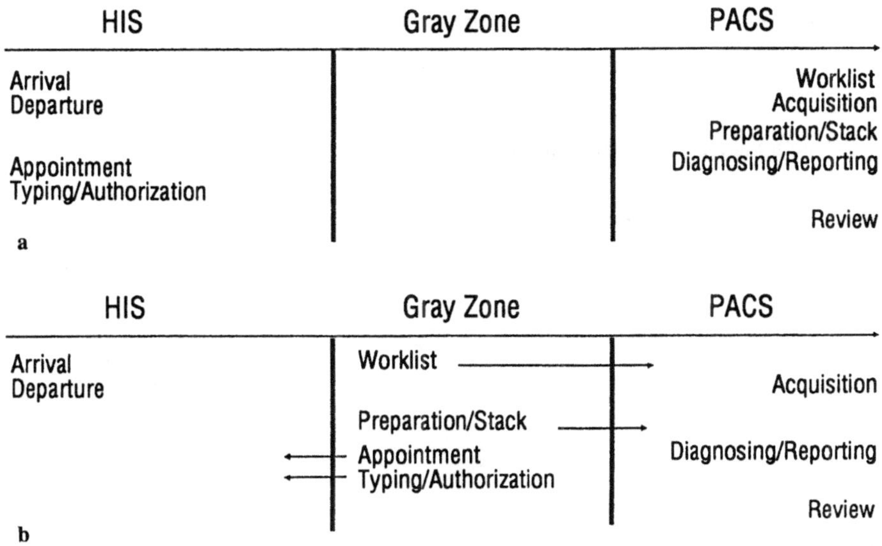

Fig. 4.8a,b. Overview of assignment of functions to information systems. **a** Ideal situation without overlap of functions. **b** Realistic situation with overlap of functions. *Arrows* indicate where a choice has to be made

In exceptional cases, the natural demarcation lines found coincide with the boundaries of commercially available systems, which means that there is no problem at all with the assignment of functions and data to the several (sub)systems. However, in practice, one has to deal with overlapping functions and relating data (Rienhoff and Greinacher 1988). In Fig. 4.8 both situations are depicted. In the most common situation (Fig. 4.8b), one has to make choices (indicated by arrows in the diagram). Of course, several other constellations are possible, some of which will be dependent on the local situation, for example.

The data have to be demarcated in a way which corresponds to the functional demarcation scenario. For performance reasons, some data entities are stored redundantly.

4.3.3.4 Some Important Aspects of HIPACS Data Base Design

Early computer applications focused on physical possibilities, and the storage of data was based upon equipment features. In the mid-1970s, the emphasis moved towards the separation of the technical aspects of data storage from the meaning of data and the data base was introduced. From the point of view of application, a data base consists of a description of the data (metadata) and a set of functions to manipulate the data (data base

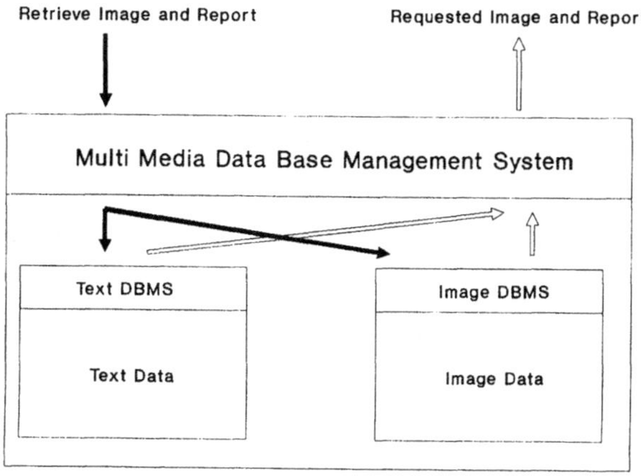

Fig. 4.9. Flow of data through a multimedia data base management system (*DBMS*)

management system, DBMS). In HIPACS, the same idea of hiding the physical aspects is applicable and the following characteristics will play a role in data base design here:

1. The HIPACS data base must be capable of managing data from different media, e.g., image data, text data, and probably also voice data in the future. It has to be a multimedia data base.
2. Data will be stored within several separate data bases. The corporate (logically one) data base is called a distributed data base.
3. Image data in a HIPACS will be stored in a hierarchical storage structure, namely a layered data base.

These characteristics will be treated in more detail below.

Multimedia Data Base. Within a multimedia data base, the multimedia DBMS splits up the data base actions into (a) actions to be handled by the alphanumerical part and (b) actions to be handled by the image data part of the DBMS. Only one set of metadata exists, and this includes the description of image data as well as textual data. In case of the retrieval of an image and its related report, for example, the retrieve request is received by the multimedia DBMS (Fig. 4.9). The multimedia DBMS splits the request into a textual and an image part, which will be sent to the textual and image data base, respectively. The text and image DBMS handle the request and send the ordered data back (presently, of course, via different hardware). Both parts are combined again at the multimedia DBMS and transferred to the requesting application.

Distributed Data Base. Within a distributed data base, data can be located at different places. A distributed data base may be chosen for its advantages in performance, reliability, and costs, or for political reasons. Disadvantages of

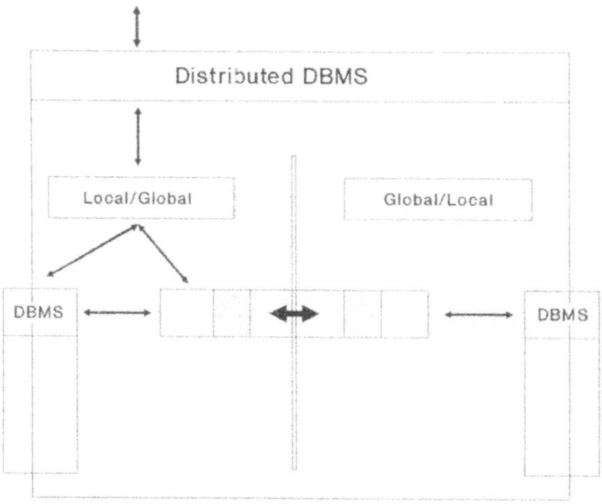

Fig. 4.10. Flow of data through a distributed data base management system (*DBMS*). The two DBMS are shown on the *left* and on the *right*; the *horizontal bar* in the middle is the guard; the *shaded area* indicates an adaptation module

the system are its complexity and difficulties with consistency, particularly of redundantly stored data.

A distributed data base is outlined in Fig. 4.10, with the two data bases shown on the left and the right. If a data base request comes in at the left side, for example, it will be handled by a local DBMS. The first task of the DBMS is to split the request into two parts, one which refers only to locally defined data and one which refers to globally defined data. The locally defined part is handled as in a normal data base, that part of the local data base has been drawn outside the frame. The globally defined part will be processed by a guard. Only this guard interacts with the remote data base in a commonly defined language. An adaptation module will be needed to convert the local language into the global language.

Note that it is not necessary in a distributed data base for data to be stored redundantly. If data are not present at the local site, they are requested from a remote site.

Layered Data Base. Within a layered data base the (image) data will be stored at storage equipment with different access time and capacity characteristics. The issue is not in the description or the handling of the data, but in the assignment of the data over the layers; an intelligent system has to organize optimal location of the data. One main difference between layered and conventional caching systems is that movements between layers are initiated from outside. The data base actions are routed by the layered DMBS to the proper layer. Once received at that layer, the DBMS of that particular layer performs the actual DBMS actions.

HIPACS Data Base. As discussed above, a HIPACS data base contains all three aspects, distributed, multimedia, and layered. A data base for HIPACS

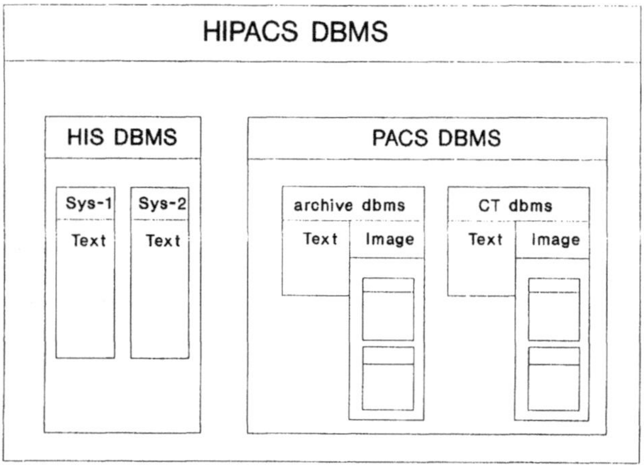

Fig. 4.11. Structure of a HIPACS data base management system (*DBMS*; CT, computed tomography). See text for details

can be designed top-down as illustrated in Fig. 4.11. Note that in this example the integrated HIS (including an RIS) was taken as starting point. The HIPACS applications interact with the HIPACS DBMS. This can be seen as the level zero data base. The HIPACS DBMS splits the requested actions into actions to performed by the HIS data base and actions to be performed by the PACS data base, and combines the results on the way back. The PACS and HIS data bases are level one data bases.

In Fig. 4.11, the HIS data base consists of two data bases, indicating that one logical data base can actually be implemented on several machines. The PACS data base consists in the first place of data bases at several locations, e.g., the archive and the computed tomography unit. Most local PACS data bases will be multimedia data bases. The DBMS of the archive, for example, splits the actions of a multimedia DBMS into calls to the text data base and calls to the image data base. The image DBMS, however, does not handle the requested actions itself, but routes the requests to a certain layer. The DBMS of the layer finally performs the actual DBMS action.

4.3.4 Conclusions and Prospects for a Second Generation PACS Concept

We have now worked through the concept of an integrated HIPACS, i.e., a PACS integrated with other information systems in the hospital, especially HIS and RIS. The necessity of such an integration has been elaborated, both from the user's point of view and from the image management point of view. The main advantages of an integrated HIPACS are functional integration, data integration, and user-acceptable responsiveness. With respect to the optimization of image management, the strategy of prefetching plays an important part.

For designing PACS interfaces with HIS and RIS, the use of a top-down approach seems to be the most promising. First the specifications of a global HIPACS are drafted. These consist of functional requirements, performance requirements, and a data model. Then the theoretical demarcation line(s) are determined. The number of lines are, for example, dependent on the local situation of the relationship between HIS and RIS. The most difficult step consists in adaptating to the real multivendor environment. In case of overlapping functions, choices have to be made with respect to the assignment of functions and corresponding data to the different systems.

The HIPACS data base may be considered to combine three types of data base, distributed, multimedia, and layered. Using the experiences gained in first generation PACS projects, and keeping in mind the design strategy explained in this chapter, the following recommendations with respect to integration can be made for a second generation PACS:

1. Only an integrated PACS can meet all the requirements.
2. Integration of PACS and HIS, RIS, and other systems will become easier if the interface(s) are well defined and standardized. Of course, standardization of such aspects as concepts, functionalities, data entities, and communication tools is a prerequisite.
3. Instead of trying to implement a hospital-wide PACS from the start, it appears to be better to adopt a stepwise approach, i.e., start with a partial PACS. This automatically implies that for quite some time a so-called hybrid situation exists, i.e., storage of both conventional film in archives and digital images in PACS. The integration and management of film and digital images becomes a specific problem here.
4. More research must be carried out into prefetching in order to make optimal use of HIS and/or RIS information in image management.

References

Bakker AR (1990) An integrated hospital information system in the Netherlands. Clin Comput 7(2): 91–97

Bakker AR, Ball MJ, Scherrer JR, Willems JL (eds) (1988) Towards new hospital information systems. North-Holland, Amsterdam

Bakker AR, Kouwenberg JML, Ottes FP (1989) HIS and PACS integration aspects. In: Barber B, Cao D, Qin D, Wagner G (eds) Proceedings of the MEDINFO 89. North-Holland, Amsterdam, pp 377–381

Bijl K, Koens ML, Bakker AR, de Valk JPJ (1987) Medical PACS and HIS: integration needed. In: Schneider RH, Dwyer III SJ (eds) Proceedings of the medical imaging conference. SPIE 767: 765–770

Collen MF (1988) HIS concepts, goals and objectives. In: Bakker AR, Ball MJ, Scherrer JR, Willems JL (eds) Towards new hospital information systems. North-Holland, Amsterdam, pp 3–9

Gane C, Sarson T (1979) Structured system analysis. Prentice Hall, Englewood Cliffs, NJ, USA

Greenes RA, Brinkley JF (1990) Radiology systems. In: Shortliffe EH, Perreault LE, Wiederhold G et al. (eds) Medical informatics. Computer applications in health care. Addison Wesley, Reading, MA, USA

Griesser GG (ed) (1977) Realisation of data protection in health information systems. North-Holland, Amsterdam

Griesser GG, Bakker AR, Daniëlsson J, Hirel JC, Kenny DJ, Schneider W, Wassermann AI (eds) (1990) Data protection in health information systems: considerations and guidelines. North-Holland, Amsterdam

Griesser GG, Jardel JP, Kenny DJ, Santer K (eds) (1983) Data protection in health information systems: where do we stand? North-Holland, Amsterdam

Heemskerk van Holtz PRB (1988) Data handling in a nursing unit. In: Daly N, Hannah KJ (eds) Proceedings of the third international symposium on nursing use of computers and information science. Mosby, St Louis, USA, pp 796–803

Kaihara S, Watanabe R (1988) HIS scope. In: Bakker AR, Ball MJ, Scherrer JR, Willems JL (eds) Towards new hospital information systems. North-Holland, Amsterdam, pp 19–25

Leguit FA (1989) Leveling or interfacing; what are the choices? In: Barber B, Cao D, Qin D, Wagner G (eds) Proceedings of the MEDINFO 89. North-Holland, Amsterdam, pp 343–347

Lehr L, Lodwick G, Nichilson B, et al. (1973) Experiences with MARS (Missouri Automated Radiology System). Radiology 106: 289–294

Lodder et al. (1989) An entity-relation model of an image information system. BAZIS internal report (in Dutch)

Lodder H, van Poppel BM, Wilmink JBM, Bakker AR (1990) Coupling in perspective. In: Schneider RH, Dwyer III SJ (eds) Proceedings of the Medical Imaging IV Conference. SPIE 1234: 676–680

Louwerse CP, Kouwenberg JML (1984) Data protection aspects in an integrated hospital information system. Computers and Security 3: 286–294

Mani R, Jones M (1973) MSF: a computer-assisted radiology reporting system. Radiology 108: 587–596

Mattheus R (1989) Picture archiving and communication systems: a digital image management system. MIM News 1: 38–44

Mattheus R (1991) The European efforts of standardization in medical imaging. In: Huang HK, Ratib O, Bakker AR, Witte G (eds) Proceedings of the NATO ASI workshop on PACS in Medicine, Evian, France, October 1990. Springer, Berlin Heidelberg New York

Rienhoff O, Greinacher CFC (eds) (1988) A general PACS-RIS interface. Springer, Berlin Heidelberg New York (Lecture Notes in Medical Informations, vol 37)

Shortliffe EH, Perreault LE, Wiederhold G et al. (eds) (1990) Medical informatics. Computer applications in health care. Addison Wesley, Reading, MA, USA

Van de Velde R (1987) Subject databases for hospital information systems: the appointment system. In: Serio A, O'Moore R, Tardini A (eds) Proceedings of the MIE, Rome, 1987

Wheeler PS, Gitlin IN (1979) Computers in radiology: a viewpoint of pitfalls and payoffs. Proceedings of the sixth conference on computer applications in radiology. IEEE, pp 1–4

Zachman (1982) Business system planning and business information control study: a comparison. IBM Systems J 21(1): 31–53

5 Networking

5.1 Image Network Technology

D. Meyer-Ebrecht, A. Keizers, W.J.J. Stut Jr., and F. Vossebürger

5.1.1 Introduction

The initial stimulus for the development of digital picture archiving and communication systems (PACS) was the desire for a digital alternative to the X-ray film archive. Digital image archives, however, are not enough, the nonphysical, digital transport of images is also necessary. Therefore, the introduction of such a system has to go hand in hand with the installation of digital image communication systems in order to do justice to the expression PACS.

The digital archiving of images will certainly be an advantageous substitute for a traditional technique, while the digital communication of images will open up new dimensions for dealing with image material. For example, a network of data transmission lines will link the various image sources with the archive's mass stores and with digital diagnostic consoles, and there will no longer be any restriction on local dependence. Furthermore, the equipment used for image evaluation – diagnostic consoles or digital light boxes – can be installed in a less restricted way and be adapted appropriately for the given work routines. Another advantage is that the final users of the diagnostic information, e.g., surgeons and radiotherapists, can have direct and immediate access to the original image material. Finally, the increasing degree of specialization and isolation in terms of diagnostic methods based on specific types of images will be counteracted by the fact that the reunion of various types of image material at the individual place of work will be facilitated.

Networks for image communication correspond structurally to the local area networks (LANs) which are established nowadays within the office automation domain. However, the data volume of digital images is in conflict with a direct takeover of that technology. The thousandfold greater volume of the data sets to be transferred requires a correspondingly higher transmission capacity of the network in order to be able to transmit the images as fast as the work. A comprehensive statistical evaluation of the image data volumes required at image workstations during reporting sessions showed, for example, a peak data flow of 11 Mbit/s and an average data flow of 3 Mbit/s between each workstation and the respective storage resources. With respect to the transmission frequency of conventional LANs, e.g., the 10 MHz claimed for Ethernet, this does not seem to be extraordinarily high. However, the physical bandwidth, i.e., the pulse frequency of the carrier signal on the transmission lines, is often mistaken for the average data rate of a message transfer. Usually an LAN needs a sophisticated protocol to solve conflicts in the case of concurrent transmission requests. The execution of the protocol has to be performed by means of dedicated network software. The processing time of these programs reduces the effective transmission data rate to a value which, depending on the number of communicating devices, is about one order lower than the frequency of the carrier signal.

The discrepancy between wish and reality will finally become evident if we further consider that the required data transmission rate has to be multiplied by the number of workstations operated at the same time. The incorporation of techniques such as caching, prefetching, or specialized network management (which will be described in Sect. 5.2) into the PACS environment can lower the requirements of the PACS network. However, even LANs of the next generation, e.g., the fiber optic LAN fiber-distributed data interface (FDDI) with a carrier frequency of 125 MHz, will probably not solve the communication bottlenecks in a full-scale PACS.

Because of the significance of an appropriately fast image transmission, it will be reasonable, if not unavoidable, to develop networks which are specialized for PACS applications. At first glance this seems to be contradictory to standardization attempts in the network domain. We believe, however, that specialization will lead to economic solutions for networks which offer the faster data transmission rate required for image communication in hospitals. In the following, we will present the results of a quantitative investigation carried out to define image network requirements. Furthermore, we will review state-of-the-art LANs and their limitations. Finally, we will describe the specialized PACS network ImNet and evaluate its behavior in a PACS environment.

5.1.2 Quantitative Requirements

One of the central design issues for PACS is the data communication network. An analysis shows that two different types of data are handled in a PACS. The first type is image data, the volume of which is extremely large, the second type is alphanumerical data, which is characterized by short data sets. A subdivision of the data into these two types seems to be efficient because of the very different kinds of management, use, and flow they each require. This offers the possibility of handling both types of data in an optimized way. Alphanumerical data sets such as patient data and reports may be stored in standard data bases. Data bases must preserve the integrity

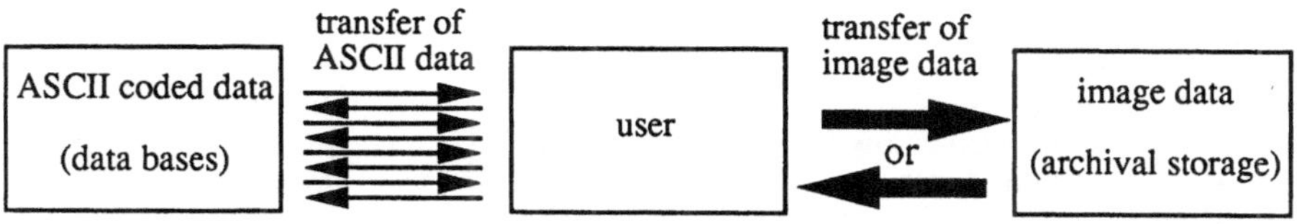

Fig. 5.1. Two-layered concept of data management separating the data into ASCII data and image data

of the stored data and permit access to the data via keys or relationships. One characteristic of the alphanumerical data is that data sets may be appended, which means that new information may be added. In contrast, image data are generated at one time, stored, and afterwards requested in the original. Any modification of the primary image is forbidden by law.

Coming back to data transfer, we can describe the flow of alphanumerical data as communication of users with a data base. Short sets of data (requests and responses) between the users and the data bases in both directions are exchanged very frequently. In contrast to the dialogue-type communication with alphanumerical data, image data transfer is always a burst of traffic in one direction. If we separate the management of images and the flow of image data into two different layers, the management layer, which can be integrated into the data base for alphanumerical data, must keep information for locating the images in the image layer, whereas the image layer only contains the images themselves. Image communication, on the image layer, only consists of commands like "GET_image", "SEND_image" and image transfers.

Using the described two-layered concept (Fig. 5.1), we may separate our investigation of data flow for these two data types. As networks for alphanumerical data have been running successfully in the domain of office automation for years, we will concentrate on the flow of image data here. Together with radiologists from the Department of Radiology at the University Hospital Aachen, we conducted an investigation of the flow of image data in order to build an image data flow model of a PACS. This investigation allows us to describe the image demand of the radiologists and other users at the radiology department.

Radiological examinations are routinely ordered by various departments of the hospital. The type of examination and the department which orders it define the reporting place of the examination. At all reporting places, the radiologists do the reporting during one or more so-called sessions throughout the day. In a session, a certain number of cases are examined. Each case consists of a number of images which belong to a certain patient. The images can be characterized according to attributes like size, image source, ordering department, and age.

The quantitative knowledge about the coherences mentioned above may be used firstly to build a model of the image flow in a PACS installation and secondly as an input to a simulation program in order to evaluate if

Table 5.1. Image production at a typical radiological department

Modality	Time required for examination (min)	Examinations per day per station (*n*)	Image size[a] (Mbit)	Images per examination (*n*)	Stations (*n*)
CT	40–45	14	3	10–30	3
MR	55–60	10	3	20–40	1
CR	10–15	40	48	2	6

[a] Image size is 512 × 512 × 12 bit for CT and MRI, and 2048 × 2048 × 12 bit for CR.

any given network will satisfy the performance. Based on our investigation at the Department of Radiology at the University Hospital Aachen and on general figures of image production and image use (as available at BAZIS, Leiden, the Netherlands), we assume the following workload for a prototypical radiology department.

Image Production. At a radiological department, computed tomography (CT), magnetic resonance imaging (MRI), and computer radiology (CR) acquisition stations may be connected to a PACS. Table 5.1 shows the acquisition stations and the assumed image production patterns of each station during a day.

Image Study. When an examination is to be reported, old images may be needed. New images together with old images, if appropriate, form a so-called case. We assumed that for CR reporting, in which normally two new images are used, the probability is 50% that in addition two old images are needed. The differences in studying cases depending on the different modalities are shown in Table 5.2. Some cases have to be studied several times (e.g., by residents, by senior radiologists, and during discussions with the referring physicians). Based on the above-mentioned production numbers, we can assume the figures presented in Table 5.3 for reporting sessions. These figures imply the image data flow towards the image workstations of the prototypical radiological department presented in Table 5.4.

The total amount of image data to be transferred towards the workstations over the day is around 80000 Mbit. Assuming the data transfer takes place during an overall working period of 8 h, it will require an average transfer rate of around 2.75 Mbit/s. It should be noted that these figures represent a very conservative estimate. Neither the image flow to other departments of the hospital is included nor the image flow from image acquisition stations (image sources) to image storage modules (ISM) is mentioned. Furthermore, the assumptions stated above only include the modalities CT, MRI, and CR. Other modalities such as digital subtraction angiography (DSA), gamma cameras, ultrasound scanners, and scanning laser ophthalmoloscopes are not taken into account at all. Furthermore,

Table 5.2. Characteristics of the study of images for different modalities

Modality	Study time/case (s)	Images/case (n)
CT	60–300	10–30
MR	60–240	20–40
CR	30–120	2 new images (+ 2 old images in 50% of all cases)

Table 5.3. Reporting data for different imaging modalities

Modality	Cases/day[a] (n)	Study frequency[b]	Studies/day[c] (n)	Time/study (min)
CT	42	3	126	4
MR	10	3	30	4
CR	240	2	480	2

[a] Cases per day for all acquisition stations.
[b] Number of times each case has to be studied.
[c] Number of cases per day × study frequency.

Table 5.4. Image data flow towards the workstations

Modality	Studies/day[a] (n)	Images/study (n)	Image size (Mbit)	Image data volume/day (Mbit)
CT	126	20	3	7560
MR	30	30	3	2700
CR	480	3	48	69120

[a] For all acquisition stations

when calculating the network transfer rate necessary in a PACS, the delay time to get access to images is an extremely important point which we have to take into consideration. Evidently, it is unacceptable for the users of a PACS to wait more than 5 s for an image ordered from an ISM. With a data volume of up to 48 Mbit for a thorax image and the assumption that searching for the image in the archive and the transfer from the ISM to the workstation will each take half of the total delay, we need a network with a transfer rate of 20 Mbit/s. However, if more users are simultaneously requesting images, they may contend for the same ISM and network channels. Depending on the delays that occur at an ISM, the network transfer rate must be significantly higher in order to meet the required performance. For example, to offer the above transfer rate to ten users, the transfer rate has to be multiplied by ten, which results in a network transfer rate of some 200 Mbit/s.

Table 5.5. Efficiency of Ethernet and Token Bus (Data Communications 1987)

Institution	Method	Date	Type[a]	Effective data rate[b]
Advanced computer Communications	Test	January 1987	Token Bus	1.76 Mbit/s
National Bureau of Standards	Simulation	Spring 1986	Ethernet and Token Bus	1.5 Mbit/s
National Bureau of Standards	Test	End 1986	Ethernet	962 kbit/s
Computer Machinery Corporation	Test	January 1987	Ethernet	592 kbit/s

[a] All types had a signal data rate of 10 Mbit/s.
[b] Rate for user data (layer 4 of ISO/OSI model).

5.1.3 Present State of LANs

In this section, we will give a rough overview of existing standard networks with respect to PACS applications. Today's standard networks for digital data transport are rather inefficient. Because of their topology and the transport protocols used to control the data transfer, only a small part of the signal rate is utilized for the transfer of user data. A number of investigations illustrate this (Table 5.5). The effective transfer rate on level 4 of the ISO/OSI model (user data transfer) is only about 6%–17% of the signal rate on the physical transport channel. Transfer rates of this order are sufficient for applications dealing with alphanumerical data, but for the transport of image data, they are far too low, as explained above. The reasons for the low efficiency of the standard networks becomes clear if one looks at the different procedures used by the media access control (MAC), which coordinates permissions to use the network for data transfers. The best known representatives of standard networks are those defined in IEEE 802.3–802.5 which use coaxial cable as a transfer medium, and FDDI, which is based on fiber-optic cables.

5.1.3.1 IEEE 802.3: Carrier Sense Multiple Access/Collision Detection

Ethernet (Digital Intel, Xerox 1982) is the best-known network using the carrier sense multiple access/collision detection (CSMA/CD) standard. All stations are directly connected to a single cable, which forms the transfer channel of the network, and the stations always listen for incoming messages. If a station wants to transmit data, it first has to wait for silence on the cable, which means that no data transfer of other stations is in operation (carrier sense); it then starts putting its data onto the cable. Since it is possible for more than one station to begin to transmit data at the same time, collisions may occur when the transfer starts. A collision will be detected at the latest after the maximum *round trip propagation time* of 46.4 µs, as defined by this standard, i.e., with a signal rate of 10 Mbit/s a total of 464 bits could be sent before the collision is detected. After a collision has occurred, which is detected by each station itself (collision detection), a *jamming* signal of 48-bit length is sent to make sure that all stations recognize the collision. To handle this collision situation, each station first stops sending data and then waits for a randomized or predefined time before making the next attempt to transmit data (multiple access). The round trip propagation time together with the jamming time form the so-called *slot time* with a length of 51.2 µs.

After the first 72 bytes have been sent without any collision detection, the transfer may be safely continued. The total network is then locked for other workstations for an *interframing time* of 9.6 µs, which starts when the transfer has finished. The interframing time is defined as the time between the end of one transfer activity and the beginning of a next one, and is intended to guarantee the detection of the transfer end to the receiver workstation. While a transfer takes place, and each transfer is limited to 1526 bytes, new requests for transfer may come up. The probability of collisions increases when huge amounts of data, belonging to different transfer tasks, are transferred. Because of this uncontrolled, randomized media access with collisions, the network will work less efficiently the larger the data sets for the transfer tasks are. For the transfer of image data, which do indeed represent transfer tasks with extremely large sets of data, this type of network will fail in a PACS application.

5.1.3.2 IEEE 802.4 Token Bus

All stations that are connected to the bus, which is a coaxial cable, always wait for a special data packet, a so-called token. The token is addressed to only one of the network's stations at a time. There are two types of tokens: the *free token*, which signalizes to the station the right to use the bus for data transfer, and the *used token* which signalizes to the station that it will receive the following data. A station receiving the free token either holds this token to initiate a data transfer or passes it directly to a next station. When the station initiates a data transfer, it places a used token on the bus, which addresses the receiver of the data. The user data are placed on the bus behind the token. All stations receive the used token, but only the addressed station identifies itself with the address and receives the data. After the data transfer has finished, the sending station gives the free-token to the next station. The rotation of the free token through all stations of the network gives every station the chance to transfer data.

The effective data rate to all active users is around 18% (see Table 5.5) of the signal rate of 10 Mbit/s on the bus. This rate results from the amount of data, limited by this standard, which can be transferred in one transfer cycle. After each data transfer cycle the free token has to be passed on, to give the next stations a chance to complete their transfer tasks. In this way, all stations continue their transfers. On the one hand, this standard gives all stations the same part of transfer capability of the bus, but on the other hand the free token has to rotate through all stations of the network, even if only one station has a transfer task. This rotation of the free token costs quite some time which lowers the effective transfer rate.

5.1.3.3 IEEE 802.5 Token Ring

The stations of the token ring are connected with one neighbor on the receiver side and one on the transmitter side via the coaxial cable. The network forms a ring which allows the data to run in only one direction through it. Like the token bus protocol, the token ring protocol uses a special data packet (token) to signalize the transmission right to the stations of the network. The station holding the free token may use the ring for transport. All data transmitted onto the ring will cycle once around. All stations receive the data, analyze the address which is included in a used token before the user data, and copy the data if compatible with this address. After the data have returned to the transmitting station, this station has to remove the data from the ring. While doing this, it compares the removed data with the data transmitted before to check for transmission errors. After all data have been removed, the transmission is finished, and the free token has to be given to the next station. As with the IEEE networks described above, the amount of data which can be transferred in one transfer cycle is limited by the token ring protocol. Because the media access procedure, the token ring principle, is equivalent to that of the token bus, the effective data rate of the token ring can be assumed to be almost the same as that for the token bus.

5.1.3.4 Fiber Distributed Data Interface

The FDDI is a proposed standard of the American National Standards Institute (ANSI) for a token ring using fiber-optic cables. FDDI was originally proposed for two primary areas of application: first, as a high-performance interconnect among mainframes, associated mass storage, and peripheral equipment, and second, as a backbone network for lower speed LANs (IEEE 802.3/4/5) as explained above.

The data rate for the transmission of protocol and user data is 100 Mbit/s. FDDI offers a packet-switching transfer mode as well as an optional circuit-switching transfer mode (FDDI-II). The packet-switching mode is almost the same as that described for the token ring. By contrast, the circuit-switching mode enables the user to allocate 6.144 Mbit/s increments of the total bandwidth of the ring's signal rate to use them as isochronous channels. Up to 16 of these isochronous channels can be assigned, covering a bandwidth of 98.304 Mbit/s. Each of these channels can be a full duplex path for data transport between the corresponding stations allocated to this channel. The bandwidth which is not allocated for isochronous channels may be used for data transport in the packet-switching mode. Concerning the required data rate for PACS applications, not even the line-switching mode of FDDI-II delivers more than about 50% of the data rate required overall for image data transmission. Extensions of the network are possible by installing multiple FDDI rings connected via bridges. This, however, entails a new dimension of complexity and a further reason for inefficiency.

5.1.3.5 Conclusions

In every case, only one physical data channel can be used for multiple connections, so that the effective data rate has to be shared among the active users, and a fixed effective data rate cannot be guaranteed. The expansion of the network with more network devices will decrease the data rate available for each active user. A considerable data rate gets lost due to the complicated protocols. Collision reparation in case of Ethernet costs additional signal rate.

The effective data rates of these networks (shown in Table 5) are too low for the image data transfer required in a PACS. However, these networks may be useful for the transport of image-related alphanumerical data. Figure 5.2 shows an estimation of the effective transfer time versus the number of active users (n) for this type of networks.

5.1.4 Network Requirements for PACS Applications

Networks for PACS applications will have to satisfy extraordinary requirements if they are to succeed! Digital images with data volumes in the order of several megabytes require extremely high transfer rates from a network if the waiting times for the user are to be kept acceptable, delays of more than 1 s may already be annoying in many situations. To achieve this aim, the overhead, i.e., the sum of all data except the pure user data, should be kept as small as possible. The network also has to be very flexible in its configuration. It should be evident that the network can be adapted to its surroundings, not the other way round. The network should be integrable in given structures of organizational forms, even when they change. This requirement cannot be reached with simple network topologies such as bus, star, or ring.

The network should be built up of a small number of modules only, to keep the task of installation and maintenance simple. The modules themselves should be clear in their functionality, and the interface between the modules should be simple to keep the complexity of the network at a low level. The network should be easily adaptable to different peripheral re-

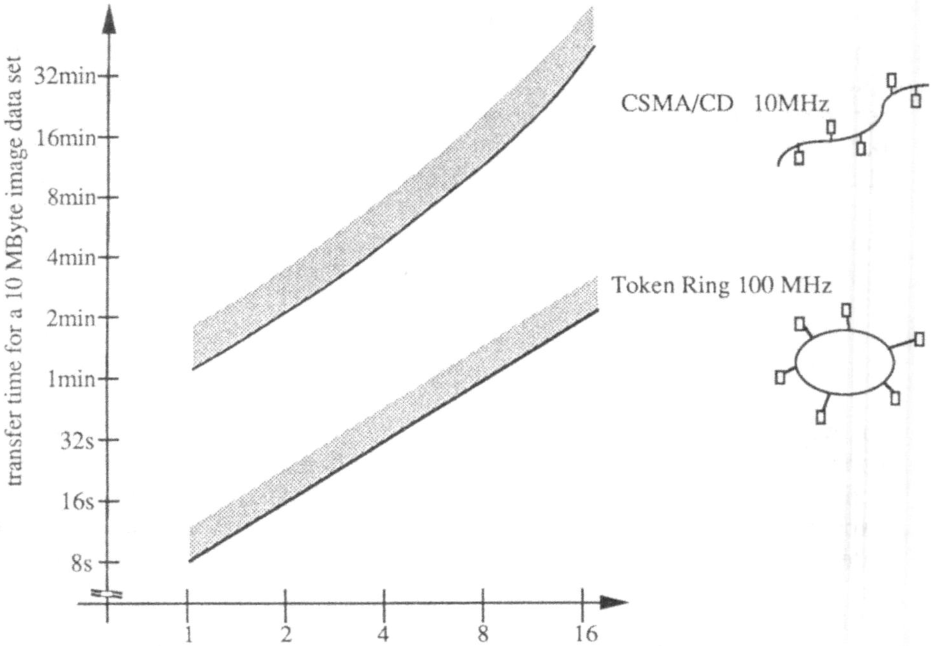

Fig. 5.2. Typical characteristics of standard LANs with respect to image transfer times versus the number of concurrent transfers. In both cases an effective data rate of 10% of the physical data transfer rate has been assumed

quirements, such as result from the various image data sources, image workstations, and image archives from different vendors. Connections to previously installed PACS subsystems which use different networks for data transfer must also be integrable. Adaptability is one of the most essential requirements on a network for PACS. Further, the possibility to build connections to public networks may be important for future PACS applications. PACS installations in different hospitals and doctors' practices should be connected via networks like ISDN to allow applications such as teleconsulting. The progress of technology also has to be taken into consideration, e.g., the availability of components with increased data transfer rates. In today's networks, the transfer rate is fixed when the network is installed, and a change in the transfer rate involves modifications to all connected stations. New networks, therefore, should offer the flexibility to adopt new technologies even in parts of the network.

A more general requirement concerns reliability. Reliability is a criterion for the acceptability of any technology, especially for a network. The breakdown of a network in a PACS may lead to the breakdown of the whole PACS system. Because errors can occur in any system, a system like a network should be able to recover itself from error condition to normal operation (at least to emergency operation) as fast as possible. To prevent network breakdowns, it is necessary to avoid tasks of the network control from the stations connected to the network. The network has to be an autonomous system to be operational independent of the operational status of the connected stations. The network control has to be implemented in a decentralized manner to avoid a total network breakdown by the breakdown of a central control system. A decentralized control will keep the remaining parts of the network fully operational when others recover from breakdown situations. Also a decentralized control keeps the network operational when reconfigurating parts of the network, which will probably often be done in the installation phase of the PACS when connecting new stations. A further requirement is obtainability. Obtainability includes the probability of getting a transfer channel to an addressed network station. The obtainability grows with the number of possibilities of connecting two optional stations in the network.

Another requirement is real-time behavior. The real-time behavior is a relative dimension, depending on the time in which a user normally expects the system to react, e.g., students learning to use radiological images within a PACS may tolerate a waiting time of several minutes for an image, whereas a doctor at an emergency station can not accept a time of more than a few seconds. To realize such a real-time behavior, the network must support priorities when establishing transport channels to different transport tasks.

5.1.5 ImNet: Specialized Image Network for PACS

The key to an increased overall data transport efficiency is the separation of management data communication and image data communication, as explained above. For the latter ImNet, a novel type of fiber-optic network, has been developed (Fasel 1990; Meyer-Ebrecht et al. 1987; Vossebürger 1991). Its hyperstar topology, asynchronous data transport mechanism and distributed network control allow multiple simultaneous image transfers at an effective speed of 80% of the physical data rate (ImNet/1: 16 Mbit/s, ImNet/2: 125 or 175 Mbit/s).

5.1.5.1 Network Physics

ImNet is based on fiber-optic data transmission technologies. Coded as a light pulse, digital data may be easily transported by means of glass fiber lines over a distance of many kilometers, even with effective data rates of more than 100 Mbit/s, so that the a digital X-ray image or a complete set of CT images can be transmitted in less than 1 s. In addition, glass fiber lines are immune to external electromagnetic interference and do not emit any electromagnetic fields on their part.

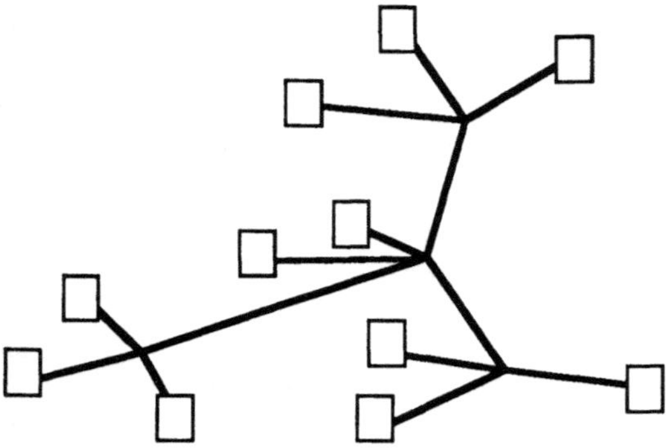

Fig. 5.3. Topology of ImNet

Using a fast transmission medium, several measures have been taken to improve the net data throughput in contrast to conventional LANs. ImNet's topology concept disentangles image data and nonimage data flows, makes multiple use of the data rate offered by the medium, and distributes the network control. Its data transport mechanism allows a close asynchronous direct memory access (DMA) coupling of image equipment connected via this network. Its routing and control mechanism supports a simple and efficient protocol on the lower ISO/OSI layers.

5.1.5.2 Topology and Switching Concept

Topology

A first essential step towards simplifying the complicated communication tasks in a PACS was to disentangle the heterogeneous data flows into pure image data flows and management data flows (Meyer-Ebrecht and Wendler 1983). This corresponds to the partitioning of services in PACS as described in Chap. 7.2, where the most important service, i.e., image archival, is split up into archival management services, image data storage and retrieval services. A strictly separated network layer then exclusively communicates images. Networks which are dedicated for this task can be optimally adapted to the special communication requirements of image equipment and thus be more efficient than general purpose LANs. ImNet has been designed particularly for that purpose.

In contrast to the well-established bus or ring topologies of conventional LANs, ImNet employs a so-called hyperstar topology, i.e., an arbitrary tree structure of star switches (see Fig. 5.3). This type of topology avoids the problem of the transfer of a message between two nodes occupying the whole network. Instead, only those transmission links are occupied which constitute the desired transmission path. Simultaneous transmissions are

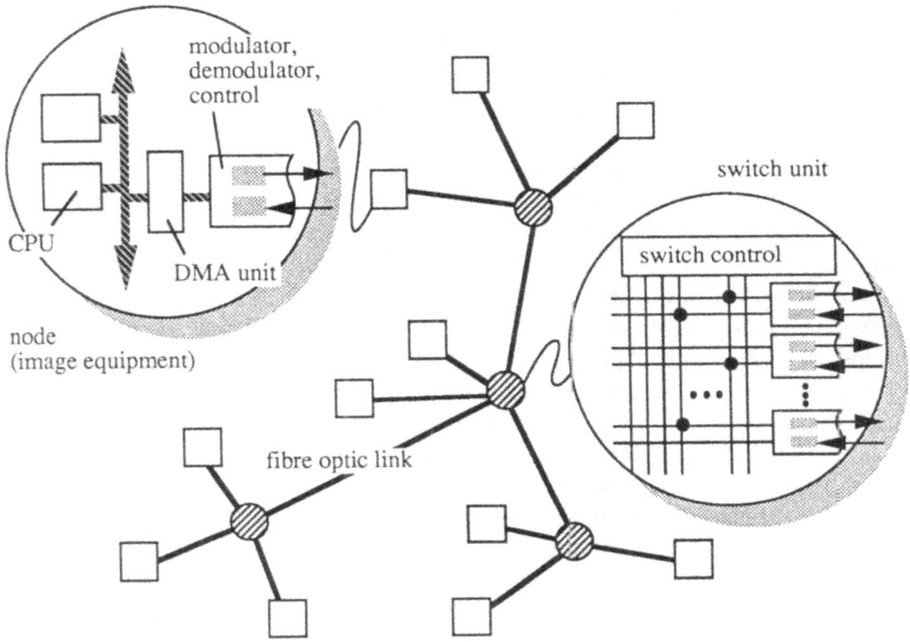

Fig. 5.4. Elements of ImNet

permitted as long as they do not use identical links between two star switches in the same direction. Thus multiple use of the transmission capacity can be made. Communication bottlenecks can be overcome by adapting the topology to the image data traffic, i.e., individual star switches may be dedicated to logistic clusters of image equipment, or by installing parallel links between star switches. A network installation may grow without leading to a collapse due to traffic overloads.

ImNet consists of only two different types of elements: switch modules, which autonomously establish individual message data paths between two optional arbitrary nodes (image equipment modules connected to the network) for the duration of a message transfer, and transmission links, which connect image equipment modules to switch modules or switch modules among each other (Fig. 5.4).

Data Transport Mechanism

Two types of information propagate over the network: messages (data blocks), which carry images and related data, and control commands (data words), which initialize or terminate a message transmission. The network operates in different modes for these two types of data. Control commands, which are dropped by any node, are computed by the routing and control mechanism of each switch module on their flow to the destination node. For message data blocks, the network applies the line-switching principle to connect two nodes as closely as possible during the message transfer. Thus messages which contain complete images packed up according to the ACR/NEMA standard (ACR/NEMA 1985) can be transmitted as continuous data streams rather than parceled out into some thousand pieces as required by the protocols of conventional LANs.

The transmission links have full-duplex capability. For message data they work in a half-duplex mode to achieve an asynchronous operation at the highest possible data rata. Data are transferred 16 bit-wise, asynchronously, with an internal organization into 2 kB frames. For an efficient asynchronous operation, a hardware handshake is performed which is independent of the propagation time on the transmission lines. This is achieved by means of the so-called sliding window method which lets the entire transmission path behave according to the first in first out (FIFO) principle.

The transmission links are equipped with twin-line fiber-optic cables. They are terminated by electro-optic transceivers and modulator/demodulator modules which offer a simple asynchronous parallel interface (either 16 or 32 bit wide). Because of the asynchronous operation of the transmission channels, a standard DMA input/output (I/O) module of a given image equipment computer system will suffice for hardware interfacing. A message can be transferred in one stroke by means of one single DMA operation. Therefore, the network driver software of the image equipment module can be made up by a simple shell added to the DMA driver which only has to take care of the initialization and termination of a message transfer. As a result of applying distributed line switching to asynchronous transmission channels, the network can be operated with a rather trivial protocol on the network-specific lower protocol layers. Instead of the image equipment adapting to the network's behavior as was necessary with conventional LANs, the network rather adapts to the image equipment's internal processes and does not bother the image equipment with network-specific processing tasks. So the transfer of a complete message can be done either at the image equipment's DMA rate or at the network's transport rate, whatever is lower. The effective transport rate, in turn, is 80% of the physical data rate on the transmission medium!

5.1.5.3 Routing and Control Mechanism

The image equipment's protocol activities in establishing a path through the network merely involve asking for a path and terminating it by means of exchanging a set of control information with the network. The control mechanism of the network distinguishes between control command frames and message data frames, as mentioned above. It is the purpose of control commands to synchronize the nodes and to provide the network with routing information. Every control command will be acknowledged by a response of the control command type. This task has to be provided by the network driver software of the image equipment modules, a negligible task compared with the transmission of several megabytes of image data.

The control commands carry all the information required to establish or to release the requested image data paths. Control commands dropped into the network by the image equipment modules will be recognized and analyzed by the local intelligence of the switch modules. The routing mechanism is inherently collision-free. The queuing of concurrent transmission requests is done by the switch modules. In this way, a completely distributed control of the network has been achieved, i.e., the image network does not need any supervisor or communication manager, and it operates independently from the superimposed management data LAN. Modifications or extensions of the network do not require any reconfiguration procedure. Nodes or switch modules which fail or which are out of operation do not affect the remaining network. Thus the concept of "graceful degradation" is supported by ImNet.

5.1.5.4 Simulation of an ImNet-Based PACS

The concept of ImNet was developed on the basis of an analysis of the overall requirements of image traffic. A more accurate description of the image data communication, i.e., statistical coherences of the traffic parameters, can only be given by observing a PACS in operation. If we want to evaluate the performance of a new PACS component piror to its application under real conditions, a simulation may help. ImNet has been simulated by BAZIS (Leijden, the Netherlands). The main objectives of such a simulation are to investigate and finally to optimize various parameters which influence the performance of a PACS installation concerning the image data transport. These are:

1. The configuration of PACS image equipment and the connecting network
2. The protocols which control the transfer of image data
3. The technical parameters of the image equipment and of the network

The data transfer with ImNet always works in three steps. First, the source image equipment orders a data transfer channel from the network. The switch modules establish a channel to the destination image equipment and signalize the result. In a second step, this channel can be used for the data transfer like a point-to-point connection to the destination image equipment. After the transfer has been finished, the channel has to be released by the ordering image equipment.

An image data transfer will make use of two data transfers on the network. The first data transfer contains the so called *request message*, while the second one contains the *response message*. An image will be fetched from the source image equipment by sending a *GET_image* request message to the source and afterwards receiving a GET_image response message, which includes the image. To transfer an image to any destination image

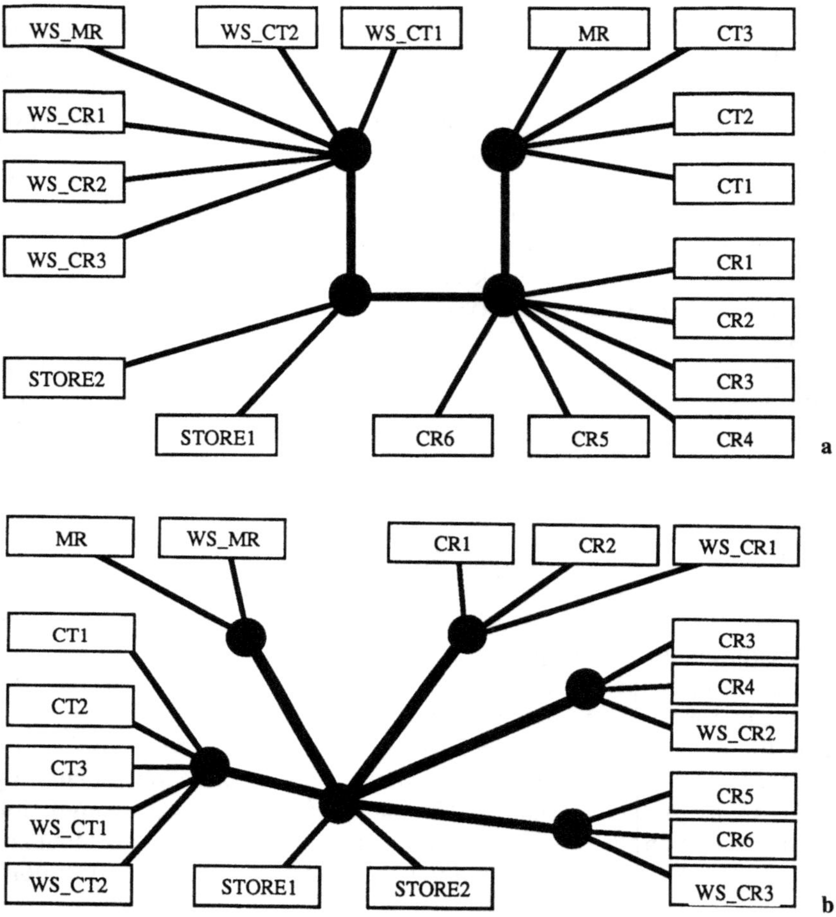

Fig. 5.5a,b. Two simulated configurations. (*solid cricles*, switch modules; *rectangles*, image equipment; *CT*, computed tomography; *MRI*, magnetic resonance imaging; *CR*, computer radiology; *WS*, workstation; *STORE*, image storage modules). **a** Configuration A, in which the acquisition stations (*CT*, *MRI*, *CR*) and the workstations are placed in different groups. **b** Configuration B, in which the stations are grouped by modality

equipment, a *SEND_image* request message including the image data will be sent to that image equipment. A SEND_image response message, which will be received from that image equipment later, includes the result of the image transfer.

For the network simulations, a workload is defined as described in Sect. 5.1.2. Further, it is assumed that new images will be sent to ISMs directly after the examination of a patient. In order to focus on the performance of the network itself, all the image equipment is assumed to be ideal, which means first that there is no delay for preparing the data for transport, and second that all the image equipment offers at least the transport rate of the

Table 5.6. Average waiting time per case for the various users (workstations) depending on the configuration

Configuration	Workstation					
	CT1 (s)	CT2 (s)	MR (s)	CR1 (s)	CR2 (s)	CR3 (s)
A	17.7	19.2	20.9	23.2	23.8	24.3
B	15.6	14.7	25.4	20.3	22.1	21.7
B[a]	14.3	12.8	15.5	22.1	22.7	22.9

[a] Segment size 1 MB.

network. In reality, image equipment will need time to move the data from magnetic or optical stores into a fast random access memory (RAM) before a data transfer via network can take place. Furthermore, the transfer rate of real image equipment may be less than that of the network, which becomes particularly interesting when raising the network tranfer rate above that of individual image equipment components.

Figure 5.5 shows two of the simulated configurations. In configuration A (Fig. 5.5.a) the acquisition stations (CT, MRI, CR) and the workstations (WS_CT, WS_MRI, WS_CR) are put into different groups. In configuration B (Fig. 5.5.b) the stations are grouped per modality. When making a report, a CT case consists of 10–30 images and an MRI case consists of 20–40 images, with an image size of 512 × 512 × 12 bits each. A CR case has either two or four images of 2048 × 2048 × 12 bits data each. Requesting the images belonging to a case means to request all necessary images one after the other, in the process of which each image transfer consists of two message transfers, as explained above.

Simulation Results

The simulation showed that the length of the waiting time depends on whether there were interfering image requests. All the sets of image equipment which are connected to the same switch module share the same network channel to the storage modules. Since this network channel can be used by only one image equipment system at a time, the image requests coming from this cluster of image equipment are served one after the other. For example, with a transfer rate of 8 Mbit/s (which was the effective transfer rate of the first realisation of the ImNet concept), the time needed to transfer a CR image of 6 MB is at least 6 s. A single CT or MRI image at least needs 0.375 s. The waiting time for a case of CT or MRI images increases significantly if the transfer of a CR image interferes.

Table 5.6 shows the waiting time per case for all users and for both configurations. Since a network channel between two switch modules can be simultaneously used for image transfers in opposite directions, in configuration B an image transfer from a workstation may overlap with an image

Table 5.7. Average waiting time per case for the various users (workstations) depending on the transfer rate of the network

Transfer rate (Mbit/s)	Workstation					
	CT1 (s)	CT2 (s)	MR (s)	CR1 (s)	CR2 (s)	CR3 (s)
8	15.6	14.7	25.4	20.3	22.1	21.7
16	4.9	5.2	7.5	9.5	10.0	9.9
32	2.3	2.3	3.1	4.5	4.7	4.7
100	0.7	0.7	0.9	1.5	1.5	1.5

transfer from an acquisition station from the same cluster. In general, the waiting times in configuration B are shorter, but due to the coincidental occurrence of interference, the waiting time for the user at the MRI workstation has increased. To give an example, another simulation in configuration B shows the results when using a segment-oriented transfer protocol. Instead of sending the total image in a single step, an image may be split into segments that are sent one after the other. The network channel has to be established again for each segment. After the segment has been sent, the network channel is closed and the next segment may be transferred. That segment, however, may belong to another image that has been requested by another user. The use of segments decreases the waiting time for an individual CT or MRI image significantly. However, Table 6 shows that the effect on the waiting time for a CT or MRI case is less significant. This is due to the fact that, for example, a CT case consists of 10–30 images; if a CR image split into six segments of 1 MB interferes, the waiting time for the CT case may still be increased by 6 s! The average waiting time for a CR user has also increased, since splitting the large CR images into segments increases the expected number of interfering transfers.

Apart from modifications in the configurations and transfer protocol, changes in the parameter of transfer rate have been studied. After a connection has been established, the image data are transferred at different transfer rates. Table 5.7 shows the simulation results. The average waiting time for a case and for the various users depends on the transfer rate. The simulation was performed with the model shown in configuration B. Note that the model assumed no delay at the image equipment. It is remarkable, that a doubling of the transfer rate diminishes the waiting time by a factor of more than 2. After a connection between two corresponding sets of image equipment has been established, the actual time needed to transfer the data is reduced by exactly one-half. However, as a result of the shorter data transfer times, fewer image transfers interfere. Consequently, the total time spent at the transfer phase, including the time needed to establish the connection, is further reduced.

The results from the above-mentioned simulation of ImNet indicate clearly which modifications may be made with ImNet in order to keep the performance of the network and of the PACS at a high level. Bottlenecks inside a PACS installation, which happen to arrise at components such as ISMs or transmission links, necessitated by the steady growth of a PACS, can be overcome by simply installing more of the same critical components. Besides permitting the installation of multiple ISMs, which makes it possible to keep most of the transfer local (compare the simulation in configurations A and B), ImNet allows the installation of parallel network links to enlarge the transfer capacity.

The use of higher transfer rates (ImNet/2 permits effective rates of 100 or 140 Mbit/s) will lead to significant reductions of the waiting times. It is, of course, only possible to have full benefit from this transfer rate if the PACS modules can transfer data at that speed. The bottleneck for the image data transfer will then be shifted from the network into the PACS modules, where the preparation for an image data transfer, e.g., copying the image data from disk to RAM, takes more time than the following transfer via the network. A simulation of ImNet/2 with the idealistic assumptions made for the image equipment, therefore, only gives information of the network itself. Figure 5.6 shows the contrast in pure transfer time, for the transfer of 10 Mb data via the different network types in relation to the number of concurrent transfers. To gain insight into the behavior of a PACS with fast networks, models for real image equipment have to be included into the simulation model. Therefore, at BAZIS, several other models have been developed, including a model for an optical disk jukebox.

5.1.5.5 Interfacing Image Data Terminal Equipment

The second generation of network components has now been developed. The first generation – ImNet/1 – was commercialized by IMTEC Image Network AB (Uppsala, Sweden) in 1987 (IMTEC 1987). Its technology was limited by the physical data rate of the fiber transmission channels to 16 Mbit/s. The transport data rate was 13 Mbit/s. Positive experience, which was gained in particular with an early installation at the Aachen University of Technology (interlinking an MRI system, CR equipment, a laser ophthalmoloscope, and several image workstations at the University Hospital and image facilities 2 km apart) motivated an upgrading of the network hardware. Figure 5.7 shows the present stage of the network. ImNet/2, equipped with recently developed high-speed components, now operates at a physical data rate of 125 Mbit/s and a transport data rate of 100 Mbit/s. Effective use is made of the network speed by means of DMA interfaces to the VME/VSB bus, to the NuBus (Apple Macintosh II) and, via a so-called generic gateway, to slower computers of imaging modalities. The striking effect for the user is a decrease in the transport time to below 1 s for a reasonable image data set of 10 Mbyte, i.e., a couple of X-rays or a set of CTs!

The network software follows the ISO/OSI seven-layer concept. The lower four layers are specific for ImNet. They are implemented on the

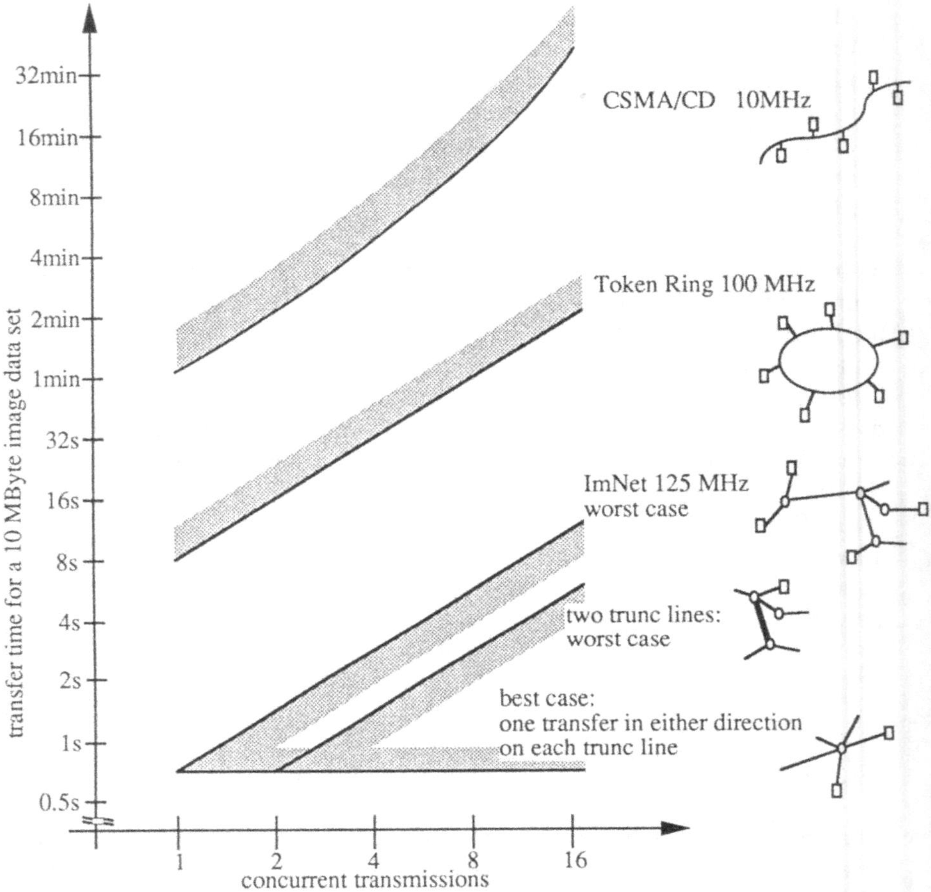

Fig. 5.6. Typical characteristics of ImNet for image transfer times versus number of concurrent transfers in comparison with standard LANs (cf. Fig. 5.2)

interface boards by means of programmed hardware and/or a dedicated processor, hence freeing the host from speed-critical protocol handling. The higher protocol layers follow the ACR/NEMA proposal (ACR/NEMA 1985). Because of the separation of image data (travelling via ImNet) and management data (travelling via conventional LANs), their implementation covers only a GET_image session and a SEND_image session.

5.1.5.6 Interfacing Public Networks

There is an obvious need to communicate images over long distances. Critical diagnostic situations, for example, provoke the wish to consult

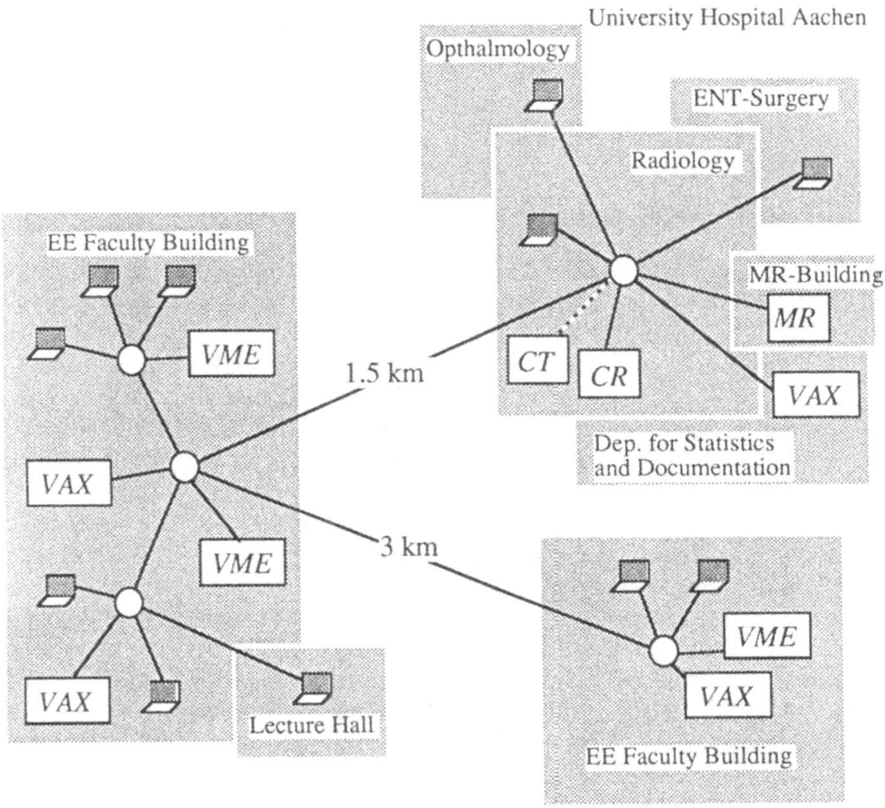

Fig. 5.7. Current stage of development of pilot network

experts practising at distant institutes. The international standardized public network Integrated Services Digital Network (ISDN) will make it possible to interconnect LANs with transfer rates of up to 140 Mbit/s with the introduction of broad-band network (ISDN-B). Its use for long distance image transfer makes it possible for the first time to get fast access to a patient's images, which have to be retrieved from widely spread stores, placed for example in hospitals or private institutes. It will also offer new possibilities in PACS applications. Digital processing of medical images can raise the efficiency of diagnostic examinations in comparison with the use of the raw image material. Because of the enormous complexity of specialized computer systems for fast image processing, only a limited number of systems exist and they are often located at specialized research institutes. A transfer time of less than 1 s, for a single image or a sequence of small images allows us to make use of these specialized computer systems via networks, even in situations where time is critical.

5.2 Network Management

R. MATTHEUS and J.G. TIBERGHIEN

5.2.1 Why Network Management?

5.2.1.1 Introduction

Since a large amount of data must be transferred within the hospital, very fast networks may be chosen in an attempt to solve the image communication problem. The volume of data creates problems, for example, on the level of the interface, in the bus structure, and at the storage level. To achieve a fully functional picture archiving and communications system (PACS) in clinical routine, a PACS architecture and network management must be chosen which make the whole system acceptable to medical specialists and which bring improvements over the methods currently used. Networks are becoming more and more complex, and the PACS networks in particular are tending to become increasingly heterogeneous. Careful management of these networks is, therefore, a crucial factor if efficient and reliable network operation is to be maintained and if the performance of the network in terms of speed, quality, and quantity of the services provided to the users is to increase. A heterogeneous network environment means more components likely to fail, more potential software, hardware incompatibilities, and more critical connections to monitor and to maintain. Network management is concerned with increasing the performance of the network, while maintaining efficient and reliable network operations. It also interacts with the hierarchical storage control systems in this environment.

The Urgent Need for Network Management. Today it has become evident to key decision makers in companies that networks are essential to competitive strength. Networks are used to link the large numbers of computers with in corporations, and thereby allow access to information on demand. This development is also taking place in the medical field, where patient data are distributed to the departments by means of networks. In this way, medical specialists can make significant decisions that are timely and well-informed. Departments within the hospital share data across the networks. Medical accuracy is improved, and medical information is used more efficiently. Networks greatly speed up decision making and enable a quick response to be made to the demanding needs of doctors.

In the PACS environment, we are dealing with image data which call for dedicated solutions. Over the last few years, the concept of distributed computing has gained wide acceptance. While centralized computing still has its place, the primary advantage of distributed computing is to put systems at the hands of the doctors who need to use them. The best system for an application can be selected according to the local needs. However, there are also some complexities associated with these advantages that relate to networking in a distributed computing environment. Typically, second generation PACS networks in such an environment include systems of all types and sizes from different vendors. These networks must support various types of applications. Further, the networks are dynamic, new systems may be added, and this also calls for management tools. Traffic control, redundancy, security, safety, monitoring, and back-up techniques are essential in a clinical PACS environment.

Network Functionality. One can see some analogy between the responsibility for keeping the network running and maintaining a highway system. The data circuits and the routers are the roads, the data packets are the vehicles that use the roads. Applications use the data packets, routers, and data circuits to get the job done, much like people use their vehicles and the roads to get somewhere. Just as the responsibility for maintaining the roads is controlled by a number of people in several departments, so network management rests with many people. Highways are maintained by the government, while other roads are managed by towns or by governments. There even are privately maintained roads that are occasionally opened to public traffic.

Networks are like people in that each one differs from the others. The management style of a network will reflect the style of the hospital which runs it. The network architecture and management will reflect the hospital structure and the working procedures. Profiles on the level of patient flow, data organization, medical specialist flow, and geographic situation need to be introduced.

5.2.1.2 The OSI Model

In 1979, the International Standardization Organization (ISO) developed a reference model for communications: the Open Systems Interconnection (OSI). The OSI subdivides communications into seven layers; a specific function is carried out in each layer and various procedures define the communications within and via the layers. The physical layer describes the medium for communications, e.g., the cable. The data link layer describes how signals are to be transmitted, and how failures are to be tackled. The network layer describes how an emitter and a receiver communicate; priorities and modes of communication are also described here. The transport layer is responsible for the end to end communication. The session layer describes how the information is to be grouped before it can be represented. The presentation layer describes the syntax to be used to make the information readable to the receiver. The application layer describes how the various devices co-operate to perform an application. The network manager is part of layer 7. The network manager is not involved in the way the images are transmitted through the network. The network manager simply decides who enters in the network first, and is aware of what is going on in the network and in its nodes.

5.2.1.3 *Factors That Affect Performance*

Various factors such as capacity, propagation delay, number of bits per packet, local network protocols, offered load, and number of stations have an effect in one way or another on the performance of the network. It is not within the scope of this book to discuss these items in detail, but we will try to give an idea of what is needed to control a image networking environment.

The local network protocols are divided into the physical, the medium access, and the link layers. The physical layer keeps up with transmissions and receptions with little delay. The medium access layer may have a significant effect on the network performance. The link layer will add some overhead bits to each frame and some administrative overhead such as virtual circuit management and acknowledgments. We can consider the first three factors listed above to be characterization of the network, and they are generally treated like constants. The local network protocol is the focus of the design effort. The next two factors, the offered load and the number of nodes (e.g., acquisition unit, imaging computer, and storage) are generally treated as the independent variables. It is important to be concerned with determining performance as a function of these two variables. By means of the network architecture and management approach, we can change these variables which will be important for image networking. The network management influences all the nodes in the network (e.g., storage, display, and hard copy) and is certainly not limited to the network only. Functions such as routing due to failure of a node (hard copy unit) is also the responsibility of the network management process.

Examination Type. Images are central objects in a medical environment. For the PACS, it is essential to consider a group of images as one entity. A clinician will look at a single patient's examination which will consists of several images. This group of images can be characterized by eight parameters. Based upon these eight parameters, minimum requirements can be calculated for image computers in terms of resolution, manipulation functions, and storage (Table 5.8).

Statistics. Different data types may be defined in a PACS network: (a) image data (b) image-related alphanumerical data, mostly in the image header, (c) patient-related data, and (d) control commands. The image data may be grouped into classes. Owing to the different nature of the types of data, and to the different requirements of management and flow, the network can be partitioned into message, image data, and medically related data.

Various factors are important in image flow:

1. Where and when are the image data produced or used (location, modalities, clusters)?
2. What is the size of the data sets, depending on image size and modality and relation to the archived sets?

Table 5.8. The eight parameters of examination type and four additional parameters acquired at the radiology department of the University Hospital Brussels (VUB) in 1991. Modality clusters can be easily distinguished[a]

M	E	N (*n*)	S (*n*)	R	C	T (min)	G (MB)	F	A (MB)	B (KB)
CT	Body	34	21	512	12	30	17	2	34	9.6
	Head	20	15	512	12	30	10	2	20	5.6
MRI	Body	80	13	256	12	40	10	1	10	4.2
	Neurological	128	13	256	12	40	16	1	16	6.8
	Bone	173	25	256	12	55	21.6	1	21.6	6.7
	Cardiological	19	19	256	12	35	2.3	1	2.3	1.1
US	Body	8	4	256	8	20	0.5	3	1.5	0.42
DR	Body	8	8	4096	12	15	256	2	500	291.2
DSA	Cardiological	400	20	512	12	20	200	1	200	170.6
	Cardiological	100	20	1024	12	30	200	1	200	113.7
	Vascular	400	20	512	12	30	200	1	200	113.7
PET	Neurological	20	5	256	8	40	1.25	2	2.5	1.06
	Cardiological	20	5	256	8	40	1.25	2	2.5	1.06

CT, computed tomography; *MRI*, magnetic resonance imaging; *US*, ultrasound; *DR*, digital radiology; *DSA*, digital subtraction angiography; *PET*, positron emission tomograply; *M*, {CT,MR,US,DR,XR,DSA} modality source; *E*, {body, head, neurological, cardiac, abdominal, vascular, bone} examination; *N*, maximum number of images; *S*, maximum number of marked images; *R*, {64,128,256,512,1024,2048,4096} matrix $n \times n$; *T*, average examination time in minutes; *C*, {8,12} contrast resolution in gray level; *G*, generated image data for one examination (MB); *F*, frequency of the examination (Examination/5 years); *A*, total image data (MB); *B*, throughput of network segment (KB/s)

[a] The eighth parameter of examination type, which is not mentioned here is: D, {2,3,4} display technique (depending on acquisition), where 2 is a two-dimensional image (x,y), 3 is an image in a three-dimensional set (x,y,z) and 4 is an image in a dynamic three-dimensional set (x,y,z,t)

3. When are these data to be transferred and for what reason?
4. Where is the medical specialist located?

In addition to the examination type, four other parameters are relevant for planning networks, storage, display units, and rules for the network management (Table 5.8). Image generation (G) takes place in a certain time frame (T). This allows the calculation of the minimum throughput of that network segment (B), considering the amount of archived images. The modality types (M) and more specific combinations with the examination type determine the throughput of the network segment (B). This is a first indication of the relation between medical knowledge about examinations and the characteristics of the network, the architecture, and the control techniques.

Network statistics concerning the response times of PACS implementations focus too much on all the examinations from all the departments taking place each moment and at every location. Technically, this is hard to realize, and in a hospital environment it is not even needed; an X-ray of the foot will be of little interest to the neuroradiologist reporting on a computed tomograph (CT) of the brain. Different types of useful statistical information can be obtained, depending on the way a hospital works. The data reflect the organization of the hospital, e.g., models for radiologist flow, patient flow, image fnow, and retrieval rules.

Medical clusters and subclusters can be defined on the basis of statistical information. These clusters and subclusters are a profile description of the type of examinations, the medical specialty, and the numbers of examinations. This information indicates very well the difference between requests for radiological examinations, e.g., oncological and neurological consultants

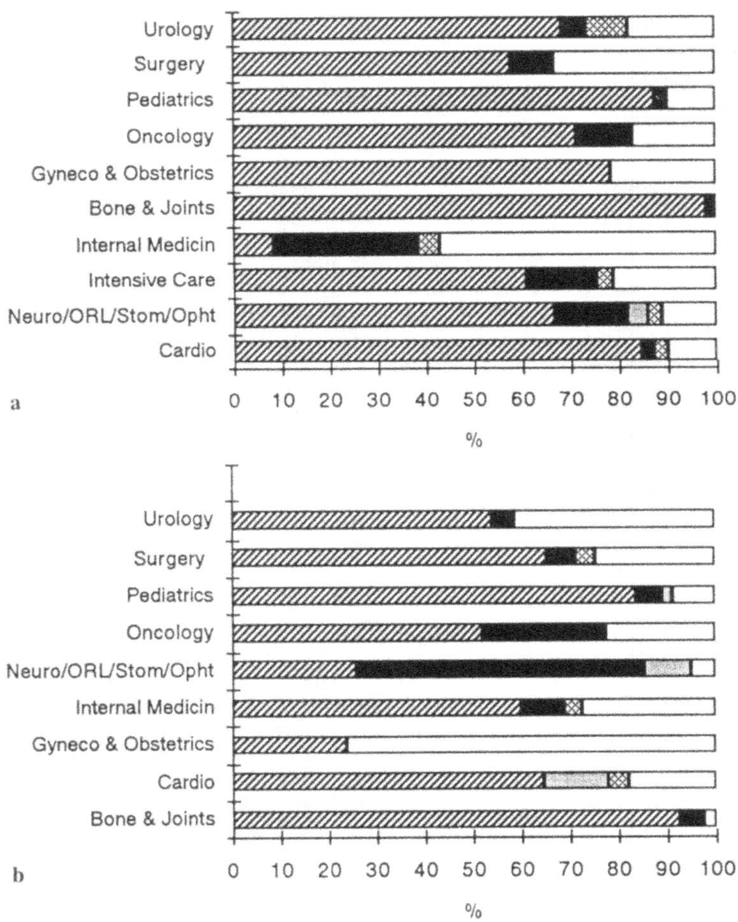

Fig. 5.8a,b. Percentage of radiological examinations for various medical specialties using different imaging techniques (*white shading*, ultrasound; *crosshatching*, digital subtraction angiography; *dotted areas*, magnetic resonance imaging; *black shading*, computed tomography; *diagonal lines*, conventional X-ray). **a** Inpatient data. **b** Outpatient data. Data from the University Hospital Brussels in 1991

perform more CT examinations than others. A difference can be found between consultation clusters and hospital clusters, for example, in internal medicine (Fig. 5.8). For PACS network management and architecture, this is useful information, as it gives an indication of where image servers are needed and about their size, as well as indications for the phased approach, which help us to establish where the PACS is most useful. It gives information about where and when the images will be needed, and what the impact on the other activities will be.

Data on the number of preexisting examinations of the same patient indicate that only a small percentage of the old images are retrieved (Fig. 5.9). The number of patients in a department, related to the time, gives an activity distribution function of the department or the subdepartments. Reporting, which takes place with a minimum delay of 30 min, can also be related to the hospital cluster and provides information to the network management unit, including hierarchical storage management.

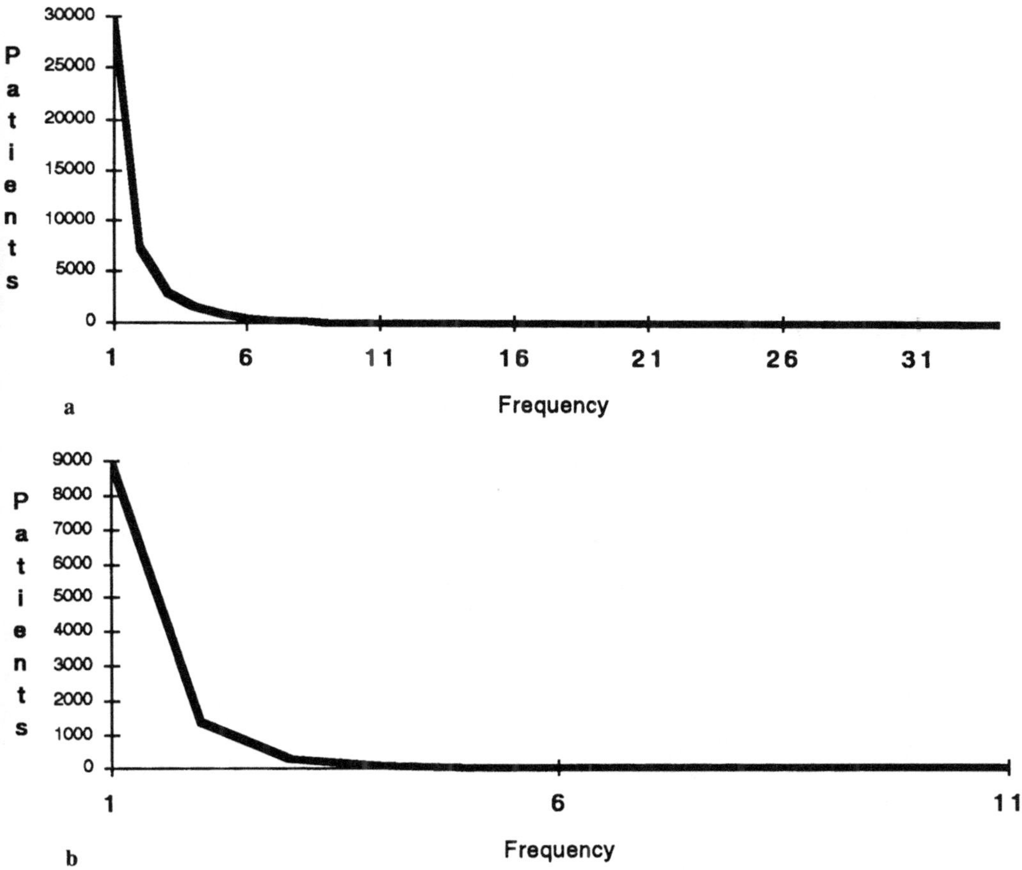

Fig. 5.9a,b. Frequency with which patients are reexamined using the same imaging technique. **a** Data for computed tomography brain scans. **b** Data for conventional chest X-ray. Information was collected from the University Hospital Brussels in 1991

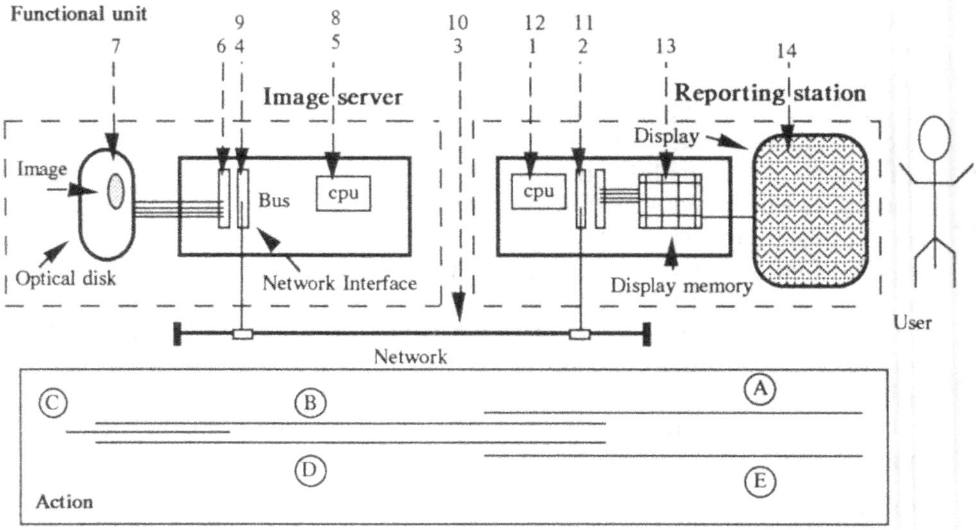

Fig. 5.10. Actions involved in requests from a user on a reporting station when the image is located on an image server

Table 5.9. Actions involved in the image transfer with an indication of the component which will define performance on that level

Action	No	Time defined by
Doctor queries patient images	*A*	
Process in reporting station initiates messages	1	Processor speed
Host system software transfers message to NIU	2	Bus type
Images are requested on the image server	*B*	
Reporting station NIU transfer message to image server	3	Network speed/bus
Images are read from disk	*C*	
NIU transfers message to system	4	Bus type
Process in image server initiates reading from disk	5	Processor speed
Data is accessed from disk	6	Disk access
Data is read from disk to controller	7	Disk transfer speed
Process on image server initiates image transfer	8	Processor speed
Data is transferred from controller to NIU	9	Bus type
Image is transferred to reporting station	*D*	
Image server NIU transfer data to reporting station	10	Network speed/bus
Image is displayed	*E*	
NIU transfers data to system	11	Bus type
Process on reporting station initiates image display	12	Processor speed
Data is copied to display RAM	13	RAM/bus type
Image is written on CRT	14	Lines on CRT

NIU, network interface unit; *CRT*, cathode ray tube; *RAM*, random access memory

End-to-End Performance. Response time is one of the key factors determining the acceptance of PACS in clinical routine use. This response time is not only defined by the network, but also by a whole range of different functional units. Figure 5.10 shows an image request from a reporting station to an image server. The different specifications of the actions involved define the performance of the end-to-end communication. Table 5.9 shows an example of functional units which may influence the end-to-end performance.

5.2.2 PACS Architecture

5.2.2.1 Introduction

The way the nodes are connected together by a communication network can be defined as the PACS architecture. In true distributed processing, each computer system is chosen to handle its local workload, and the network has been designed to support the system as a whole. A network architecture is mostly defined by the way the interconnections between nodes are defined. The open system approach is also an important factor for the PACS architecture. To give an idea of the evolution and a classification of PACS environments, four different architectures are defined here.

5.2.2.2 Architectures

Closed line. A closed line is modality dependent and only aimed at connecting devices of the same modality together, possibly with a viewing station. The so-called second consoles of the modality are also connected by means of these techniques (Fig. 5.11).

Central line. In a central line, a central computer system is added to the first architecture with a local storage, data base, archiving possibilities, display and a PACS reporting node (Fig. 5.12). It is possible to interconnect

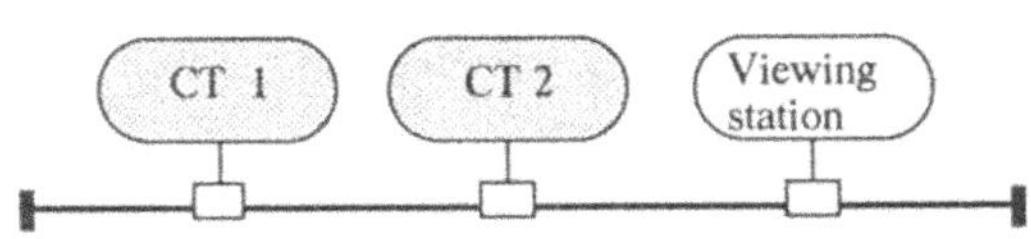

Fig. 5.11. A closed line architecture with two CT units and a viewing station

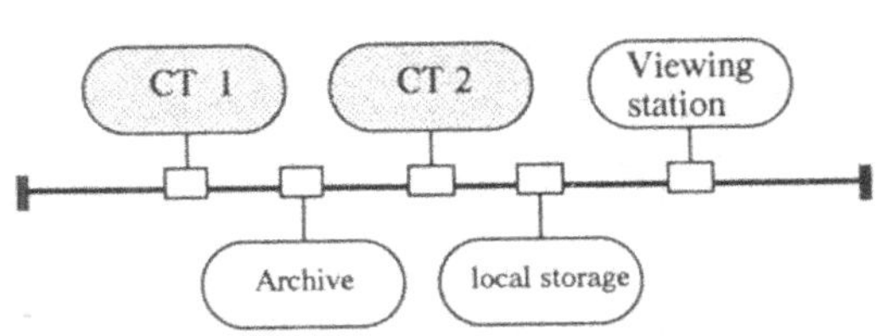

Fig. 5.12. A central linearchitecture

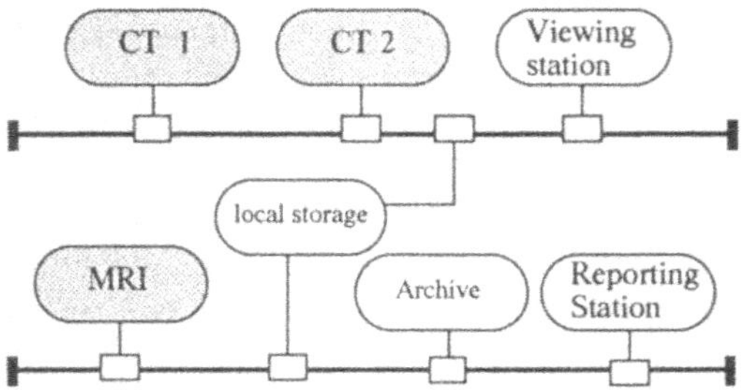

Fig. 5.13. A distributed network architecture. A computer is used for the integration of two networks or more

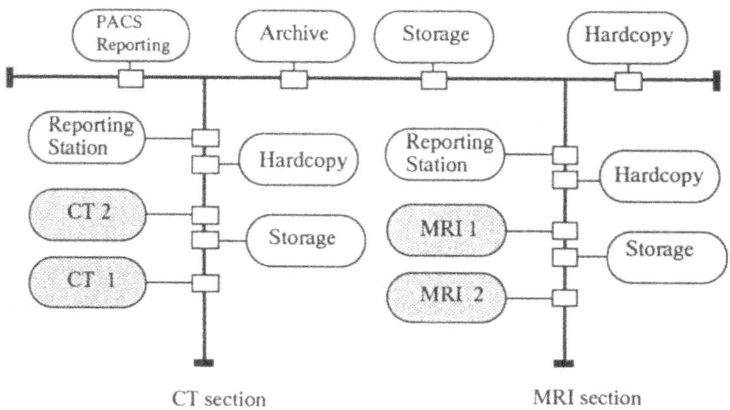

Fig. 5.14. A distributed PACS network. The two departments on the figure are interconnected via the PACS backbone

devices from different modalities. The openness of the computer depends on the degree of possible connections.

Distributed network. In a distributed network, there is the additional possibility of making use of distributed processing on the different computers in the network as well as heterogeneous networking possibilities (Fig. 5.13).

Distributed subnetworks. Each subdepartment (e.g., magnetic resonance imaging, MRI, CT, and emergency department) has its own small PACS environment with local storage, reporting consoles, hard copy units, and a gateway or bridge to the backbone of the PACS network, which interconnects all the subnetworks (Fig. 5.14). This approach allows the image flow to be distributed over the network, making traffic on a single subnetwork possible without interfering with the traffic on the other subnetworks. This PACS architecture allows fully heterogeneous networking even with multivendor PACS components. A phased upgradable approach is possible, starting with one of the PACS subnetworks. This is technically more relevant and also more cost effective, while the educational requirements are more easily met with this type of phased approach; medical specialists need to be educated to a minimum common technical level.

5.2.3 PACS Network Management Kernel

5.2.3.1 Introduction

In general, the term network management covers a wide range of tasks. Network design and configuration, for example, are network management tasks in the preoperational phase. Network monitoring and control, including error detection, fault diagnosis, and dynamic routing, are network management tasks with a real-time aspect. In a PACS network for a hospital environment, some of these tasks are not needed or of much less significant, whereas others become very important. The tasks can be expanded to the global communication needs.

In fact, careful traffic management becomes mandatory for a PACS network in order to ensure a reasonable response time to the network users. A standard data transfer in a PACS network is an examination which includes many images. The size of such a data transfer is several orders of magnitude larger than a typical data transfer in a local area network. The existing local area network technology uses protocols which are not suited for image transport. Therefore, it is necessary to control the image traffic in the network explicitly, i.e., access conflicts are not left to be resolved by the transport layer, but are arbitrated by a software module. In addition, the network traffic can be distributed in time, because knowledge about patient, radiologist, and image flow is availabe. This knowledge can be exploited for careful planning and scheduling, for example, by organizing overnight prefetching of images from the central archive to the local archive.

Software modules may be implemented to perform an explicit traffic management strategy, although this will lead to several problems. First, the traffic management modules cannot automatically adapt to changing circumstances such as a reconfiguration or extension failure of a network segment. Second, when the PACS environment grows, it becomes very hard to upgrade and to maintain the traffic management modules as a result of their ad hoc nature.

It is a fundamental requirement to make the domain knowledge and the traffic management strategy clear. A first advantage of this approach is that the traffic management can automatically adapt to a changing context. A second advantage is that the experimentation with different management strategies is facilitated, which is essential since each hospital is different.

5.2.3.2 Basic Components

Many of the existing systems for networking tasks in a non image environment can be classified as expert diagnosis systems. All these systems collect the expertise gathered over the years by human experts in a rule base. A PACS environment is, however, much more heterogeneous than, for example, a wide area telephone network, i.e., image stations and storage of different types from different vendors, which means that the traditional, rule-based approach is not appropriate because of the knowledge acquisition effort involved in capturing expertise about all these different devices.

A network model is needed in the first instance as a means to represent the state of the network and further as the basis for analyzing the decision-making processes. In a PACS environment, traffic management is a prime issue. Up to a certain point, traffic management can be static, i.e., for handling the network configuration and the knowledge of image flow, patient flow, and radiologist flow in a hospital environment, but beyond that point, decisions on which transfers should be served first have to be made dynamically, taking into account the current state of the network including pending request and actual disk usage.

Configurations may be proposed by the system and evaluated by means of a simulation. This also constitutes an important aspect of a PACS network and relates to decisions on such matters as network architecture, where to connect new devices, and where to add extra storage capacity. The combination of a network model and an explicit model of the traffic manager (TM) can result in a discrete simulation suitable for evaluating the performance of a possible configuration. This can be the foundation for a PACS configuration or reconfiguration tool. It is even more important to note that this can be the basis of a tool to tune the TM for optimum performance. Instead of changing the network model, the TM model can be modified, and the resulting performance can be evaluated using the discrete simulation.

5.2.3.3 Kernel

Key components in a PACS network management system will be the network model, the monitor, a TM, a flow manager (FM), a simulator, and configuration and strategy managers (Fig. 5.15). The combination of the generated network model and the simulator allows us to test and experiment with different traffic management strategies and different network con-

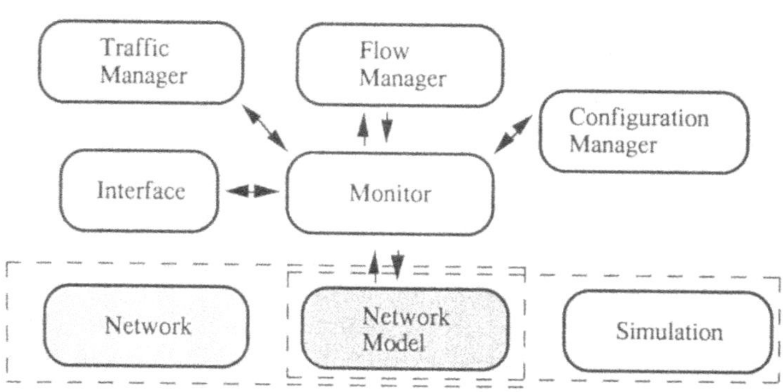

Fig. 5.15. Components of the network management kernel

figurations. The image flow controlled by the FM creates and alters image transfers, whereas the TM sequentializes these image transfers over the network and is required to clarify the traffic management strategy and the domain knowledge used in it. Extensive use of strategy rules is made by the FM and the TM. These rules are the explicit representation of bits and pieces of common sense and/or domain knowledge related to management of the PACS network. These strategy rules are the profiles of the hospital environment.

5.2.4 Network Model

The network model is a key module in the PACS network management. It is a knowledge-based model of the various network components, their properties and interrelations, the network architecture, and the model of other objects and events in the PACS environment such as images, image transfers, and examinations. In short, it constitutes a complete and consistent description of the operational network. The link between the real network and the network model is rather special. First, consistency between the real network and the network model is assumed at all time. A reconfiguration of the real network, for example, implies that the network model is to be edited, but this is not necessarily a constraint. Adding a component to the network usually involves more than connecting a piece of hardware. Different address tables, for example, may need to be updated to keep the network operational. It is possible to develop a dedicated interface that handles the graphical issue of the network, as well as all necessary updating of addresses and tables in the real network, which are automatically derived from the editing step.

In addition, the functionality that is typically attributed to a network monitor is integrated in the network model. In the one direction, data from the real network are stored with the network model where they are available to the other modules. A typical example here is logging the activity in the network. This information is made available to the network users or to the other modules in the network management system through the network model. In the other direction, the controls needed to implement the decisions of the other modules are passed to the real network through the network model.

5.2.5 Traffic Manager

5.2.5.1 Introduction

One of the main tasks of the TM is to sequentialize the image transfers in the network by implementing a specific strategy based on priorities of image transfers. The traffic management strategy, for example, describes when and where an active transfer is to be interrupted to give way to another transfer. This is similar to a policeman controlling the traffic in the streets. The TM takes care of real-time problems.

5.2.5.2 *Functions*

Among network segments, a hierarchy is defined. Each segment is connected to its single supersegment by means of a bridge. The highest segment in the hierarchy, i.e., the segment which has no supersegment, is called the backbone of the network. Accordingly the TM of a segment's supersegment is referred to as the supervisor of this segment.

TMs receive transfer requests, i.e., requests from image stations to transfer an image, originating from stations located upon the TMs' segment. More details about such a request, e.g., source, destination, and priority are filled in by the FM. These completed transfer requests, also called transfers, are stored in transfer queues. All logic storage units (see Sect. 5.2, 6.2) such as image stations and TMs have transfer queues. A queue of a TM is called the queue to its supervisor. The decision to store a transfer in a particular queue is made according to the queueing strategy of the TMs. For each image transfer, one TM, the so-called master of the transfer, is responsible for activation of the transfer. The master of the transfer is also set according to the TMs' queueing strategy.

A TM manages the queues of modalities on its segment and the queues of TMs on its subsegments, i.e., the segments lower in the hierarchy which are connected via a bridge to its segment. This means the TM is responsible for serving the transfers of these queues in the correct order. The queueing strategy of TMs defines the way a transfer is put on a queue managed by the transfer's master. TMs constantly investigate whether transfers waiting in the queues they manage may be executed and, as a consequence, interrupt other running transfers. The TM's interrupt strategies define various solutions, mostly based on the urgency of different transfers, to deal with this task in a satisfactory way.

5.2.5.3 *Strategy*

A strategy is a role description of the way the TM reacts and interacts on events. It is impossible to describe all the strategies, but the most important ones are described here.

A *queueing strategy* determines the master of a newly created transfer and the queue in which this transfer request will be stored, i.e., it defines the way a transfer is put in a queue which is managed by the transfer's master.

As long as a transfer request is not stored in a queue, no other TM or FM is able to see this transfer. This means that no FM can change this

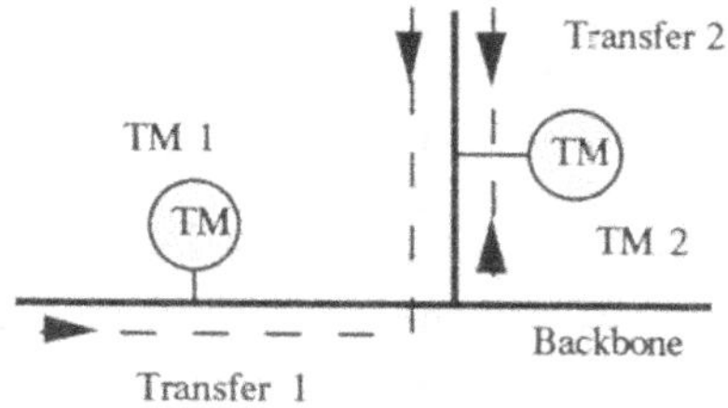

Fig. 5.16. Interrupt strategies. Transfer through the backbone and in a segment

transfer's source, destination, or priority. Therefore, each TM can manage its queueing strategy in parallel with the other tasks of FM and TM.

An *interrupt strategy* investigates whether a waiting transfer may be executed and as a consequence interrupts other running transfers. While a TM looks for the best transfer to pick out of the queues it is managing, one of these queues may change. For instance, a better transfer according to the used interrupt strategy may enter a queue, or the priority of one of the transfers in a queue may be upgraded. Then it may well be that the best transfer of that moment is not chosen to be sent into the network. This is not dramatic, since during the next cycle the TM will notice the changes and send the best transfer into the network. Notice here the similarity to the consider next-best transfer subtask. A worse problem occurs when a TM has decided to put a transfer into the network and that transfer changes before it is taken out of its queue. For instance, a FM may at the same time have decided to change the transfer's source or destination, or even to delete the transfer.

Another problem that might occur when implementing the TM and FM as loosely coupled processes is that various TMs may decide at the same time to put a transfer in the network. The result would be more than one transfer going over the same segment, and the TM would no longer sequentialize the traffic over the network. For example, suppose a TM decides to put a transfer in the network when there is no transfer on the path from the source to the destination of the transfer (Fig. 5.16). TM1 chooses to serve Transfer 1, which has to travel over the backbone and the subsegment. TM2 wants to put Transfer 2 into the subsegment. Since no transfer is running in the network, TM1 and TM2 may both conclude they are allowed to put the transfer into the network. If both come to this conclusion at (nearly) the same time, Transfer 1 and Transfer 2 will simultaneously occupy the subsegment.

5.2.5.4 Mutual Co-operation of TMs

Any possible solution to the problem of various TMs deciding to put a transfer in the network at the same time, depends on the queueing strategy implemented. For instance, suppose first that our network manager uses the nonqueueing TM strategy. The master of a transfer is the TM of the segment and of its source module, and the storing queue of the transfer is the queue of this source module. The interrupt strategy used is the interrupt if best of all running transfers strategy. To avoid different TMs putting a transfer in the network, an order of execution of the TM's interrupt strategy task has to be defined. Since every transfer a master controls can have any module in the network as its destination, every decision to put a transfer in the network can collide with an analogue decision of another TM. Therefore, the order of execution of the TM's interrupt strategy task has to be very strict: only one TM at the time can implement its interrupt strategy. In this way, no parallelism can be defined in putting new transfers in the network, even if two transfers have no common segments on their path from source to destination, they cannot be put on the segment at the same time.

Since the rate of requests to transfer an examination is not very high, it should be no problem to sequentialize the task which consists in putting the transfers into the network. It may, however, be worthwhile to consider other ways of implementing this strategy. An evident solution is mutual communication between the different TMs. A TM intending to put a transfer into the network can ask the other TMs if it is allowed to do so. In this queueing strategy, the TM has to issue its question to all the other TMs and to wait until replies have been received. Several problems proceed from this approach. All these messages have to pass bridges which may be hard to cross, they put an extra load upon the network, the danger exists that they may get lost, and the TM will have to wait for a long time before it can resume work. Therefore, the first approach seems to be more suited. Sequentializing the task of putting a transfer in the network does not solve all the problems concerning this task. The defined interrupt strategy can also cause problems.

Suppose a TM decides to put a transfer into the network when there is no transfer in its own segment (Fig. 5.17). TM1 wants to put Transfer 1 into the network, and TM2 wants to put Transfer 2 in the network. Both transfers have to pass through the backbone. Since no transfer is running in its segment, TM1 decides to put Transfer 1 into the network. Then TM2 is activated, and also puts Transfer 2 into the network as no transfer is running on its segment. In this situation, TM2 interrupts Transfer 1, because it is occupying the backbone. The next time TM1 is activated it might put Transfer 1 into the network again because there is still no transfer running in its segment. This time Transfer 2 will be interrupted. This process will keep going on and TM1 and TM2 will keep interrupting both transfers as a result of the bad interrupt strategy.

Suppose our network manager uses the direct queueing TM strategy. The master of a transfer is the highest TM in the hierarchy on the path of the transfer, and the storing queue of the transfer is the queue of this source module or of a corresponding TM queue. The interrupt strategy used is the interrupt if best of all running transfers strategy. To avoid different TMs putting a transfer into the network, one has to define an order of execution of the TMs interrupt strategy task. Note that the way the masters of transfers

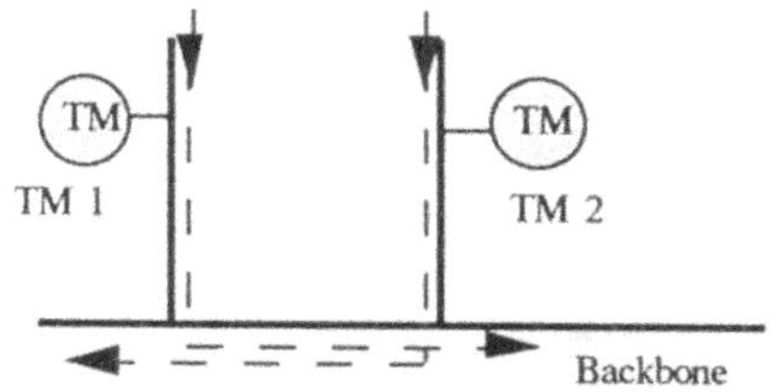

Fig. 5.17. Mutual co-operation of TMs. Transfer through the backbone on two segments

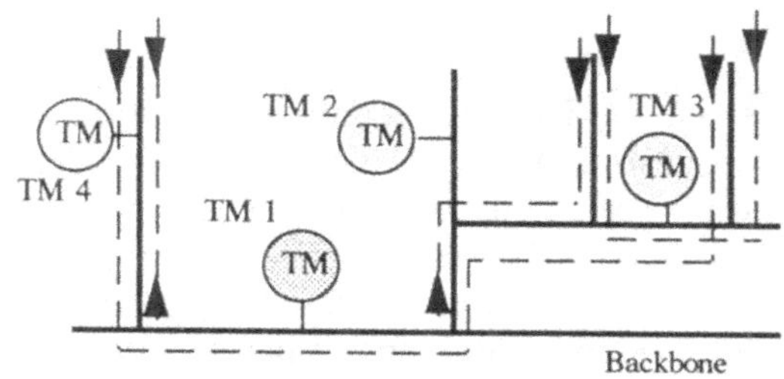

Fig. 5.18. A hierarchy of TMs

are defined introduces a hierarchy among TMs. A TM is only responsible for those transfers which pass its own segments and the segments lower in the hierarchy of the network.

The subsegments of a segment can be seen as a subtree of segments (Fig. 5.18). Each TM is able to put a transfer into its own segment and into the segments of the subtrees of its segment. It cannot put a transfer into any supersegment or into a segment of subtrees of supersegments. This relationship defines a hierarchy between TMs, equalling the hierarchy of segments (not all TMs are shown in Fig. 5.18). This hierarchy can be used to define an order in which the TMs will execute the interrupt strategy tasks. Since no TM located on the subtrees of the network can put transfers into the network which have to pass the same segments, those TMs may execute their interrupt strategy task together. Notice that this does not apply to TMs situated on the same subtree of the network and, therefore, those TMs have to be synchronized. The proposed order of executing the interrupt strategy tasks of the TMs is:

1. TMs on the same level in the hierarchy of the network can work together. For instance in Fig. 5.18, TM2 and TM4 are able to put a transfer into the network at the same time.
2. The order in which the different levels of the network are visited can be from top to leaves or from leaves to top.

Figure 5.19 shows an example of the order in which to execute the processes.

Another solution to the synchronization problem of the different TMs is mutual communication between these different TMs. Unlike the TMs in the first example, a TM does not need to broadcast its request to all other TMs in the network, but can rely upon the hierarchy of TMs to do so. It only needs to broadcast its request to the TMs higher up in the hierarchy,

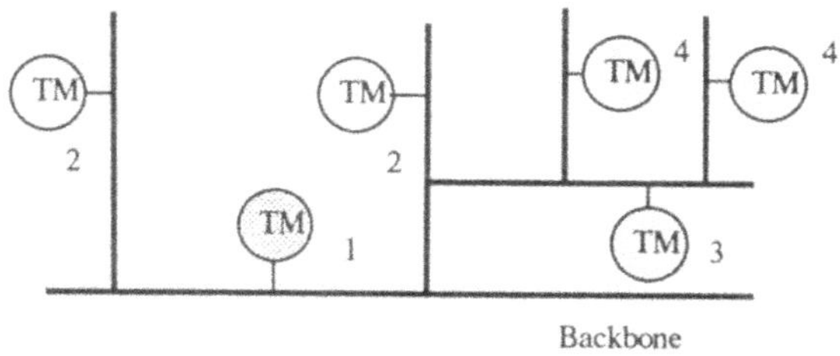

Fig. 5.19. Example of the order of execution of TM interrupt tasks. The number next to a TM shows the order of execution. Equal numbers indicate processes which run together

because these are the only TMs that can decide to put a transfer into its own segment. This may reduce the time the TM has to wait for the replies to its request, and there is less load on the network than in the first example. For this reason, this kind of implementation might be suitable.

A *combine strategy* tries to find transfers which have need to transfer the same examination and combines them into a single transfer. First of all there is a technical problem. What we neet to define in a combine strategy is the concept of a transfer with multiple destinations. The destinations of such a transfer are not always located in the same segment, and most of the time the transfer has to pass bridges. If not, the combine strategies cannot be implemented. Another problem we have already met concerns a FM trying to modify the source or the destination of one of the combined transfers or tries to remove one of these transfers. We refer to the discussion of the TM's interrupt strategies for more detail.

5.2.6 Flow Manager

5.2.6.1 Introduction

The FM is responsible for the distribution of images over the network's storage levels in order to achieve a better distribution of image transfers over the network and reduce the TM's work. The FM, for example, organizes prefetches of images from the central archive to local storages or to network segments to prevent excessive traffic in the network backbone at peak hours. For the same reason, it also prevents deleting images from storages local to a segment when the image is likely to be needed in the same segment later on. To achieve all this, the FM stores knowledge on image flow, patient flow, and radiologist flow, all of which are very specific to the hospital environment.

5.2.6.2 Functions

The FM is responsible for many tasks, one of which is to decide where every examination should be stored and to issue images to the network's storages in order to minimize network traffic when the examination is needed later.

The FM also ensures that urgent transfers are served before less urgent transfers and that reasonable response times are achieved for all transfer requests. Further tasks of the FM are ogranizing prefetches at nonpeak hours, minimizing network load at peak hours, and monitoring the load factor of the system's storage media to prevent overflow. The FM transports images from one storage level to another if, for example, the storage capacity of an image acquisition device reaches the saturation point. Just like for the TM, the implementation of the FM is distributed, i.e., on each segment of the network, a single FM is in charge.

FMs receive transfer requests from stations located in their segment. In turn, they send completed transfer requests, i.e., transfers, to the TM of their segment. Various types of transfers are defined. A transfer request originating from an acquisition station will result in an acquisition transfer, one originating from a consultation station will result in a consultation transfer, and one requested by a reporting station in a reporting transfer. Other transfer types are copy transfers and copy before delete transfers, which copy or move examinations to other storage devices. A transfer is assigned a priority level by the FM. Knowledge about types of transfers, their importance, and their frequencies, for example, is required for such a decision. Some very important transfers are given the status of emergency transfers. Priorities and the status of emergency transfer are assigned to transfers to allow the TM to distinguish between urgent and less urgent transfers.

To be able to decide where an examination has to be stored each time, in order to minimize network traffic for its later retrieval, the FM needs information about patient flow and examination flow. With this knowledge, a FM assigns a source and destination to a transfer. Examinations can be sent to or taken out of logic storage units. These are logic storage devices which group a set of physical storage devices, i.e., disks, all storing examinations for a common purpose. The logic storage units are the image stations (acquisition, consultation, and reporting stations), local stores, local archives, central stores, and the central archive. Local stores group devices which store the acquisitions made by the acquisition stations in their segment. Local archives archive examinations which are expected to be needed in the near future by modules of their segment. Central stores store examinations which are dubious to be needed in the near future, and the central archive archives examinations which are of no interest in the near future, e.g., after a period of 6 months an examination can be stored in the central archive.

To distribute images over the network's storages in order to minimize network traffic for later retrieval of the examination, copy transfers are created by the FMs. To ensure that reasonable response times are achieved for all transfer requests, FMs adjust the priority value and the emergency status of waiting transfers. Adjusting of source and destination of transfers is also a task of the FMs. Monitoring the load factor of the storage media in the system to prevent memory overflow can be achieved in different ways, as the next section will show. The organization of prefetches at nonpeak hours to minimize network load at peak hours requires the hospital appointment system and common sense. For the time being, prefetching is performed manually in the prototype.

5.2.6.3 Strategies

A *modify s/d strategy* modifies the source and/or destination (s/d) of transfers. Since each FM only examines the transfer requests of examinations stored on modalities local to the FM's segment, all FMs can apply modification strategies in parallel. Nevertheless, FMs and TMs have to coordinate their activities. We refer here to the discussion of the TM's interrupt strategies for more detail. We wish to complete this discussion with the following remark: One of the defined modify-s/d strategies, the modify source transfer on source queue of finished transfer strategy, is fired immediately after an examination has been transmitted, in other words when the transfer is completed. This means we are unable to predict when the FM's process will be fired, and if we want to put an order to activate one of the different processes, we have to take into account that some processes are likely to be activated at undefined times. If the activation of such a process is of no danger to the functionalities of other processes this process can be activated, otherwise the process has to be delayed, if possible.

An *update-priority strategy* updates priority values of transfers. No problems are expected in updating priorities of transfers. If decisions are taken based on the old priority value of a transfer, the changed situation will be noticed and restored in the next cycle.

A *check-capacity strategy* investigates whether storage devices have run out of free space and takes appropriate action. The problems expected in implementing the check-capacity strategies are not due to problems of concurrency, but rather to the definition of the strategies themselves. The defined check-capacity and remove-examination strategies always ensure that there is enough free space left on a disk to store the planned examinations plus an extra amount of free storage to store unexpected examinations. Now the simulations can show that the available free space is still unsufficient, and that, as consequence, the strategies have to be changed. This kind of problem can be predicted and solved by the strategy manager.

A *remove examination strategy* states how many, which, and in what way examinations have to be removed from storage devices. There is a risk that different FMs will decide to remove all the occurrences of an examination at the same time, as illustrated in Fig. 5.20. Module 1 and Module 2 both store the same examination. At the same moment, FM1 and FM2 both decide to remove this examination. Since FM2 sees that a copy of this examination is still available in Module 1, it does not copy the examination to another disk before deleting it (such a copy transfer is named a copy before delete transfer). In the same way, TM1 does not make a copy before delete

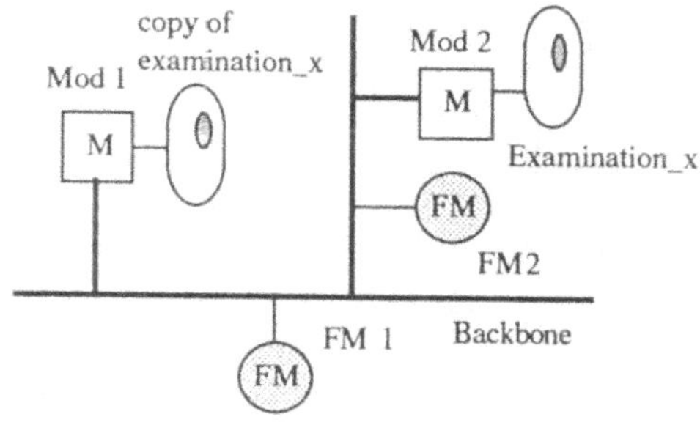

Fig. 5.20. Remove examination strategie

transfer, since the examination exists in Module 2. Both occurrences of the examination are thus deleted, and no copy is left in the network.

The solution to this problem is again sequentializing the FM's processes to remove examinations, in other words only one FM at a time is allowed to execute its remove examination strategy, or to leave the different FM to communicate among themselves. Using the latter solution, each FM will have to broadcast the question to all other FMs in the network if it is authorized to remove an examination and will have to wait until all answers have been received.

5.2.6.4 Co-operation of TMs and FMs

Another problem occurs if a TM decides to put a transfer into the network at the same time as an FM changes the transfer's source or destination or even deletes it. Ways to avoid this problem are forcing the TMs and FMs to communicate with each other, putting a lock on a transfer, putting a lock on a queue, or locking the FM itself or part of its functionalities. An FM that wants to change the source or the destination or to remove a transfer can ask the master of this transfer if it is allowed to do so. It then has to wait for the reply before it can take further action. Using this approach, there is a risk that the communications may get lost.

Another approach is to put an order of execution on the different processes (being a TM/FM or a task of a TM/FM). This is in fact what happens in the prototype system. A process is fired and, after it has finished, its job a new process is started. The sequential order of the processes in the prototype may be too strick, and it is, therefore, desirable to investigate if more processes can be executed in parallel. For example, suppose an FM's modify s/d strategy or remove examination strategy wants to change a transfer which is ready to be put into the network by a TM's interrupt strategy. Since each FM only examines the transfer requests of examinations stored on modalities local to the FM's segment, the following remarks can be made concerning the different queueing strategies. The nonqueueing TM strategy defines the master of a transfer as the TM of the segment on which the source of the transfer is located. So the TM responsible for the transfer is located on the same segment as the FM responsible for the modification or the removal of this transfer. We can therefore, conclude that a TM and an FM located on the same segment are not allowed to run their corresponding interrupt, modify s/d, or remove examination strategies at the same time. The other FMs can do their tasks in parallel with this TM without risking interference.

The direct or gradual queueing TM strategy, on the other hand, does not always define the master of a transfer as the TM local to the FM that is able to modify this transfer. A TM can be the master of a transfer originating from each module situated on its segment or a segment lower in the hierarchy of the network. This means that with a given TM, no FM on the same level or lower in the hierarchy is allowed to run its modify s/d or remove examination strategy together with the interrupt strategy of this TM.

5.2.7 Simulator

5.2.7.1 Introduction

A simple, high-level, discrete-event simulator can be used taking the network model. It associates user profiles with the different network components and mimics the activity taking place on the real network, taking into account the traffic and flow management implemented by the TM and FM modules, respectively. The combination of the network model and the simulator allows us to test and experiment with, for example, a global traffic management strategy in a kind of detached mode where the real network is not needed nor put into effect. It actually allows experimentation with different hypothetical network configurations and/or with different hypothetical traffic management strategies. Running a simulation over a specific network model will result in a log file which can, for example, be analyzed to detect bottlenecks or evaluate overall performance in terms of throughput and response time.

5.2.7.2 Functions

A simulation starts with an interactive phase where the user is invited to associate so-called profiles with the different image stations in the network. For acquisition stations, for example, this profile takes the form of a list of specific types of examination which are expected to take place in that station. For viewing stations, the profile takes the form of an appointment list stating which patient is expected for a consultation with the doctor working with that station.

The *new request* function polls all stations in the network to check if they have a new request for an image transfer. A viewing station, for example, is expected to request the images of the last examination of the patient at the time the consultation starts. An acquisition station is expected to produce a request for an image transfer to some storage after an examination is finished. The time for such a request can be computed from the time the examination was supposed to start and the expected duration of a specific type of examination. When a station has a new request for an image transfer, the FM is responsible for completing that request, i.e., to assign a priority and to decide on source and/or destination for the transfer. The completed request is than queued by the simulator as prescribed by the TM.

Active image transfers check the image transfers which are active on the different network segments, i.e., check whether they have been completed or not. This involves a simple computation taking into account the current time, the time the transfer became active, the expected duration of a transfer, and the interrupts that may have occurred. The duration of a transfer can be computed from the transfer size, which is in turn computed from the characteristics of a specific patient examination and from an empirically derived throughput rate which depends on the type of the source and destination of the transfer.

The function *new image transfer* checks for each of the network segments if another transfer must be given the active status. The TM prescribes under which conditions this must happen.

All of this activity in the network is logged in a history, which is basically a file containing the following data for each image transfer in the network: the time of request of the transfer, the source and destination, the priority, the time the transfer was served, the possible interrupts and restarts for this transfer, and the time of conclusion of the transfer. Analysis of such a log can show bottlenecks which may either result from a bad configuration or from a bad traffic management strategy.

5.2.8 Case Study AZ-VUB

The VUB–PACS/IMACS project is being executed in distributed upgradable phases. In a first step in 1985, a limited scale PACS system was installed consisting of a local network with two CTs as acquisition units and two 512 × 512 screen-reporting consoles and storage possibilities. This was a typical example of a closed architecture. In early 1989, we decided to shift towards a totally distributed approach and this resulted in the creation of small PACS islands for medical subsections, i.e., the distributed subnetworking approach (Fig. 5.21).

The CT-PACS consists of two CT units (Siemens), a prototype three 1024 × 1024 screen reporting station (Siemens), and local storage and archiving possibilities (2 GB). A hard copy unit (3M) is shared by the two CT units and the reporting console. The installation of the laser hard copy unit with the CT-PACS is an example of a usable image management environment. The Multimodality unit (MMU) is used to connect the two

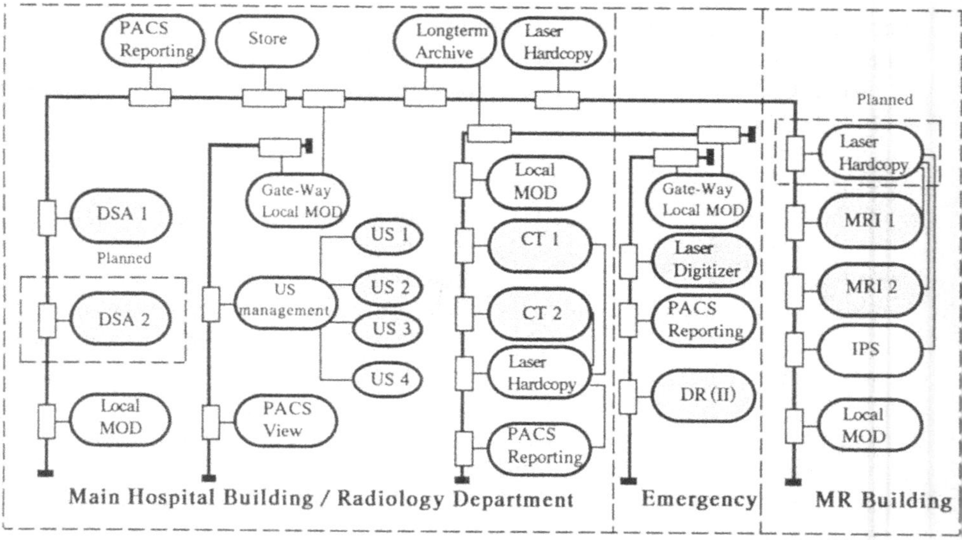

Fig. 5.21. PACS architecture at the University Hospital Brussels in 1991

CTs and the PACS network (serving the reporting console). Images are routed to the digital subtraction angiography (DSA) section when the hard copy unit is out of service. The MR-PACS section consists of two MRI units (Siemens), two powerful image processing stations with array processors, local storage, shared hard copy (3M) and archiving possibilities (3.2 GB).

At the emergency department, the PACS section consists of a laser-digitizer (Dupont), a two 1024 × 1024 screen reporting console (Dupont), and a prototype digital fluoroscopy (DRF) (CGR-GE) system based on image capture on the image intensifier tube. Evaluation studies are continuing for the PACS emergency. The medical results are promising, but there are technical problems at the level of integration of the patient identification on the laser scanner and the throughput of a set of images.

The DSA (Philips) system is integrated in our network, and a logical step planned for next year is the connection of the DSA (Siemens), which was installed early 1990. This will result in the creation of our DSA-PACS section, with local storage, reporting, and hard copy units.

The ultrasound (US) management application allows the user to archive, retrieve, and manipulate echo images. Examinations can be compared locally. The system allows the retrieval of the echo images together with the report. This US unit is based on standard Macintosh hardware, and allows the connection of up to four US units.

In 1991, a test at the orthopedics department with a 1024 × 1024 viewing station (Imlogix) will be set up with a personal computer-based image server (Macintosh). These subsystems are linked to an acquisition backbone network in the radiology department via Ethernet. This backbone network consists of a buffer storage (MOD), optical archiving, a multimodality reporting console, and a hard copy unit (3M). The distance currently covered by the network, linking MRI, emergency, and radiology, is 300 m. An optical fiber network with a length of 1.5 km was completed at the end of 1990. This network, consisting of 20 parallel fibers, will not only serve the PACS, but also a number of other hospital informatics projects. It will allow for further extension of the PACS system towards the nursing units. Ethernet, TCP/IP, and Decnet will be used via this fibers until other protocols and interfaces become more cost effective (FDDI). Experiments are also being considered which could extend outside the hospital premises (e.g., to a radiologist on duty, who may then give advice during the weekends on the basis on images sent to his home or to less experienced radiologists on duty inside the hospital). A project for interhospital communication based on ISDN and B-ISDN is under study.

Terminals are integrated on the different acquisition modalities containing the control functions to request image transfer. On each modality, the radiologist can select the various functions archive, report, special study, and temporary storage. The messages on the control layer are sent to the network management process. The image manipulation and reporting console communicates at image transfer, control, and security level. The communication with the optical disk image data base takes place in time-sharing mode via message structure at the control level and by batch processes created by the control layer on the image transfer level (making use of statistical information). Images are converted to the SPI (ACR-NEMA) format. The network manager shell described in the previous section is implemented using KEE on an HP 9000 workstation. KEE is a knowledge representation system build on top of a common LISP. Various functional network components such as image stations, storages, and viewing consoles are modeled as KEE units. Other objects and events in the PACS environment such as images, image transfers, and examinations are also modeled as KEE units. All these units are organized in inheritance hierarchies. Figure 5.22 shows a fragment of our knowledge base, i.e., the classification hierarchy of image stations encountered in a PACS environment. Knowledge of the types of transfers, their importance and their frequencies, for example, is necessary to make such a decision. The different priority levels can be those currently used in the system, but a decision on priority levels can also be one of the factors that make up a specific traffic management strategy.

The management level performs the logical management of the stored images and handles all the supervisory and administrative tasks. In addition it performs the logical link of image to related nonimage information such as patient data. The security level forms the top layer, which supervises the different tasks, notes the history of events and controls logging and password information. This hierarchical structure of the network allows its workload to be optimized and enables us to handle image transport 24 h a day. The network shell uses various input parameters and handles corre-

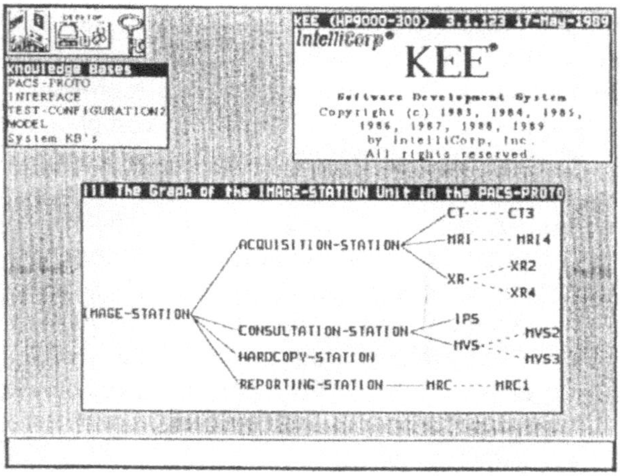

Fig. 5.22. Screen dump of the network management user interface. Classification hierarchy of image station

lations between the workloads and the report and image generating functions at the radiology and emergency departments (number of images per hour or per day). This processing of the information and of other statistical data such as appointments and priorities creates a constant and continuous throughput function instead of a highly variable and discontinuous function and enables us to use the PACS environment in clinical practice.

5.2.9 Conclusion

Modular network architectures capable of reacting to growth and changes in traffic patterns are essential. Partitioning the network into subnets will reduce bandwith requirements and increase response time by distributing network traffic. A hierarchical decomposition will make it easier to use transmission techniques with an optimum choice at each level. As an additional benefit, this design strategy offers the possibility to start the introduction of PACS into a given environment by establishing the local subsystem first. In subsequent steps, the integration of a complete PACS could be performed, accompanied by a step-by-step training of personnel and a gradual change in the routines. Maintenance and monitoring tools are necessary in this multivendor environment to control failure of components and manage the environment to the unit level.

5.3 Potential Benefits and Critical Issues of Prefetching*

B.M. van Poppel, H. Lodder, P.H. Elsakkers, M.L. Koens, and A.R. Bakker

5.3.1 Introduction

Quick delivery of the images will be one of the main demands which have to be fulfilled by the second generation of picture archiving and communication systems (PACS). The provision of an acceptable response time is a major problem because of the relatively large amounts of digital data involved in the representation of a radiological film image in electronic form. The current film archive must be replaced by its electronic counterpart, since only thousands of optical disks, stacked in jukeboxes, can provide the storage capacity required for the tremendous amount of digital data. These jukeboxes, however, can only deliver the images at limited speed; typically it takes up to several minutes. Presently, three main strategies (which complement each other) have been proposed for shortening these unacceptable waiting times, i.e., image compression, high-speed networks, and prefetching. In this chapter, we will elaborate prefetching.

The principal elements of prefetching are a fast storage with limited storage capacity and a rule-based system. Images which will in all probability need to be retrieved in the near future should be placed in the fast storage. The waiting time can be reduced if a maximum percentage of images can be retrieved from the fast storage instead of the slow one. The rule-based system has to bring about that only the relevant images are transferred to the fast storage in the proper period of time. Patterns of previous image retrieval behavior are used to evaluate which images are expected to be relevant. This image management strategy is called prefetching. The rule-based system will be referred to as the prefetch algorithm or, for short, the algorithm. Prefetching does not influence functionality. For the user, there is no visible difference between the slow archive and the fast buffer being used to read the images and subsequently present them on the screen. The only difference for the user is that the images appear fast when prefetching has been effective.

In the early 1980s prefetching was proposed, in addition to image compression and high-speed networks, as a contribution to the problem of retrieval waiting times. One of the first proposals can be found in Bakker (1984). Some first research on prefetching by BAZIS can be found in van Rijnsoever (1984) and Bakker et al. (1987). Within the Dutch PACS project, as far as we know, the first hospital information system/radiology

* The authors of this chapter would like to thank G. Bavelaar and R. Raps of Leiden University Hospital for their support on the data base queries. Our thanks are also due to K. Bijl of BAZIS for many fruitful discussions.

information system (HIS/RIS) coupling with PACS was realized and demonstrated during the EuroPACS meeting in April 1988 in Leiden and Utrecht (Lodder et al. 1988). Through this coupling, some appropriate data were pushed to the PACS for prefetching. However, the image management of this prototype PACS did not use that information, so prefetching had to be applied in its manual form; van Poppel et al. 1989). Prefetching is currently being applied in the Hokkaido PACS in Japan (Irie et al. 1990). In Hokkaido, old (reference) images are sent during the night to a faster storage device. From the start, prefetching has been one of the design issues within the PACS at the AZ-VUB, Brussels, Belgium (Mattheus 1987). More recently, research on prefetching started at the Georgetown University Hospital, Washington, USA (Levin and Fielding 1990) and at the University of Arizona, Tucson, USA (Sheng et al. 1990). Prefetching has been identified as a design issue at the Bowman Gray School of Medicine, Winston Salem, USA (D'Lugin et al. 1990). Some first steps towards a design of prefetching are presented by van Poppel and Lodder (1990a) and the implications for standardization have been indicated at the standardization workshop held on Crete in May 1990 (van Poppel and Lodder 1990b). The first thorough pilot study on the potential effectiveness in a real hospital situation has been carried out as far as we know within the AIM/HIPACS project (van Poppel and Lodder 1990c). Since the first propositions were made, there has been a growing interest in the concept within the PACS research community. Its theoretical basis has been further elaborated, and prefetching is being successfully applied in some (operational) PACS systems. Currently, prefetching is believed to be a vital component in the achievement of the required performance.

In this section, a series of prefetching aspects will be discussed. Firstly, a model of prefetching will be presented, which will serve as a guideline for the design of the prefetching algorithm within PACS presented subsequently. Two groups of parameters of the algorithm will be discussed, namely, events which initiate the algorithm and parameters with which the relevant images are to be selected. Some possible events and parameters will be proposed. A method for evaluating the effectiveness of the algorithm will be proposed. The potential effectiveness of an algorithm has been studied, and a selection of the first results of a pilot study at the Leiden University Hospital will be presented.

The prefetching chain is activated by events occurring in the HIS (some in the RIS). The final reallocation of images from a slow storage to a fast storage, however, takes place within the PACS. One of the design issues is the assignment of prefetching components to HIS/RIS or to PACS and the development of a preferably standardized interface. In the transition phase from film images to digital images, the current film folder management system, e.g., a bar code tracking system, has to be integrated in the PACS image management system, preferably by a standardized interface.

5.3.2 A Model of Prefetching

5.3.2.1 The Amount of Image Data

The problem of achieving a suitable response time stems mainly from the tremendous amount of digital data involved in comparison with the capabilities of current network and storage technology (cf. Chap. 2, Sect. 2.1). To illustrate this comparison, let us look at some typical data. An examination performed using a nondigital modality (excluding computed radiography, CR) is represented by about 11 MegaByte (MB) of digital data. The annual production of an average hospital of 850 beds equals about 1 TeraByte (TB) (1 TB = 1 000 000 MB). If the images are stored for 10 years, about 5000 optical disks of 2 GigaByte (GB) each would be needed. Most radiology departments destroy film which has not been used for a certain period, e.g., 10 years, but because examinations are sometimes used again, some older films are also present, which leads to the necessity for a larger file room (van Poppel and Lodder 1990c). If the two most recent years of image data are placed (on-line) in jukeboxes, a dozen jukeboxes with a capacity of 90 disks would be needed. In comparison, in an extended HIS, only several 2 GB of data are stored. Handling of disks (on-line and off-line disks) would take several minutes and, besides that, jukeboxes and networks are not presently capable of transmitting the image data from one examination in a few seconds.

5.3.2.2 Hierarchical Layered Storage Structure

As indicated above, prefetching can reduce the waiting time by delivering the images to the user's workstation from a fast storage device instead of from the slow jukeboxes. In this case, two storage layers are involved. For a PACS three layers are proposed (van Rijnsoever et al. 1984):

1. The archive
2. A fast storage near the workstations, called local storage
3. A central buffer placed between these

In Fig. 5.23, the properties of the successive layers of a three-layered structure are indicated by the triangles. The archive has huge storage capacity with limited speed, the local storage is fast but has limited storage capacity. The central buffer has intermediate properties. One can think of optical disks in a jukebox for the archive, of winchester disks for the central buffer, and of parallel transfer winchester disks for the local storage. The local storage could also be realized as random access memory (RAM). At this point one should note that the speed of computer peripherals does not grow as fast as their capacity. This is one of the main reasons why it is not believed that we only have to wait for high-speed storage devices to solve

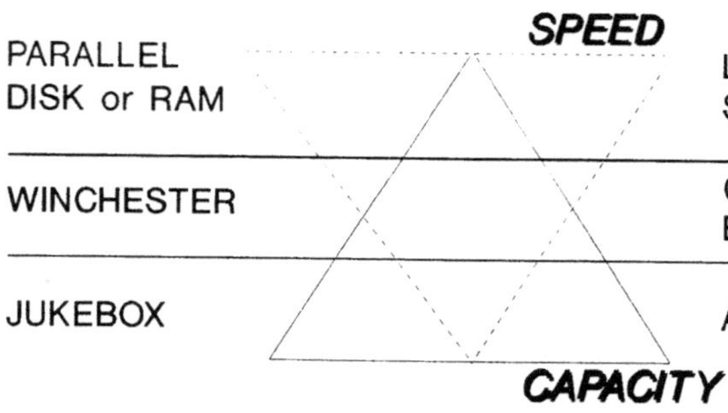

Fig. 5.23. Hierarchical layered storage structure

the performance problem; moreover, such high-speed components will be very expensive (van Poppel et al. 1990).

One of the issues for future research will be to determine the dimensions of the successive storage layers. However, this chapter focuses on the algorithm aspect of prefetching, and some first calculations (van Poppel et al. 1989) on the capacity needed may indicate the order of magnitude. Note that the needed storage capacity depends heavily upon the required image resolution and the required number of gray values (per pixel). The required local storage has been estimated, for an 850 bed hospital, at several gigabytes and the central buffer storage at several dozen gigabytes.

5.3.2.3 A Model of a PACS with Prefetching

In Fig. 5.24, an outline of a PACS with prefetching is shown. First the hardware components will be discussed. Several types of workstations have been projected, each designed for a specific task. The extended workstation (EWS) is designed for the radiologist. Images can be presented on six to eight screens in high resolution. The EWS offers sophisticated image processing functions such as histogram equalization. The simple workstations (SWS) are meant to be used by the referring physicians.

The SWS has two to four screens on which images will be displayed in a lower resolution than on the EWS. Image manipulation functions are supported, but the SWS has no advanced image processing capabilities. The output-only station (OOS) is meant to replace the (simple) lightboxes, which can presently be found throughout the hospital. It is a one-screen monitor on which only the basic image functions such as zoom and window are available. In general, the requirements such as number of screens, resolution, and image processing capabilities will decrease from EWS to OOS. The fastest storage layers, called local storage (LS), have been projected near the acquisition units, the EWS and the SWS. The acquisition

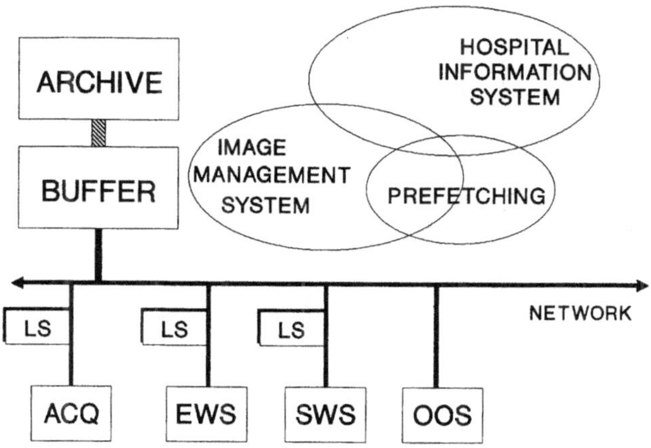

Fig. 5.24. A model of PACS hardware and software. At the *top left*, the archive is shown; the *bottom line* shows the end user devices: *LS*, local storage; *ACQ*, acquisition units; *EWS*, extended workstation; *SWS*, simple workstation; *OOS*, output-only station

units and viewing devices are connected by a network via the central buffer to the archive. Notice that no LS has been projected near the OOS because of the relatively small amount of data needed to represent one image in the resolution of this type of station.

To control and run the above hardware, computer programs will be needed. A part of the PACS software will be the image management system (IMS), which controls the occupancy of the storages. The HIS is needed to provide access to textual patient data and to HIS functions (Lodder et al. 1990; Koens et al. 1988). The position of an RIS with respect to HIS and PACS is discussed in Sect. 4.3. Prefetching can be positioned between the IMS, responsible for he physical transfer of images, and the HIS as supplier of the events on which the image transfers have to start. Besides that, HIS data will be needed to evaluate which images are relevant.

5.3.2.4 An Outline of Prefetching

The principle of prefetching will be explained by discussing the retrieval of images. A two-layered storage structure has been chosen for simplicity (Fig. 5.25). The user who interacts with the information system via a workstation is found at the top of the figure. This information system has been called hospital integrated PACS (HIPACS), because at this moment we are not concerned about assigning specific components to the PACS or to the HIS. The slow but large storage containing all images is shown at the bottom of the figure. The fast storage with limited storage capacity is placed below the workstation.

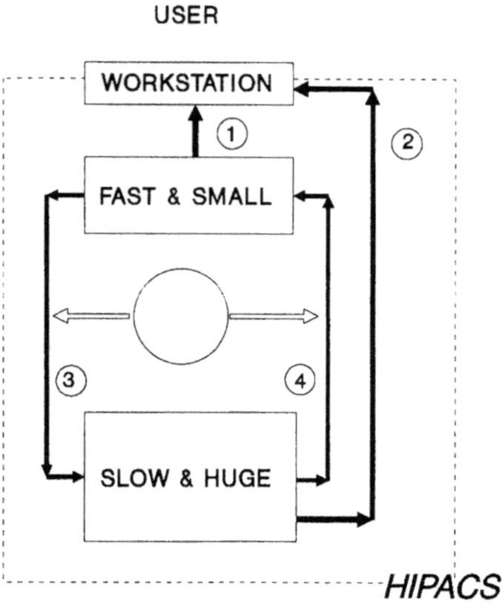

Fig. 5.25. Outline of prefetching. For details, see text

Without prefetching, all images will be retrieved from the slow storage. With prefetching, a number of images will be retrieved from the fast storage. Prefetching can reduce the waiting time if we succeed in providing a high percentage of images to be retrieved from the fast storage, in other words, flow 1 should be greater than flow 2. Before the user retrieves an image we have to try to place this image into the fast storage. The prefetch algorithm evaluates which images are expected to be retrieved and which are not. The algorithm looks ahead to the medical usage of images and is initiated by certain events occurring in the hospital.

5.3.2.5 The Functions Prefetch and Retrieve

A next step towards the design of an information system is to analyze the data, the processes, and their relations. The two processes in which prefetching plays a part, namely the retrieval of an image and the reallocation beforehand, will be analyzed. This analysis leads to a scheme in which the two processes are related (Fig. 5.26).

The primary task of the prefetch component is to take care that as many relevant images as possible are present in the fast storage in a relevant period of time. The prefetch process is initiated by events occurring in the hospital and reflected in the HIS (or RIS) data base. When such an event takes place, e.g., an admission, the algorithm is activated. After activation, the algorithm starts to perform its task, to evaluate which images are expected to be needed within the near future. For this evaluation, various types of HIS data will be needed. At the end, a number of images will be

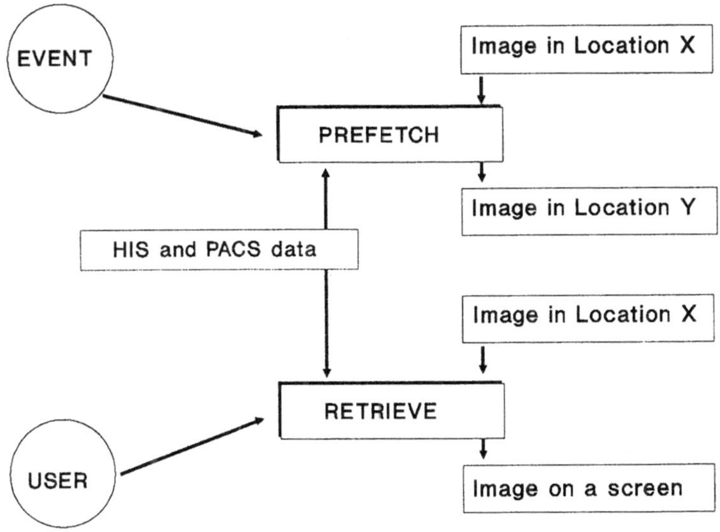

Fig. 5.26. The processes prefetch and retrieve: basic scheme

reallocated from the slow storage to the fast storage or vice versa. Note also that the removal of images from the fast storage layer, by the release of occupied storage space, has to be managed by this process. The generalized formulation reads the reallocation from a certain storage to another storage.

Images can be retrieved by authorized persons throughout the hospital, for example, a radiologist, a referring physician, or a technician. The retrieve function is initiated by the user, and after the identification of a certain patient, the pictorial index belonging to that patient will be shown. The pictorial index may be the image in reduced size and in low resolution, but might also be an alphanumerical description. After the desired images have been selected from the pictorial index, they will be retrieved from a (certain) storage and displayed. This function will make more explicit use of image data (pictorial index).

When decomposing these two main processes, prefetch and retrieve, it appears that both of them lead to image reallocations. The first one moves images between storage layers, and the second one from a storage layer to a screen of a workstation. Because of the similarity of these two image reallocations, this will be defined as a common activity within these processes. Notice that the prefetching chain is activated by transitions within the HIS data base. With respect to the design of the HIPACS data base (cf. Sect. 7.1) note that the data base management system for the HIPACS data base will not only provide the user with images, but will also control the image transfers between the storage devices. The final reallocation of images however, takes place within the PACS.

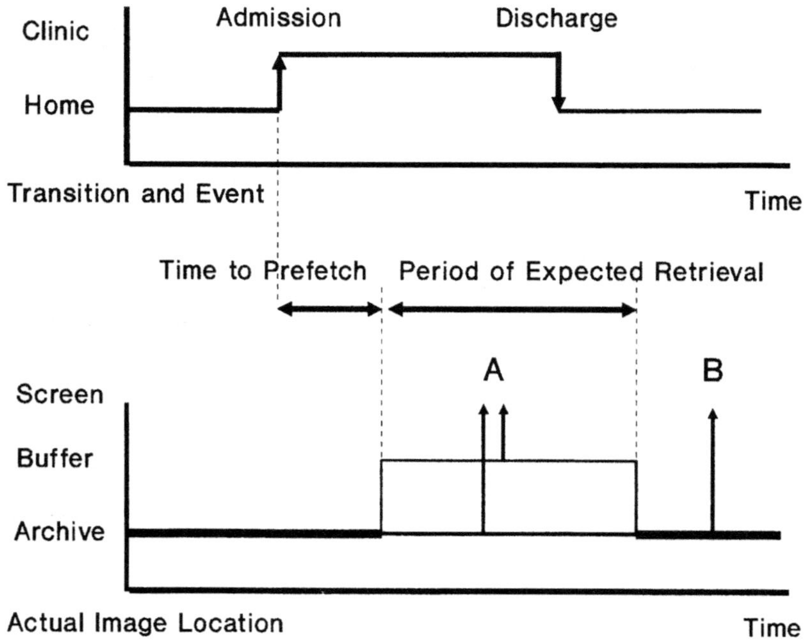

Fig. 5.27. Events and image transfers. The images requested at moment *A* are partly retrieved from the fast buffer and partly from the slow archive. For details, see text

5.3.3 The Algorithm and its Effectiveness

In this section, the algorithm will be discussed in more detail, and some suitable parameters will be proposed. Finally, some attention will be paid to the quantitative measurement of the effectiveness of a particular algorithm.

5.3.3.1 Dynamic Aspects of Prefetching

The prefetch algorithm has the task of controlling the flow of images by anticipating their expected usage. In this section, we will consider the time aspects, using an example. Figure 5.27 shows the dynamic aspects of the prefetch process. At the top, the initiation by the events are shown, while the bottom part presents the actual image locations as a function of the time.

In the upper diagram, two states have been put on the vertical axis, i.e., patient at home and patient at clinic (inpatient clinic). The transition from patient at home to patient at clinic is the event *admission*. The counterpart is the event *discharge*. These events can be detected in the HIS (in the admission/discharge/transfer, ADT, subsystem). An event can be defined as a transition between states. In the lower diagram, two storage locations have been put on the vertical axis, i.e., the central buffer and the archive; only two layers are considered for simplicity. In the beginning, the patient is at home and all images of that patient are in the archive. At the moment the patient is admitted, the prefetch algorithm will be activated, resulting in the advice to place a set of images in the central buffer for a certain period of time. Within this period of time, an enhanced retrieval probability is expected. It is assumed that some images will still be in the archive, and that other images are placed in the central buffer. Notice that the images can be found only some time after the occurrence of the event in the central buffer. A (minimal) amount of time is needed to apply the rules of the algorithm, to distribute the scarce buffer capacity, to organize the image transfers, and to perform the transfers themselves. These steps will be discussed in Sect. 5.3.5. At monent A, images can be delivered from the central buffer to the screen and, in an optimal situation, no images have to be fetched from the archive. The moment B is found outside the period of expected enhanced probability, and subsequently the waiting times can be considerably longer. A second remark concerns the termination of the period of enhanced retrieval probability. This termination can be determined by the event *discharge*, although it is possible to finish the period in another way, e.g., by specifying a certain number of hours after the admission. In a real HIPACS where many events have to be handled, there will be growing complexity. Furthermore, with respect to the images which are retrieved the question arises of whether the specific set of images retrieved is comparable to what can be expected in analogous cases, or is it an extraordinary retrieval.

In the above, the following important aspects have been indicated: the choice of the event (because there must be enough time to perform the image transfers), the proper expectation of the period of enhanced probability, and the evaluation of the probability with which an image is expected to the retrieved (in that period of time). When prefetching is applied to the LS (one particular LS of the many present), then the algorithm also has to evaluate the proper LS.

5.3.3.2 Proposed Events and Their Corresponding User Functions

In Fig. 5.28 a number of user functions and related events are shown. Because of the dominant time aspect in event-driven processes, the user functions can only be executed in a predefined order. At the top and bottom of the figure we find the arrival and departure of a patient. The flow of the patient himself is symbolized by the open arrows at the outer left-hand side since a patient may visit the hospital more than once. For inpatients and outpatients, different terms are used for the event *arrival* (or *departure*): inpatients are *admitted* and outpatients *check in* with the referring physician. The transition from *not patient in the hospital* to *patient in the hospital* is caused by the event *arrival*. Between *admission* and *discharge*, three possibilities exist with respect to images:

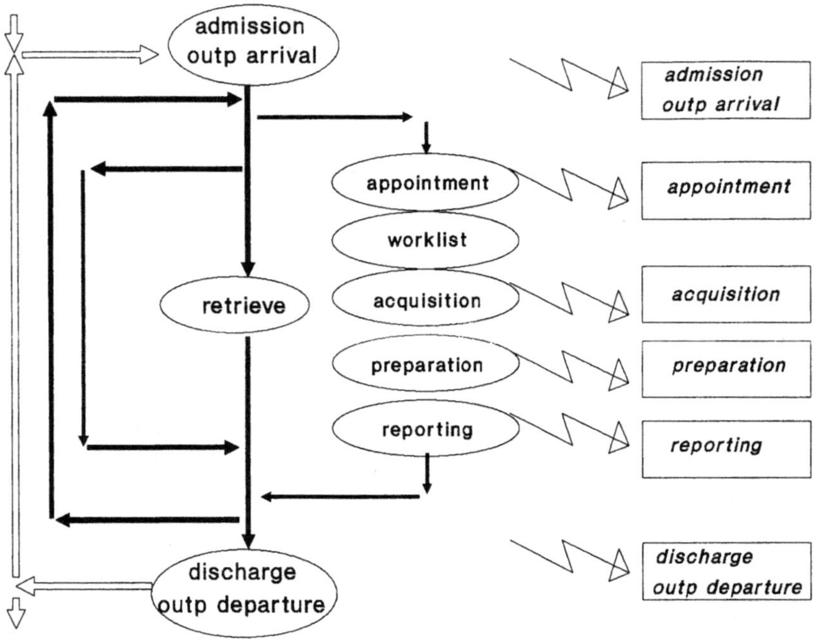

Fig. 5.28. User functions and related events. For details, see text

1. No action.
2. The retrieval of an image.
3. The execution of a radiological examination, which is composed of the following five functions: appointment, work list, acquisition, preparation, and reporting.

Certain events may be associated with these user functions (described extensively in Sect. 4.3). The following events with the resulting image transfers are listed as a first proposition:

1. Admission/outpatient arrival: select and transport the relevant part of the image history to the central buffer or/and to the clinicians workstation.
2. Discharge/outpatient departure: release occupied storage space at the central buffer or at the local storage.
3. Appointment: relevant images can be transferred to local storge located at the radiology department. If the radiologist's schedule has been organized, the routing to his workstation can be prepared.
4. Preparation: prepare a stack of images for transfer to the radiologist's workstation.
5. Report (authorization): images can be sent to the requester. Storage space at the radiology department can be released.

6. Acquisition: As soon as the acquisition has been taken place, (a copy of) the images can be sent to the archive.

5.3.3.3 Proposed Selection Parameters

In other publications, the following parameters have been mentioned for the purpose of selecting the relevant part of the images of a patient (Bakker et al. 1986; Levin and Fielding 1990):

1. Type of examination
2. Requesting specialism
3. Date of the examination
4. Report of the examination in condensed (or coded) form
5. Status of the examination (e.g., authorized, reported)
6. Previous use of the image

5.3.3.4 Specifying a Quick Response

As stated in the introduction, the realization of a quick response is one of the major problems in designing a PACS. It is strongly emphasized that the requirement of a quick response refers to a certain pattern of usage or to a certain user, e.g., should the response time be specified per single image or should it be specified as the average time (per image) for the set of images of one patient. Therefore, the response time requirement has to be specified in detail. This is illustrated by the following examples. It can be expected that in an intensive care unit other needs will exist than in an ordinary clinical ward. At the department of oncology, the emphasis lies on comparing historical images in order to assess the development of a tumor. For emergency patients, an extra requirement can be expected, as emergency patients are more often transferred to other wards in the first hours after their arrival. Images should follow the patient on his or her way through the various departments. Besides these differences within a hospital, significant differences between hospitals and in different countries will surely exist.

5.3.3.5 Measuring the Effectiveness

The effectiveness can be expressed as the ratio between the number of retrieved images and the number of images that could be supplied from the fast storage. This ratio is called the hit rate:

Hit rate = (number of images supplied from the fast storage)/
(number of images retrieved)

Applying this definition to Fig. 5.25, the hit rate is: (arrow 1)/(arrow 1 + arrow 2). The hit rate has enabled us to quantify the effectiveness: a certain algorithm can be classified as an effective algorithm if the hit rate exceeds 90% (Bakker and Kouwenberg 1984). The final response time of a HIS/PACS using prefetching will depend upon a balance between the dimensions of the PACS architecture, e.g., the capacity of the fast storage, and the effectiveness of the algorithm.

5.3.4 Pilot Study of Potential Effectiveness in Leiden University Hospital

The potential benefits of prefetching have been studied in a real hospital environment using a large test set of over 1800 events. The actual locations of over 17000 accompanying visit film folders (comparable to examination film folders) have been determined with the lending subsystem. The following algorithms have been proposed, executed on the test set, and evaluated:

1. Age of the examination: prefetch visit film folders younger than *n* months
2. Type of the examination: prefetch the *n* most recent visit film folders of the same type as the new examination
3. Length of the history: prefetch the most recent fraction (F) of the history

The properties of the test set have been studied in order to propose indicators for the application of prefetching, e.g., the test set has been divided into classes, each class representing a specific number of historical visit film folders, and the algorithm has been executed on the separate classes rather than on the test set as a whole (van Poppel and Lodder 1990c). Since the aim of this chapter is to introduce prefetching, only a small part of the above-mentioned study will be presented.

5.3.4.1 Evaluation of the Effectiveness

The purpose of prefetching is to optimize image management. Prefetching will ensure that images are placed, before that they are actually needed, in storage devices from which they can be retrieved with an acceptable waiting time. The key question is to know in time which are the required images, which is the correct storage, and what is the appropriate period of time. The algorithm should supply the answer to this question. The effectiveness can be evaluated by comparing the outcome of the algorithm with the actual retrievals of the users. To indicate the potential effectiveness and the critical issues of prefetching on a global level, we should not use imaginary retrievals of imaginary users and we should not use an imaginary algorithm; a real-life environment must be investigated. The real data have to be extracted from the HIS, particularly the embedded subsystems for radiology and visit film folder management, and brought to a laboratory environment in order to study several algorithms. Such a study basically consists of the following steps:

1. Observe the film image usage of the users
2. Execute the algorithm initiated by the event
3. Evaluate the effectiveness (calculate the hit rate)

5.3.4.2 A Suitable Hospital

The smallest unit of interest is the image. In a PACS, one image can he retrieved, and the algorithm then evaluates the expectation for retrievals in the near future per image. However, in the conventional situation, film images will not be pointed out separately. Various ways of organizing the film folders exist, and organizing the images into small units with, for example, one folder for each examination, seems suitable for a pilot study.

The translation of an image retrieval (the actual viewing of the image on a workstation) to its conventional counterpart, which can only be observed in the study, gives rise to some difficulties. The PACS image retrieval might be approximated by the presence of the film image near a viewing device. This implies that it has to be possible to determine the actual location of film images at every possible spot throughout the hospital at every point in time. The decision rules of the algorithm are based upon patterns of image retrieval. The recognition of patterns is only possible if based upon a sufficiently large amount of observations. This requires an automated acquisition of the raw data. Subsequently the raw data set is brought to a laboratory environment, and several algorithms have to be evaluated again in an automated way. Recognition of the events in the data base has to be possible. Moreover, the data to be used by the algorithm for selecting the relevant images have to be available. An integrated HIS offers the possibility to supply the needed (intercorrelated) data items, the most important of which are events, image selective data, and the actual image location.

At Leiden University Hospital, films of one visit (to an acquisition room) are stored in a separate film folder. A visit is more or less comparable to an examination. There are no patient folders. The lending of film folders is supported by a dedicated lending system, using bar codes. This lending system is integrated in the RIS (an embedded subsystem of the HIS) and in other subsystems of the HIS. Films are lent per (visit) film folder and each transfer is registered. By querying the data base at each moment, the actual location of a (visit) film folder can be obtained. Leiden University Hospital offers an exquisite opportunity for research on the algorithm, as the above-mentioned conditions can be fulfilled to a sufficient degree.

5.3.4.3 Film Folder Flow at Leiden University Hospital

The radiology department of Leiden University Hospital performs about 130000 procedures annually in about 100000 visits. A visit is to a large extent comparable with an examination. There are several specialisms organized as subdepartments within the radiology department, each of which has its own reception and secretarial office. Requests for a new radiological examination are ordered on an order form. The request consists of the requested procedures and of the medical issue. After acceptance of the request, the secretarial office orders historical visit film folders which are expected to be used during acquisition and/or reporting. These requests for visit film folders generated by the secretarial office are handled by the lending system. The result is a picking list for the file room(s) or a request for a certain borrower to return the visit film folder. Only as an exception is more historical material ordered afterwards. This can occur, for example, in the case of a discussion between the radiologist and the requester.

After scheduling the visit for the acquisition the secretarial office creates a new visit film folder namely for the scheduled patient visit. A bar code label is printed and attached to the visit film folder just created. From that moment on, the location of the visit film folder is known (Fig. 5.29). After acquisition, the visit film folders of inpatients are transported to one of the so-called demonstration rooms. In the demonstration room, they are reported by the radiologist. Clinicians can look at the film images in these demonstration rooms. Visit film folders are commonly not lent to locations in the inpatient wards. Films of outpatients are reported in reporting cabinets. Thereafter, they are returned to the archive or lent to an outpatient clinician. At a typing pool, the reports are typed into the HIS (or rather into the embedded RIS subsystem). After authorization, the reports are printed on a printer at the requester's location, and they can be retrieved by an authorized user at every HIS terminal (out of nearly thousand) in the hospital.

5.3.4.4 The Archive Management and Lending System

The three main objectives of the archive management and lending information system (ALIS) (op het Veld and Koens 1987) are:

1. To support the operational process of archive management and the borrowers
2. To corrdinate the flow of objects among the archive and the users
3. To provide HIS users with information about the actual location of objects.

The lending system is embedded in the HIS (Koens et al. 1990), and it supports various objects in a hospital such as medical records and (visit) film folders. For the visit film folder, which we focus on here, the ALIS is integrated in the RIS. The following main activities are supported by the system:

1. *Registration of the actual location of each visit film folder*. The most important success factor for the system is the knowledge of the actual location of each visit film folder. Bar code labels on each visit film folder are used to create an easy-to-use registration facility. Any transfer of a

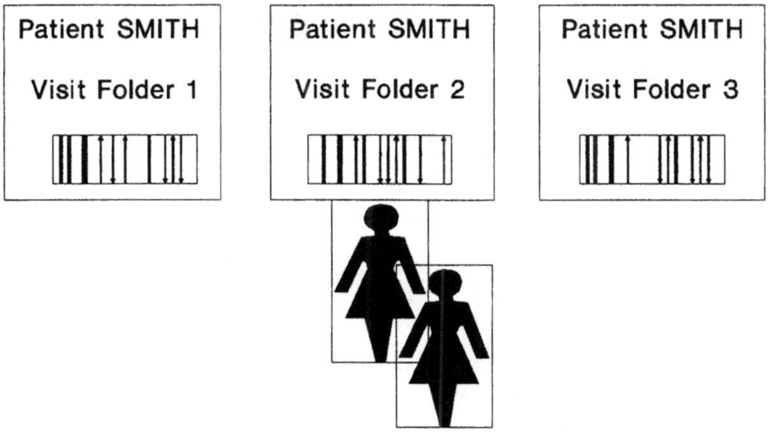

Fig. 5.29. Every visit by a patient results in a separate film folder. Each visit folder is tracked by its unique bar code. In our study, the actual location of over 17 000 folders was investigated

visit film folder is simply entered into the system by using a bar code reader. Most terminal locations within the radiology department, through which large numbers of visit film folders pass, are equipped with such a bar code reader. If a bar code reader is not available (because there is not much visit film folder traffic), the alphanumerical representation of the bar code can be entered. Stacks of visit film folders can be transferred by the accompanying picking list number.

2. *Allocation of visit film folders to the relevant location.* The second objective concerns the coordination of the flow of visit film folders throughout the hospital, which is initiated by requests. These requests can be entered anywhere in the hospital and, in our case, from the RIS.
3. *Processing of requests.* The ALIS selects the requests periodically, in Leiden University Hospital four times a day. A pickup list is produced for the file rooms, and a mailing list for borrowers who have exceeded their lending period. The receiver of a mailing list is instructed to send the listed visit film folders to a file room or to another borrower.

With the aid of the lending system, the radiology department of Leiden University Hospital is able to offer a very high service level for lending visit film folders (well above 95%). Because borrowers rely on this high service level, they return their visit film folders after usage, and they only borrow visit film folders relevant to them.

In our prefetching study the fact that at every moment the exact location of each visit film folder of a patient is known will be used for observing retrievals. In Fig. 5.30, three lending locations have been put on the vertical axis, i.e., file room, radiologist, and requester (of the examination). On the horizontal axis, the time is shown. In this figure, part of the transfer process of the visit film folders during the production of a new examination is

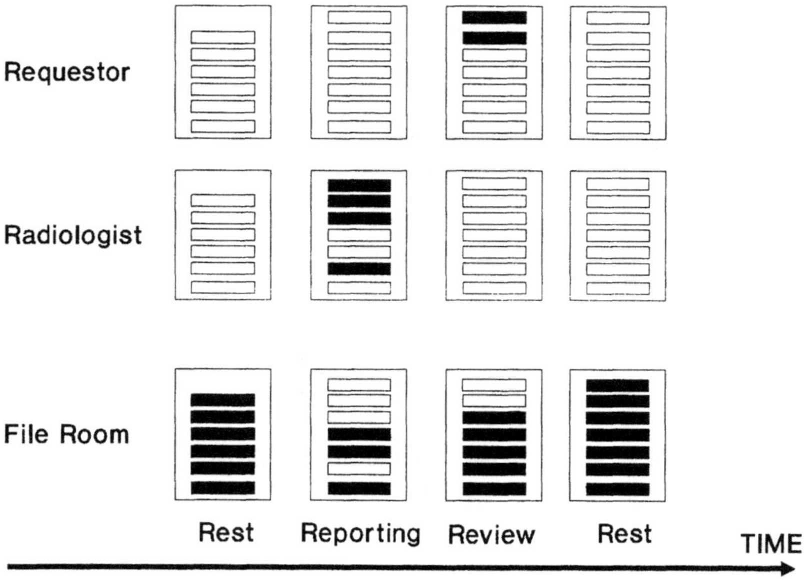

Fig. 5.30. The exact location of each visit film folder of a patient is known at each moment. For details, see text

expressed. Before the request of the new examination, all six visit film folders reside in the archive. After the acquisition, four of the now seven visit film folders are used by the radiologist. The next column shows that the requester of the examination has borrowed two of the seven visit film folders. In the end, all visit film folders will reside again at the archive. In this diagram only three locations have been considered. At Leiden University Hospital, over 200 locations have been defined at which each of the presently about 1 600 000 existing visit film folders from about 310 000 patients might reside. Of approximately 860 000 registered patients at Leiden University Hospital, about 550 000 have never had a radiological examination.

5.3.4.5 The Experimental Set-Up: Event, Algorithm, and Retrieval

The lending system offers a very detailed insight in the logistic pattern, but in a pilot study a simplification will be needed. It was decided to take only two locations into account, namely residing in the file room and being elsewhere, whereby the six file rooms have been aggregated into "the file room" and all other lending locations into "elsewhere". These two locations have been interpreted as "not in use" and "used" and may be translated to the archive or the central buffer, both of which are PACS components.

The event "new examination" is selected here (Fig. 5.31). Some time after the new examination has taken place, the point in time of interest has

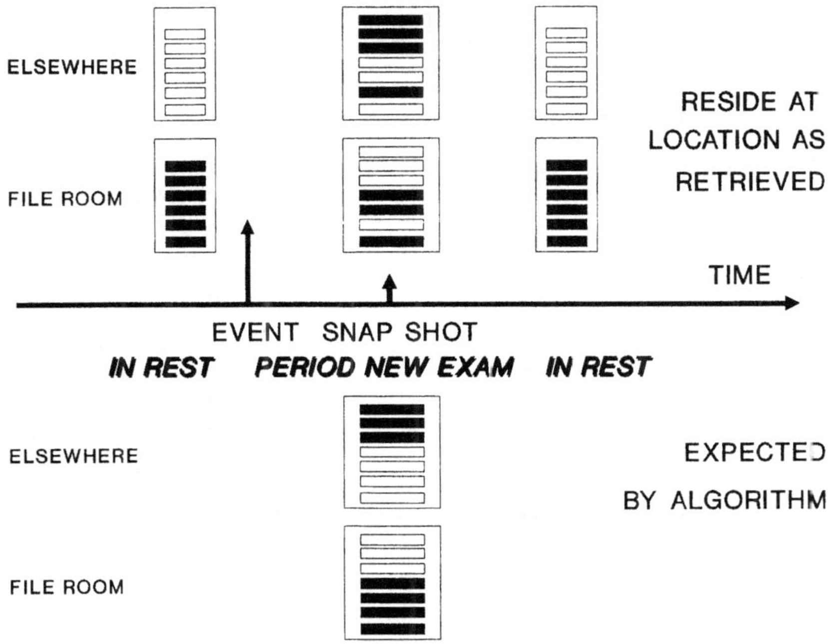

Fig. 5.31. Experimental set-up. The algorithm is executed for the event "new examination", which results in an expectation. A snapshot of the actual locations of the examination (visit) film folders is taken. A comparison of the actual and predicted locations indicates the effectiveness

been defined (the arrow marked "snapshot" in the figure). At this moment, the retrievals by the users and the expected usage by the algorithm are to be compared. Upon activation by the event, the algorithm evaluates for every visit film folder the expected location (file room or elsewhere) for the defined point in time of interest. Also at this point, the actual location of every visit film folder (aggregated into file room or elsewhere) has been extracted from the lending system.

For the selective parameter of the algorithm, the age of the visit has been chosen. The rule reads as follows: if the visit film folder is older than *n* months, then the visit film folder is not expected to be used, else it is expected to be used.

The algorithm has been run off-line in order to evaluate the effect of several values of the age parameter. To be able to perform the study in the way described above, the following data have been extracted from the HIS data base for constructing the test set: all patients having a new examination at a certain day (event), the age of all the visits, and the actual location at the point in time of interest of each visit. This point in time (snap shot) has been chosen as being during the night mainly for practical reasons.

Table 5.10. Example of data collected for the patient P1[a]

Patient number	Visit number	Visit Date	Examination	Requester	Actual Location	Interpreted
P1	1	01-08-1984	Elbow/arm	HONP	OEGST	not used
P1	2	24-03-1986	Thorax	UROK	RONHARKEL	not used
P1	3	13-06-1986	Sinus	SNEL	RONAR	not used
P1	4	13-06-1986	Long scintigram	SNEL	RONAR	not used
P1	5	25-06-1986	Thorax	AIGP	RONAR	not used
P1	6	20-08-1986	Thorax	AIGP	RONA TYP	used
P1	7	20-10-1989	Shoulder	HONP	RONHAR	not used
P1	8	25-04-1990	Thorax	LUYK	RONA TYP	used
P1	9	08-05-1990	Thorax	LUYK	RONA TYP	new exam

[a] Obtained *at* 3 A.M. on May 9, 1990, at Leiden University Hospital

5.3.4.6 Acquiring Raw Data and Constructing the Test Set

The actual location in the night following the creation of the new examination of all visit film folders in the history of those patients who visited the radiology department for a new examination were selected from the data base. In order to exclude any influences coming from a certain day of the week, and to obtain a broader statistical basis, these observations were carried out for new examinations on 5 consecutive working days. In this way, over 1800 events were detected and the actual location of the accompanying over 17 000 visit film folders recorded. For each visit film folder the following data were registered (Table 5.10). Patient number, visit number, visit date, examination requester, actual location at 3 A.M. of the visit folder according to the lending system, and interpretation. Table 5.10 shows the data collected for a patient P1, who visited the radiology department eight times before the new visit under consideration.This example can be interpreted as follows: The patient P1 has eight visit film folders when he visits the radiology department on 8 May 1990. At 3 A.M. on May 9, the actual location of all visit film folders is recorded. The two most recent thorax examinations (Thorax), performed during visit numbers 6 and 8, stay at the RONA TYP (typing pool of subdepartment A) location, together with the new thorax examination. Most probably the new examination has been reported, while the previous two have been used. After the report has been recorded on tape, all three were moved to the typing pool. If the algorithm uses 12 months as discriminant, then visits 7 and 8 should have been fetched, in contrast to numbers 6 and 8, which have actually been used.

The logistic pattern studied here is: which old visit film folders are involved in establishing a new one, or, translated to the PACS situation, which visit film folders (images) should be fetched from the archive if a new examination is performed during the period following the moment of the image acquisition.

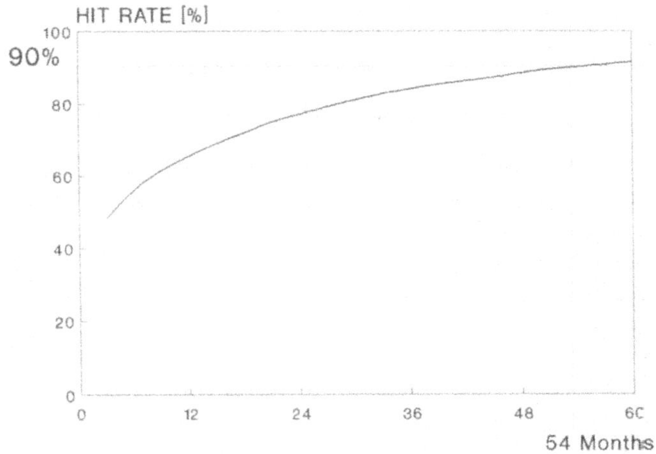

Fig. 5.32. Effectiveness (*hit rate*) of the algorithm. If the examination (visit) occurred less than *n* months ago, then prefetch. A hit rate of 90% is reached if all folders younger than 54 months are prefetched

5.3.4.7 Effectiveness of the Age Parameter

The last step in this pilot study was to execute the algorithm on the test set and then compare the expected locations with the actual ones. As discussed above, the expert rule reads: if the visit film folder is older than *n* months then the visit film folder is not expected to be used else it is expected to be used.

The algorithm was executed for several values of *n*, ranging from 3 months to 60 months with steps of 3 months, and for each run the hit rate was calculated. The results are plotted in Fig. 5.32. For example, for the value of 6 months for the discriminant, the hit rate is approximately 60%. This means that 60% of all visit film folders present outside the file room in the period following the execution of the new examination were also expected by the algorithm to be outside the file room. If the hit rate exceeds 90%, the algorithm can be classified as an effective algorithm (see Sect. 5.3.3.4). This hit rate is reached by our algorithm when 54 months is chosen.

At a hit rate of 90%, 50% of the prefetched visit film folders are retrieved later on (for further elucidation, see van Poppel and Lodder 1990c). The ratio of the visit film folders used to the visit film folders prefetched is called the utilization rate. A hit rate of 90% is therefore reached at a utilization rate of 50% with 54 months as discriminant in the age algorithm. About two-thirds of all visit film folders are indicated by the algorithm. Furthermore, we noted that in Leiden University Hospital a surprisingly high percentage of the old visit film folders are in use, more than we expected at the start of the study; this might be quite different in other hospitals.

5.3.4.8 Some First Conclusions

A pilot study of the potential effectiveness of prefetching was carried out in a real environment. Some main prerequisites for such a study are: the availability of the required data in the data base of the hospital in an integrated way; the automated processing on the extracted test set; the use of film folders per visit (comparable to examination) instead of folders per patient; and the availability of an archive management and lending information system using bar codes. The pilot study (of which only a small part has been summarized) has been successful in the sense that it has been shown that such studies are possible and offer useful results. The basis for staging follow-up studies has been laid. A follow-up study should be based on following the visit film folders (rather than taking a snapshot). Furthermore the method for measuring the effectiveness should be further refined, e.g., should the response time per image be used or the average response time per image of all the images of the one patient under consideration by the user.

The algorithm has been studied for predicting that a visit film folder is needed outside the archive (i.e., needed by one or more users) on the event "visit to the radiology department for a new examination". In a PACS, this event will probably leave too little time for image reallocations. Use of the event "appointment for a visit at radiology" will not be successful in a significant number of cases, because many patients walk in without appointment. Furthermore, we only looked at "in the archive", interpreted as "not used", and at "outside the archive", interpreted as "used". Finally, the current situation will most probably change when PACS has been introduced. At this point it is noted that the provision of the pictorial index may introduce a considerable load on the image network. The results of the age parameter have been presented in this section as an introduction; from this presentation alone the potential effectiveness can hardly be indicated. The following is partly based upon the complete study. The age parameter alone will not be sufficient for the selection of the relevant part of the patient's history. The parameter type of the examination may have powerful properties. Other parameters to be studied are: requester, diagnosis, and body region.

5.3.5 Design of the Prefetch Component

For the following discussion of the design of prefetching within an HIS/PACS, the following method has been adopted: The user, who interacts with an HIS/PACS, has been selected as the starting point. Prefetching functions and data in this nondivided HIS/PACS are detailed further. Subsequently, a scenario for the assignment of components to HIS and PACS is proposed, based upon components which are definitely to be assigned to HIS or PACS. Attention is given to the transition from the film-

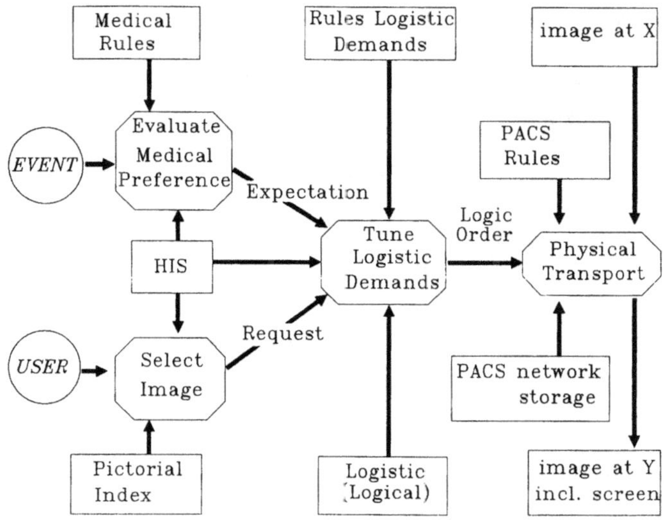

Fig. 5.33. Basic scheme of the processes retrieve and prefetch (cf. Fig. 5.26). *Octagons*. processes; *Rectangles*; data

based situation to PACS, especially to the management of images. Subsequently, a number of standardization needs are addressed.

5.3.5.1 Processes of Prefetching

In Fig. 5.33 the processes prefetch and retrieve (cf. Fig. 5.26) have been worked out in further detail. Let us first look at the process "evaluate medical preference" in the upper left corner of the figure. On the left, we see the initiation by an event. The result is the expectation that a certain image will be retrieved (with a certain probability) to a certain location in a certain period of time. This expectation will be evaluated by using rules about the medical usage of the image. For example, if the patient is admitted for surgery, then it is expected that the images of the two most recent examinations of the similar examination type will be needed. Note that the evaluation of this expectation starts upon a transition within the HIS data base, namely admission, and that this evaluation uses HIS data (not RIS only), i.e., in this example, the treating department and the age of the examinations.

Images can be retrieved by authorized persons throughout the hospital. The selection of images to be shown will not be made from the images themselves. After the identification of a certain patient, the pictorial index of the images of that patient will be shown. In the left bottom corner of Fig. 5.33, the retrieval of an image by a user is shown. It differs only slightly from the upper part: the request can be seen as an expectation with a

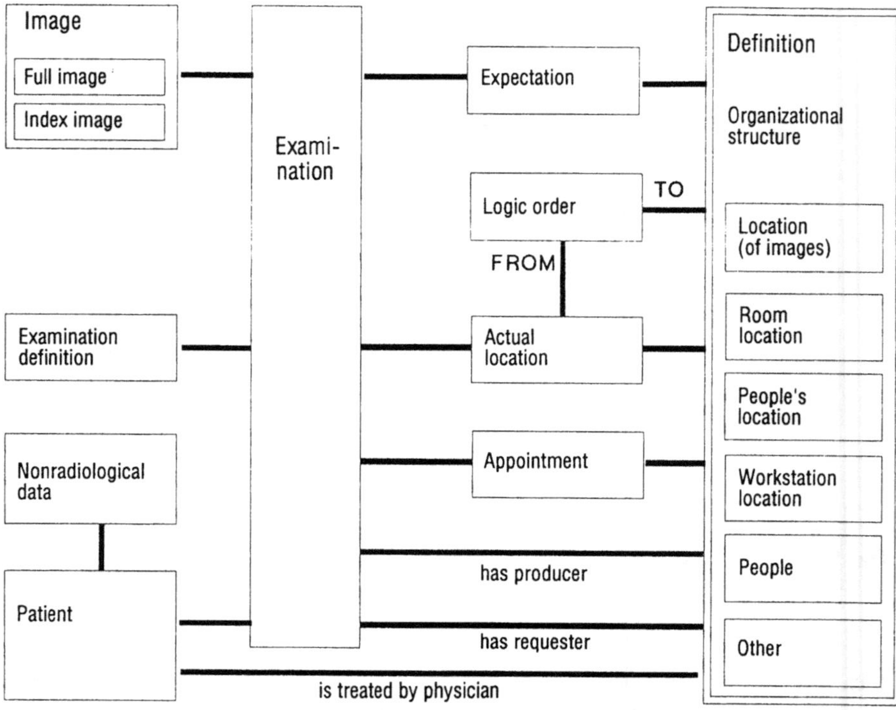

Fig. 5.34. Bachmann diagram of the data specific to prefetching

certainty of 100%. In the case of the retrieval of an image, the process "physical transport" will result in the display of the image on the screen.

This expectation initiates the process "tune logistic demands", which controls the transfer of images seen from the user's point of view. Conflicting expectations are handled here. The input of this process is information about single images. The process manages all these singles into a coherent strategy. Overcrowding is avoided by making use of the medical context, e.g., in the case of two images with the same expectation, a choice has to be made. The output is a reallocation order in logical (user) terms, e.g., move images of patient *P* to the workstation *W* in the room *R*. The strategy has been set down in the entity "rules logistic demands". The actual (logical) location of the images and the (logical) traffic is stored in the entity "logical logistics".

The next process "physical transport" takes the physical dimensions such as the number of storage layers, the access time of a layer, and the throughput of the network(s) into account. It will use rules as to how to make optimal use of the PACS configuration. A change in the configuration, e.g., a workstation off duty will be registered in this data entity. The actual occupancy of the storages and the actual network traffic is recorded in the entity "PACS network/storage". After the logic order has been translated into a physical description, it will be decided how to route the packets into which the image has been broken down across the network. The result is the transfer of an image to another storage (or screen) or the release of storage space occupied by an image. As this process knows nothing about the medical context, it will handle conflicts differently from the previous process.

5.3.5.2 Data of Prefetching

Processes and data are the two elements on which system development is based. In the previous section, we discussed the processes involved, here the data involved will be discussed. Figure 5.34 shows a Bachman diagram of the data specific to prefetching. The data entities are aggregated, as far as possible, for example, the entity "study" has been aggregated into "examination". Two attributes are proposed for the entity "image": the full image and an index image, to be used in the pictorial index (which might be alphanumerical). The entity "expectation" can be defined as the probability that a certain image will be needed in a certain period of time on a certain location. The entity "logic order" is defined as: "move a certain image to a certain location at a certain point in time". The two entities "expectation" and "logic order" are not of a permanent nature, they evaporate. The entity "definition organizational structure" contains a number of entities and their relations. The relations are rather complex and will differ strongly between hospitals. It should be noted that this aggregated entity contains entities from different levels, e.g., the logical and physical location of a workstation. As a consequence, it lies across the HIS–PACS interface.

5.3.5.3 Assignment of Processes and Data to HIS and PACS

The basic scheme presented in Fig. 5.33 and at the bottom of Fig. 5.35 can be used to address a number of design issues. In Fig. 5.35, the data entities have been left out and the following processes are visible:

1. Decide medical preference
2. Tune logistics
3. Physical transport

The initiation of this chain by an event, here, for example, for example, by the event "appointment", is shown in the middle on the left. The upper part, which shows the current film-based situation, has been added because certainly in the first years of PACS, a hybrid situation will exist. Basically, the functions are the same as in the PACS situation: at the moment the appointment is made (event), the secretary decides which historical visit film folders should be ordered from the archive. The secretary uses medical rules. This request is entered into the film folder lending system (see Sect.

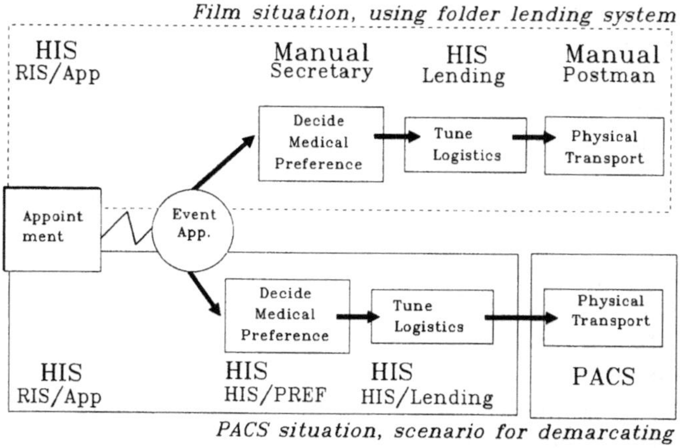

Fig. 5.35. A scenario for demarcation. The *upper half* shows the current film-based situation; the *lower half* shows the PACS situation

5.3.4.4). The lending system produces a pickup list for the file rooms, in other words optimizes the logistic process. Finally, the delivery service brings the visit film folders.

In Fig. 5.35, a scenario is proposed for the assignment of the processes to the HIS and the PACS. This scenario tries to fit closely with the film situation in order to support a hybrid image management. Furthermore, the medical part has been placed within the HIS, while the pure PACS task of physical transport has been placed within the PACS. Further research will be needed to develop a precise concept of the demarcation. It should be noted that the prefetching component has been considered. The final interface (cf Sect. 4.3) must also include the other aspects such as data integration, function integration, and data integrity.

5.3.6 Suggestions for the Second Generation of PACS

5.3.6.1 Prefetching as a Prerequisite

One can state that PACS will not be used at all if the images do not appear within an acceptable time on the screen. The provision of the required response time is a problem that stems mainly from the tremendous amounts of digital data needed to represent radiological film images. It is currently expected that the joint application of high-speed networks, image compression, and prefetching will solve the response time problem. However, the effect of image compression is limited because of juridical requirements, and high-speech image networks will not be available in the near future at reasonable costs. Prefetching combines the huge storage capacity of the storage devices needed for the tremendous amount of image data with the fast access time of storage devices with too limited storage capacity by applying knowledge about the patterns of image retrieval of the users.

5.3.6.2 Response Time

The response time requirement has to be specified from the user's point of view, which means that the specification should refer to a certain pattern of usage. It can be expected that several profiles will exist. A method for assessing the response time in relation to the working procedure has to be (further) developed.

5.3.6.3 Preliminary Results of a Pilot Study in Leiden University Hospital

The potential effectiveness of prefetching has been studied in Leiden University Hospital. The availability of an information system for visit film folder management, as one of the subsystems of an integrated HIS, was one of the key factors for success. The first results of this pilot study (in which over 1800 events were studied and the location determined for over 17000 accompanying visit film folders) are encouraging. It is suggested that future research should focus on the time span between the occurrence of the event and the reallocation, the evaluation of the overall (improved) response time, and the selection of the relevant images.

5.3.6.4 Moving to PACS Via Visit Film Folder Management

The design of prefetching only possible by knowing the patterns of usage. These patterns can be observed in a reliable way if a lending system for visit film folder management is used. As significant differences between hospitals exist, the prefetch algorithm for a particular PACS has to be tuned with the logistic information of that particular hospital. The PACS promise of fast delivery of images might be fulfilled by first implementing a visit film folder lending system. The implementation of a visit film folder lending system can offer the required information for the algorithm, and, moreover, it improves the present logistic process of visit film folders.

5.3.6.5 Design Issues and Consequences for the HIS–PACS Interface

A model for prefetching consisting of three processes in a chain has been proposed. This chain is activated by an event occurring in the HIS. The first process evaluates the expected retrieval of an image according to medical rules. The second process combines all these expectations for single images in a coherent logistic strategy. The final process takes care of the physical image transport in the PACS, not aware of the medical contents of the images. Because the start of this chain lies in the HIS and the end lies in the PACS, the HIS–PACS interface should include prefetching. We, therefore, need a clear definition of the functions to be assigned to PACS and HIS, thus specifying the interface. The definition of events which play a major role should be part of the interface as should an accurate description of the process that caused the event and of the actions which should follow the data push. Prefetching will make use of the data and events supplied by several HIS subsystems, most probably including a radiology subsystem, an ADT subsystem, and a subsystem for patient registration. A subsystem for scheduling the appointments for the admission of inpatients (or the visit of outpatients) to the hospital might be necessary. Principally the same chain of processes has been identified in the current film-based situation. In the transition phase from the film situation to the PACS situation, the current visit film folder management system has to be integrated with the PACS counterpart.

5.3.6.6 Potential Benefits and Critical Issues

It can be expected that prefetching will make a significant contribution to reducing the waiting time. Its effectiveness may be limited by its complexity, by the inability to recognize retrieval patterns, by a too short period between event and image transfer, by the unavailability of necessary data and/or events, and by an inappropriate interface between HIS and PACS. We suggest that further research should focus on the retrieval patterns, the definition *and assessment* of the response time, and the development of a standardized interface.

References

ACR NEMA (1985) Digital imaging and communication. ACR-NEMA Standards Publication No. 300-1985 Washington DC, USA

Bakker AR, Kouwenberg JML (1984) Retrieval and representation of X-ray images, a layered structure. In: Proc ADV, 7th international congress on data processing in Europe, 1984, pp 70–79

Bakker AR, Didden H, de Valk JPJ, Massar DAA (1986) Considerations on an algorithm for activation of images in a multi-layered storage system within a PACS. In: Proc PACS IV Conf, SPIE 626: 637–640

Bakker AR, Didden H, de Valk JPJ, Bijl K (1987) Traffic Load on the Image Storage Component in a PACS, In: Proc. Med Im Conf, SPIE 767: 824–830

Data Communications (1987) Newsfront: OSI throughput performance: breakthrough or bottleneck? Data Communications, May 1987

De Simone DN, Kundel HL, Arenson RL, Seshadri SB, Brikman IS, Darvey MJ, Brisbon NE (1988) Effect of a digital imaging network on physician behaviour in an intensive care unit. Radiology 169: 41–44

Digital, Intel, XEROX (1982) The Ethenet – specifications, version 2.0, November 1982

D'Lugin JJ, Boehme JM, Choplin RH, Maynard CD, Wolfman NT (1990) Optimization of image transfers from the central archive to workstations in a PACS, In: Proc Conf Med Im IV, SPIE 1234: 398–405

Fasel B (1990) ImageNet - Ein neues Datennetz für Bildinformationssysteme in der Medizin. VDI Düsseldorf, (Fortschritt Berichte VDI Series 10 No. 123)

Huang HK, Cho Paul S, Taira RK, Ho BK, Chan KK (1990) Picture archiving and communication systems in japan: 3 years later. Am J Roentgenol 154: 415–417

IMTEC (1987) ImNet specification. IMTEC imaging network AB, Uppsala, Sweden

Irie, G, Miyasaka K, Miyamoto K, Kojima T, Yamamoto I, Kudo T (1990) PACS experience at the University of Hokkaido Medical School. In: Proc SPIE Med Im Conf IV 1234: 26–32

Koens ML, Lodder H, Bijl K, de Valk JPJ, Bakker AR (1988) HIS-PACS integration: experience and future. In: Proc CAR Hilton Head Island, June, 1988

Koens ML, Weber RJ, Bakker AR (1990) HIS/RIS integration: experiences and future developments. In: Proc S/CAR Computer Applications to Assist Radiology, 1990, ISBN 0-88372-005-1

Levin K, Fielding R (1990) Methods to prefetch comparison images in an image management and communication system (IMACS). Conf Med Im IV, SPIE 1234: 270–274

Lodder H, Weperen JH, de Valk JPJ, Bijl K, Bakker AR (1989) HIS-PACS coupling: first experiences. In: Proc Conf Med Im, SPIE 914: 1141–1146

Lodder H, van Poppel BM, Wilmink JBM, Bakker AR (1990) HIS-PACS coupling in perspective. In: Proc Conf Med Im IV, SPIE 1234: 676–680

Mantelson et al. (1986) Networking design, testing and management. Data communications

Mattheus R (1987) Experimental PACS: intelligent distribution of information flow. In: Proc MIE 87: 1397–1402

Mattheus R, Osteaux M (1987) Intelligent distribution of information flow. In: Proceedings of MIE/EFMI — Rome September 21–25, 1987. pp 1397–1402

Mattheus R, Osteaux (1991) PACS and PACS research in Belgium. Springer, Berlin Heidelbery New York (NATO ASI Series, vol 74), pp 251–258

Mattheus R, Luypaert R, Osteaux M (1988) Hierarchical layers in a clinical PACS environment, Med Imag Tech 6(2): 157–158

Mattheus R, Luypaert R, Osteaux M (1989) PACS Topology, Proceedings of IMAC

Mattheus R, Moyson F, Temmerman Y, Osteaux M (1990) Hospital integrated picture archiving and communication system (HIPACS): a European project. Symposia Foundation SCAR, pp 396–404

Mattheus R, Ottes F, Bakker AR, Osteaux M (1991) HIPACS: hospital integrated picture archiving and communication system. Springer, Berlin Heidelberg New York (NATO ASI Series, vol 74), pp 325–332

Mun SK, Beason H, Elliot LP, Göhringer F, Saarinen A, Haynor D (1989) Total digital department: implementation strategy. In Proceeding of Medical Imaging III, SPIE 1093: 133–139

Meyer-Ebrecht D, Wendler T (1983) An architectural route through PACS. IEEE Computer 16(8), 19

Meyer-Ebrecht D, Fasel B, Vossebürger F (1987) Image network for PACS. In: Proceedings of the International Symposium CAR'87, Springer, Berlin Heidelberg New York Tokyo, p 558

Op het Veld WA, Koens ML (1987) Experience with an archive management and lending administration system for X-ray folders and patient medical records. In: Proc MIE 87, Rome

Sheng ORL, Wang H, Garcia HC (1990) IRES-image retrieval expert system. In: Proc Conf Med Im IV, 1990, SPIE 1234: 832–840

Van Poppel BM (1989) User's manual capacity version 2E, June 1989, BAZIS, Leiden

Van Poppel BM, Lodder H, de Valk JPJ, Wilmink JBM, Ising C (1989) Benefits of a HIS-PACS coupling in clinical practice. In: Proc CAR'89, 1989. Springer, Berlin Heidelberg New York, pp 521–525

Van Poppel BM, Lodder H (1990a) Prefetching: procedures, events and data important for data transfer from HIS to PACS. In: AIM/HIPACS report 3

Van Poppel BM, Lodder H (1990b) Implication of image management strategies for standardization. In: Proc Workshop PACS Standards in Europe, Irapetra, Crete, Greece, 1990

Van Poppel BM, Lodder H (1990c) Prefetching, In: AIM/HIPACS report 4

Van Poppel BM, Gennip EMSJ, Bakker AR, Wilmink JBM (1990) First results with the software package CAPACITY for cost modelling of PACS. Proc Conf Med Im IV, SPIE 1234: 905–910

Van Rijnsoever RC, de Valk JPJ, Bakker AR (1984) A layered storage structure for images confronted with the use of X ray images in a hospital. In: Proc applications of optical disk storage systems conference. SPIE V 490: 49–52

Taira RK, Mankovich NJ, Bouchat MI, Kangarloo H, Huang HK (1988) Design and implementation of a picture archiving and communication system for pediatric radiology. Am J Roentgenol 150: 1117–1121

Vossebürger F (1991) ImageNet/2: ein lokales Breitbandnetz für die digitale Bildkommunikation. Thesis, RWTH Aachen

6 Digital Image Workstations

Th. Wendler, K.J. Mönnich, and J. Schmidt

6.1 Workstation Design Considerations

6.1.1 User Interfaces to Picture Archiving and Communication Systems

Digital image workstations, located at various works places in the hospital, will provide the interfaces between fully digital picture archiving and communication systems (PACS) and their medical users. From the users' point of view, they can be regarded as "windows" to all the resources, documents, and data available in an integrated PACS, and radiology and hospital information systems (RIS/HIS). Advanced image workstations aim at far more than just replacing traditional lightboxes or alternators by digital technology. They will introduce new and improved ways of information handling in radiology, with the aims of increased diagnostic efficiency and improved patient care.

By definition, the *basic functionality* of a second generation PACS workstation has to support the handling and presentation of all digital documents and data of diagnostic relevance including:

- Multimodality pictorial documents and document collections (e.g., images, image sequences, acquisitions, examinations, and folders).
- Image-related data (e.g., image acquisition parameters and image annotations).
- Alphanumerical documents (e.g., diagnostic reports and clinical examination requests).
- Clinical data associated with a patient (e.g., patient history, referring department/physician, basic/actual disease, current clinical question, and suspected diagnosis).
- Patient demographic data.

For pictorial documents, an extended workstation functionality will also provide techniques for image enhancement and analysis that prove to be useful from the medical point of view. This perspective, however, will not be discussed extensively in this chapter.

For the design of workstations in a total digital PACS environment, a number of *basic requirements* appear to be vital from the medical point of view. Digital image workstations will have to:

- Allow the diagnostic interpretation of multimodality images (including large format, high-resolution radiographs as well as sequences of tomograms or angiograms) directly from the display screens.
- Guarantee at least the same diagnostic safety and accuracy as with photographic films.
- Provide capabilities for document access, handling and display which are faster and more convenient than traditional tools (at least, no additional workload has to be put on the radiologist).
- Support all relevant tasks to be performed in diagnostic radiology by different kinds of users.

This catalogue of minimum requirements will be used as a guideline for the basic design considerations discussed later in this chapter. At present, these demands cannot be easily fulfilled. From the viewpoint of medical needs and their technical consequences, the general consensus is that digital image workstation design belongs to the more difficult and critical issues in PACS development. It is critical because appropriate user interfaces which meet the requirements of various user groups and which effectively support the variety of diagnostic tasks will have a decisive influence on the success and acceptance of PACS as a whole. Total digital systems will simply not exist in radiology until the above-mentioned requirements are fulfilled by digital workstations. Some of the benefits claimed for PACS, e.g., fast, reliable, and convenient access to multimodality images, are mainly expressed by workstation design and will only become obvious to users through appropriate user interfaces.

Designing PACS workstations to meet these requirements is certainly a complex and, therefore, difficult issue. Digital image workstations have to support the wide variety of work settings found in radiology. For example, they have to assist the work of various user groups such as principal radiologists, assistant radiologists, radiological technicians, physicists, and referring physicians, all of whom have clearly different roles and responsibilities in the diagnostic process. Furthermore, a number of typical tasks established in radiology have to be supported, for example, pre-examination viewing (inspection of previous images preceding the acquisition of new ones), image quality check and authorization after the acquisition, image reading and reporting, consultation sessions with colleague radiologists, report discussion and authorization by principlal radiologists or department head, preparation of demonstration sessions, demonstration sessions with referring physicians, radiological education, and research. In some of these tasks, provisions have to be taken for multiple viewer involvement. Additionally, image viewing by referring physicians or surgeons outside the radiology department has to be considered. The complex environment of tasks and users clearly indicates the necessity for different workstation types to be installed at different locations. From the economic point of view, however, this should not result in a large number of special purpose devices. Instead, a small number of workstation types with adaptive (task- and user-dependent) functionality appears to be attractive. Some aspects of adaptive user interfaces are discussed in the second part of this chapter.

As a further element of complexity, the workstation design process not only has to consider user requirements derived from the analysis of today's film-based radiology, but also anticipate future demands that will undoubtedly evolve in the transition to the total digital information system (e.g., desires for novel ways of document handling, display, and processing induced by new technological capabilities and by changing image reading habits). Some of the difficulties with the definition of prospective design scenarios will be highlighted in Sect. 6.1.2.

From the above-mentioned list of medical requirements and design issues, a number of technical challanges become evident. The demand for fast and convenient handling of high resolution images, for example, leads to throughput requirements of processing devices which cannot be fulfilled using off-the-shelf hardware platforms. New image processing systems at the edge of technology are a prerequisite for sufficient workstation responsiveness. In an environment of developing user requirements, software concepts applied in workstation prototyping have to provide for easy and fast user interface modifications. The domain of radiology (which is a complex environment in itself) will be complemented by a sophisticated technical system. As another vital requirement, this technical complexity has to be made transparent to medical users. They have to be protected from being confronted with technology-oriented concepts that do not contribute to their goals and interests.

In recent years, many interesting workstation design approaches have been proposed in the literature and partially evaluated and used in radiology. Still, existing digital image workstations can clearly not compete yet the with speed and accuracy of film-based image handling and presentation procedures. In Sect. 6.1.2 we will indicate and discuss in depth some of the barriers that make digital workstation design a complex issue, and we will argue for a strictly usercentered design methodology to improve the situation for second generation PACS workstations.

6.1.2 Workstation Design in the Transition to Fully Digital Imaging Departments

In the late 1970s, the idea of pictorial information systems in radiology was stimulated by a technology push. Optical disk storage technology was introduced, which offered the potential for cost-effective and reliable storage of high-resolution digital images. The increased mass storage capacity made it attractive to replace photographic film-based diagnostic image archives by electronic storage systems (Kowalsky et al. 1977; Meyer-Ebrecht 1980). In those days, discussions focused on the technical realization of picture bases, image computers, and hard copy devices. Image workstations and their user interfaces were rarely considered. Some years later, in the early 1980s, the perspective of a digital communication system, and finally a total digital diagnostic imaging department was added, stimulated by a number of international conferences such as PACS I (1981) and PACS II (1982). At this time, it became apparent that digital systems would not just replace photographic films as information carriers. In radiology, films are simultaneously detectors, archive media, displays, and a means for communicating diagnostic information. A fully digital PACS must support all of these functions. Furthermore, it became clear that the integration of PACS into departmental (e.g., RIS) or hospital-wide (i.e., HIS) information systems is an essential requirement. All of these perspectives have added a tremendous complexity to the design of PACS in general and of digital image workstations in particular.

A closer look to the problems of image handling and presentation reveals that traditional tools (films, lightboxes/alternators) and digital image workstations differ quite a lot with respect to their capabilities, limitations, advantages, and disadvantages. The differences between film-based and digital systems in *image handling* are striking. Once photographic films have been accessed from the archive and drawn out of a film folder, they can be easily arranged on a lightbox. It is simple to change the orientation of images or to alter their position on the display area. Complex image arrangements can be quickly provided and modified in a straightforward manner. Concepts for film handling appear "natural", in the sense that no additional skill is needed beyond what is available from daily life. For handling digital images on display screens, in contrast, more artificial concepts must be introduced that have to be learned by workstation users. Elementary operations that appear trivial in film handling (like repositioning, erasing, or rotating images on the display screen, or putting a copy of an image into a radiologist's private folder) have to be performed with the aid of interaction concepts that are certainly more complicated. As a further element of complication, different of such interaction concepts will be offered in a multivendor environment and in the absence of standardization. Although the simplicity of film handling clearly appears as a striking benefit, it can be seen at the same time as a significant limitation and drawback. In the light of today's information technology, some of the film-based operations look rather clumsy and anachronistic (e.g., searching for particular images in a disorganized film folder). Digital image workstations will certainly offer faster and more convenient techniques for the selection and display of images and related information (ranging from structured pictorial indexes to co-operative systems that volunteer needed information).

A number of different strengths and weaknesses in image presentation are obvious. Lightboxes and alternators provide a large display space for a number of transparent films with excellent spatial resolution and dynamic range. Lightboxes are available in various locations in the hospital. It is even possible to view films without lightboxes (e.g., during the doctor's visit in the patient's bedroom). The state of the art in display technology allows a single high resolution radiograph to be presented on a cathode ray tube

(CRT) display monitor, with in the order of 2000 × 2000 picture elements and a mapping of the images' dynamic range (8–12 bit) to 256 displayed gray levels. CRT monitors are available with dimensions ranging from about 45 cm to 75 cm screen diagonal, resulting in about 7.5–4 nominally displayed lines per millimeter. Experiments indicate that this resolution is adequate for reading most image types; (investigations to determine the required resolution for various medical image types are surveyed by Arenson 1990).

If larger display space for parallel viewing of multiple images is required (as suggested by established work patterns and currently used tools), today's technical solution is an arrangement of several high-resolution monitors. This, however, may not only be extremely expensive, it tends also to be counterproductive for the design of simple, convenient, and consistent image handling models. Undoubtedly, the particular strength of electronic displays is their dynamic behavior. Therefore, the discussion on parallel/static versus concurrent/dynamic viewing procedures is of central interest for digital workstation design.

An interesting and important consideration is the question how much display space a digital image workstation has to provide for various tasks in diagnostic image viewing. A discussion of medical requirements for parallel viewing and a comparison of the capabilities and limitations of film-based and digital displays reveals the following perspectives for workstation design. From the viewpoint of diagnostic radiology, image-reading habits and work patterns have been developed which are based on the simultaneous presentation of multiple films. For a number of reasons this seems to be an essential requirement in film-based radiology:

1. Image comparisons are an important element of image interpretation. The spatial arrangement of films consists of images from current and previous examinations to track the course of a disease, images from different projections that allow the locations of objects in the three-dimensional space, images generated by different imaging modalities that offer complementary information, series of tomograms (slices) or angiograms (time sequences), or reference images with a well-defined pathology (e.g., from the teaching archive).
2. In most diagnostic work sessions, high image throughput is required. Therefore, it is often useful to separate image handling (selection and arrangement on the lightbox/alternator) and image reading. For image interpretation and reporting, the parallel arrangement can be scanned rapidly by head or eye movements. With alternators, it is possible to quickly display complete patient cases. Switching between patients takes only a few seconds.
3. In the film-based system it is slow and inconvenient to change images during the work session (e.g., searching for images in a folder and adding them to the display).
4. The parallel arrangement of images on the lightbox serves as a visual aid that helps to locate needed pieces of information, to maintain context

and orientation. In the absence of other orientation aids, this spatial information model offered by lightboxes and alternators is an important element of traditional work patterns.

In summary, these image-reading habits reflect the capabilities and benefits, but also the constraints of the film-based display system. For some cases, for example, for image comparisons, we may conclude that the parallel arrangement is one of the fastest and most convenient ways of image interpretation, making it also indispensible for electronic displays. Parallel viewing capabilities may also be considered for a smooth transition from the film-based to fully digital systems. In general, however, several authors have argued that film-based image reading habits may not necessarily be efficient with digital image workstations (e.g., Rogers et al. 1985; O'Malley and Giunta 1988). A significant reduction of parallel viewing habits and thus reduced display space requirements can be assumed, if the capabilities of digital display systems, particularly their dynamic capabilities, are considered:

1. Electronic displays allow fast and convenient changes of the presented information. This may generally lead to more efficient concurrent viewing habits.
2. Faster and more convenient image access mechanisms can be designed that are superior to film access. Users can rapidly lood at object collections, e.g., patient folders, that offer a structured pictorial inventory of the accessible documents. With dynamic displays it is also easier to get rid of documents on the screen. In general, the image arrangement may be quickly and conveniently changed during the worksessions.
3. Image sequences (tomograms or angiograms) may be more efficiently presented as stacks of images with browsing capability. Time sequences may be shown as movies. Useful combinations of parallel and sequential viewing techniques may optimize the reading of image sequences such as the filmstrip-model suggested by Beard et al. (1987), or the use of lower sampled index slices shown by Pizer et al. (1987). Computed tomography (CT) scans with different window/level setting may not be treated as separate images (as is common practice on films), if the desired settings can be obtained interactively. Three-dimensional presentations may have a dramatic impact on viewing habits for slice sequences.
4. Digital images are no longer transparent, but opaque. This allows the introduction of logical screen models, where images are allowed to overlap, resulting in more efficient usage of the available viewing space.
5. Image presentation may in some cases be restricted to regions of interest if tools are available to rapidly obtain and modify regions and if orientation aids are provided that indicate the region's position in the document. This may, where applicable, lead to significantly reduced space requirements.

6. In addition to comparisons with simultaneously presented images, new techniques may be introduced for problem-oriented image comparisons, e.g., novel image superposition technique like switching or cutting (see. Wendler et al. 1986).
7. The spatial information model available for a parallel arrangement of images may be replaced by other models of context and orientation that help to organize the information on the screen (e.g., mechanisms that allow rapid switching between survey arrangements and full resolution document presentation). The Document box shown in Fig. 6.2 is one of many examples of such mechanisms.

This discussion has indicated fundamental perceptual and behavioral differences between traditional tools in film-based radiology and the options offered by digital image workstations in the areas of image handling and display. For other areas of workstation functionality, e.g., image modifications, image analysis, or the access to related clinical information, these differences become even more pronounced. In summary, we can conclude that new technologies to support radiological image interpretation will certainly provide far more than just a functional copy of the old tools. Digital image workstations will not be electronic lightboxes/alternators! A 1:1 mapping between the film-based and the digital system is hardly possible, nor in many aspects desirable. Both systems have their strengths and weaknesses. From the perspective of film-based radiology, the current image reading habits appear optimal; however, we can predict that radiologists will develop new digital reading habits that will differ from the current ones. Stating this, we must conclude that together will digital technology changes will be introduced to the diagnostic work procedures which will probably have an impact on the organization of radiology departments. Extended access to clinical data on the one hand and better access to images by referring physicians on the other hand may also have an impact on the role of radiology in the hospital environment. Considering these far-reaching consequences, some general thoughts on a methodology for the design of workstation user interfaces appear useful.

6.1.3 Methodology for the Design of User-Friendly Digital Image Workstations

The success of workstation design is influenced by a large number of interdependent medical, technical, and human factors considerations. The complexity of this situation calls for a multidisciplinary effort involving, for example, radiologists, engineers, computer scientists, and cognitive psychologists, and for a strict and systematic design methodology. This is not self-evident in system design. It is common practice that user interfaces are created intuitively by technical designers. Insufficient background of the medical diagnostic process sometimes leads to technology-driven,

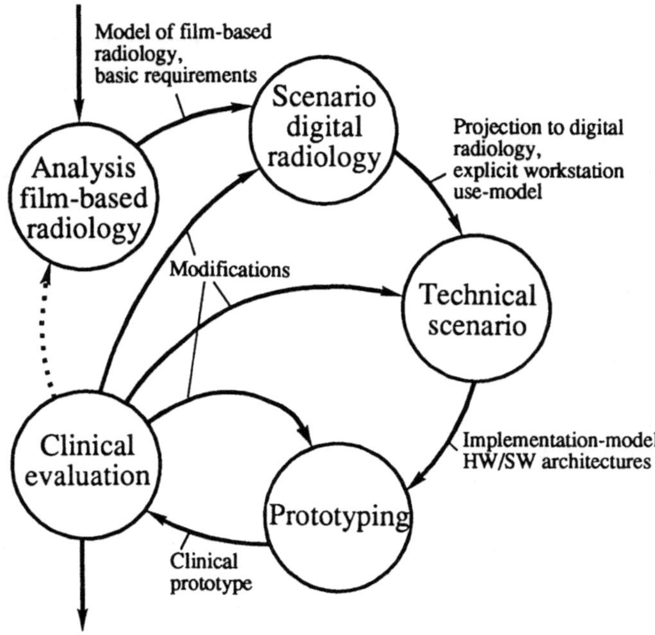

Fig. 6.1. Digital workstation design cycle

inappropriate solutions that fall short of the critical requirements of fully digital PACS. Designs tend to be burdened from the beginning with fixed technical or economical boundary conditions (e.g., frozen hardware or software platforms). Frequently, user interfaces are regarded as the last step of engineering that gives a developed technical system a nice outward appearance (a finish).

In human factors research, the notion of user-centered design has been developed as the basis for user-friendly interfaces (e.g., Monk 1984; Norman 1986). It demands an iterative design process in which end users participate from the beginning. Figure 6.1 sketches the steps of a typical user-centered design cycle for a digital image workstation. The various stages can be briefly described as follows:

Analysis of film-based radiology. User-friendliness of an image workstation can only be approached for specific users and tasks. Therefore, a thorough analysis of the current situation in film-based radiology has to be performed as the initial step of every user interface design. Such an analysis has to make an inventory of the key elements of the diagnostic process. The goals of the diagnostic process and the tasks established to reach these goals have to be identified. The staff involved in radiology (users of future systems) and their roles, responsibilities, and attitudes have to be described. The organization of radiology departments, typical data flow mechanisms, and communication structures have to be investigated. The examination types, documents, and data currently used for diagnostic work have to identified. The result of this design step should be a precise model of film-based radiology that reflects a profound understanding of the medical diagnostic process. To avoid errors, this analysis should summarize the conditions in several hospitals. As a direct result for workstation design, a list of basic and indispensible requirements for future digital systems should be formulated.

Scenario of digital radiology: the explicit workstation use model. Understanding film-based radiology is certainly a necessary, but in no way a sufficient condition for the design of workstations in a fully digital information system. Another important element is a projection of current work procedures and requirements to the anticipated digital radiology of the future. A workstation user interface scenario has to describe the assumptions of how users will perform the various diagnostic tasks in the future and what impact this will have on their habits and on the radiological process as a whole. An appropriate scenario will neither try to copy the traditional system by electronic means (the "electronic alternator"), nor will it come up with technical solutions that ignore the fundamental medical requirements. This is a creative process which has to be guided by the needs of diagnostic radiology, by knowledge about the capabilities of hardware and software technology, and by human factors considerations. A multidisciplinary cooperation appears mandatory. It will only be successful with a medical and technical understanding of PACS as a whole.

There should be an awareness that an initial scenario of a future system will only be a first draft. Design decisions will be evaluated and probably modified or revised in subsequent design steps. However, the scenario has to point into the right direction, otherwise the design process will be inefficient and may not result in a suitable system. The direct outcome of a user interface should be a document that explicitly describes the outward appearance of a digital workstation from the user's point of view, unrestrained by any internal technical operation. This description is sometimes referred to as a use model (e.g., Rubinstein and Hersh 1984; Wendler 1985), a guideline that represents hard design constraints for the implementation. The use model has to define the physical design of the display screen, the logical screen model (metaphor), the principal interaction technique, the consistent appearance of generic types of objects on the screen, the basic functionality and its utilization, and basic mechanisms for information access, handling, presentation and modification. For the design of consistent user interfaces, the use model has to address *all* of these aspects simultanously.

Technical scenario: the implementation model. Guided by the use model, hardware and software architectures have to be developed. Being aware of use model revisions and developing user requirements, the implementation model has to be more than a platform for the realization of current design ideas. It has to provide a strategy for easy extensions and modifications of hardware and software components. In practice, conflicts may occur between use model demands and technical or economical boundary conditions that may lead to early design revisions. The soundness of these technology driven revisions has to be evaluated later.

Prototyping brings the implementation model to reality.

Clinical evaluation. Prototypes have to be evaluated in clinical PACS environments. Mismatching conceptions or new design ideas will lead to various modification cycles, as indicated in Fig. 6.1.

In summary, the notion of *user-friendliness* describes a user-centered design process rather than a designed feature of a system. Such a requirement driven design process is clearly required for the success of second generation PACS workstations. An explicit use model appears as the important and interesting focal point of all designs. Section 6.1.4 will highlight some of the elements to be considered in use-models for digital image workstations.

6.1.4 Elements of Image Workstation User Interfaces

A number of general and common issues have to be explicitly addressed in all digital image workstation designs. Some of these basic design elements will be listed in this section and some options for their realization will be discussed, which reflect a workstation use model designed by the authors.

Physical Display System. A display system, i.e., a single or a set of display monitors, has to provide for the presentation of all required pictorial and alphanumerical information. For images, the display screens have to maintain the adequate quality for primary diagnosis in terms of spatial resolution, contrast resolution, perceptually adequate contrast characteristics, and flicker-free screen refresh. The display's update rate has to match the requirements of responsiveness as defined by the workstation use model. Decisions have to be taken on how many images need to be presented in parallel. This will determine the display space requirements and, at a given stage of technology, the number of monitors involved.

From the perspective of film-based radiology, a single large-size and high-resolution display screen (for about four large radiographs) with fast update rate (in the order of under 100 ms for basic and critical image handling and display operations) appears desirable. As discussed earlier, the actual space requirements in digital radiology may be significantly reduced by the design of the logical screen model. Currently available monitors offer 2560×2048 pixel displayed on 30×25 cm, or 2048×2048 pixel on a 50×50 cm display screen. The total display space offered by a workstation (regardless of how this space is distributed over several monitors) will be referred to in the following as the *viewing area*.

Logical Model of the Viewing Area. Independent of the physical realization of the display system (this may change with technology), a *logical* model

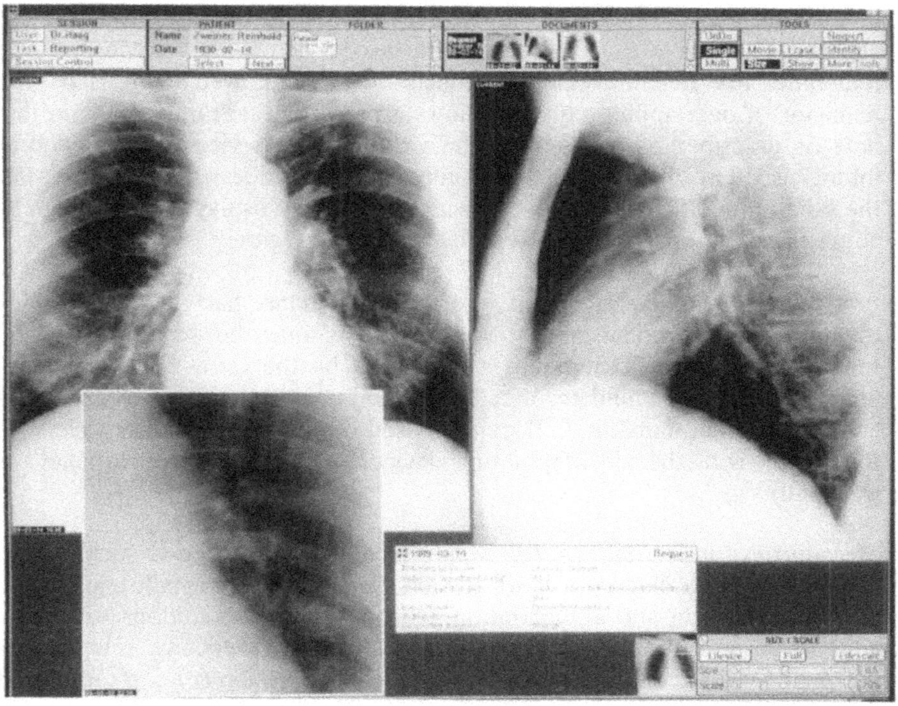

Fig. 6.2. User interface design example developed for reporting sessions. Separate interaction-"boxes" are provided for items of radiological interest (*SESSION*, *PATIENT*, *FOLDER*, *DOCUMENTS*, *TOOLS*). The screen model is based on overlapping objects which can be moved across the viewing area in real time

must be designed for the viewing area that defines what displayed objects look like, how they behave, how they relate to each other, and how they can be manipulated. Decisions must be taken as to whether objects are presented in "tiled" viewports[1] or whether they are allowed to overlap. The definition of a screen metaphor (analogy models such "desktop with movable objects" or "filmstrip") may help users to develop predictive mental models of the basic system operation.

For the design of consistent, simple, and fast image handling mechanisms, we strongly advocate defining a *single* logical viewing area, even if multiple monitors are involved. As discussed earlier, the spatial relationships of images on the viewing area seems to be an important consideration for diagnostic work. Radiologists frequently reposition images until an appropriate arrangement is reached. Therefore, the possibility of moving and positioning images easily and quickly on the viewing area is postulated as a basic requirement. Figure 6.2 shows an example of a display screen

[1] A viewport is a rectangular area of the viewing area used to display a document or part of a document.

model that allows objects of radiological interest to be easily touched (by clicking on them with the mouse) and moved across the viewing area in real time. For free movements, objects must be allowed to overlap. The behavior of overlapping objects follows a predictive, natural paradigm that may be described as paper-like. The viewing area is virtually extended to infinity, so that objects can be partially shifted outside its visible part. For the sake of an efficient usage of viewing area space, displayed objects can be conveniently altered in size and scale (display of regions).

Interaction Technique. Physical interaction elements have to be provided together with mechanisms by which objects may be manipulated and functions activated. Techniques summarized by the term "direct manipulation" have been found to offer simple and comprehensive ways of interaction (Shneiderman 1983). They are based on indicating objects visible on the screen with the aid of pointing devices (e.g., mouse, touch-panel, or trackball).

Mechanisms for Session Control. Means have to be provided to start, pause, resume, or quit a diagnostic work session. Sessions will normally start with a user identification and authorization procedure. In workstations with task-adaptive user interfaces, a task identification also becomes relevant. A nesting of tasks should be possible within a work session (e.g., a radiologist should be able to do an "image quality check" in the middle of a "reporting" task and continue reporting afterwards). In the example interface presented in Fig. 6.2, all of these session control functions are located in a separate interaction box in the upper left corner of the viewing area.

Mechanisms for Patient Selection. For patient-oriented diagnostic tasks, e.g., reporting, mechanisms to sequentially examine patient cases are of central importance. Means have to be provided to select a particular patient from a list of relevant patients. For subsequent patient selection, simplifying and accelerating functions such as *FIRST, NEXT*, or *PREVIOUS* may be introduced (see Patient-interaction box in Fig. 6.2). Patient selection may open the path to associated documents and data, e.g., patient folders, or results of laboratory tests.

Mechanisms for Authorized Document Access. All workstations need mechanisms to find documents (or document collections) in data bases and to retrieve them for viewing. The technical complexity of distributed pictorial information systems e.g., the physical location of images in a distributed hierarchy of storage devices, appears uninteresting for users and should not become visible at the user interface. Although in digital systems images and related information are not kept in folders, the folder concept may be maintained as a comprehensive construct for the access to entities of data, e.g. patient folders containing documents of a particular patient, or teaching folders as part of the teaching archive. For document access, users may easily

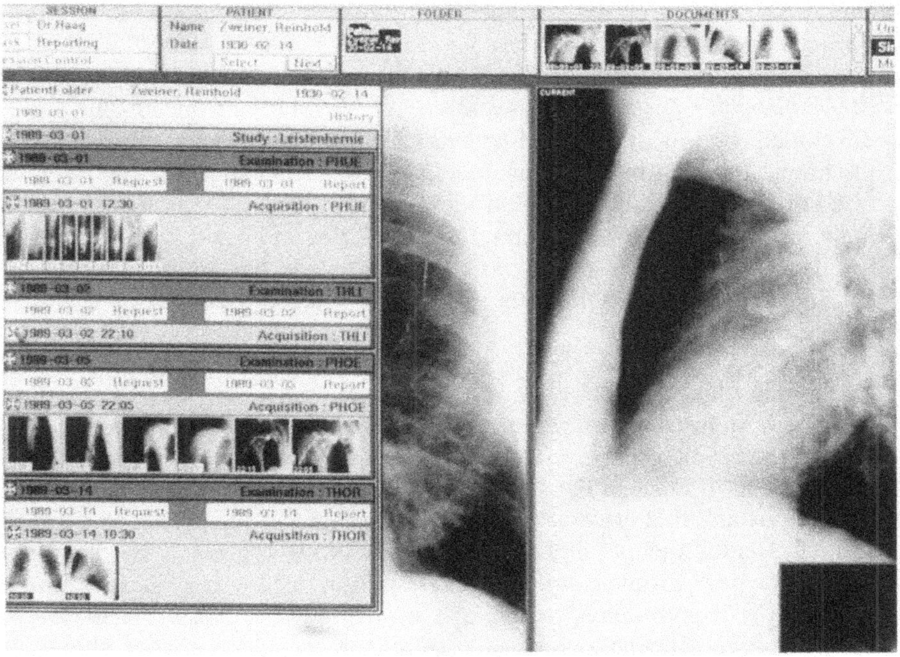

Fig. 6.3. Access to documents in a patient folder by a structured pictorial index

look into indexes of folders (Fig. 6.3) and select objects of interest. The indexes may present selected information according to user-definable entity criteria such as studies, examinations, acquisitions, anatomical description, pathological description, or acquisition date. The presentation may consist of mixed pictorial and alphanumerical items. Folders may also allow access to all kinds of nonpictorial data such as alphanumerical documents, patient history, and clinical data.

Mechanisms for Image Handling. Mechanisms have to be provided for basic document handling operations. Concepts have to be developed of how images are brought up on the viewing area, how the image arrangement can be changed, and how they can be erased again. There is also a need for mechanisms that assign documents to a document collection, e.g., to put a copy of an image from a patient folder to the radiologist's private folder or add it to part of the teaching archive. The basic image handling operations have to compete with speed and simplicity of film-based procedures.

Bringing images to the viewing area can easily be achieved via index panels. The example in Fig. 6.3 shows a structured pictorial index of a patient folder, where images are displayed or erased simply by pointing to their index items. In analogy to film handling, images on the viewing area may be easily shifted to any desired position in real time. All visible objects can also be picked up and dropped into other locations, e.g., a copy can be put into another folder.

Mechanisms for Display Modification of Single Images. Concepts have to be developed of how the visual appearance of image type objects can be modified. Frequently occurring modifications are changes in size, e.g., to obtain lifesize, scaling (magnified versions of interesting regions), gray scale mapping, e.g., window/level operations, or orientation, e.g., show an image upside down. Besides these basic operations, it has to be conceptually considered how the whole range of possible image processing operations is to be utilized by the user.

Mechanisms and Tools for the Display Arrangement of Image Collections. Display systems in general, and particularly those with logical screen models that allow objects to overlap, offer a high degree of freedom for the arrangement of images. For the efficient comparison of a number of images, it is important that users can quickly generate desired standard arrangements. Besides the parallel image configurations suggested by film-based radiology, new problem-oriented presentation techniques such as superpositions, or fast-switching techniques may be introduced. From the observation of film viewing sessions, we may also conclude that it should be possible to save complete display arrangements and to recall them later, e.g., in a planned demonstration session.

Mechanisms for the Display of Image Sequences. Time sequences or slices of images can be shown both in parallel and sequentially. For sequential operations (movie), means are needed to control movements (forward, backward, stop, movie speed, step, etc.). The combination of parallel and sequential viewing techniques appears attractive. In the interest of a consistent and predictive logical screen model, the presentation of image sequences should not be regarded as an isolated mechanism, but as a feature to be combined with all other described mechanisms. For example, within the proposed screen model, it may be attractive to display a gray scale mapped region of a dynamic time sequence movie, overlapping with any other information on the viewing area.

Tools for Image Annotation and Analysis. From the observation of film-based radiology, it is desirable to annotate images (put marks on them or add comments). Moreover, mechanisms have to be provided to extract features from images by measurements such as distance, angle, area, and volume.

Mechanisms for Access, Handling and Display of Nonpictorial Documents and Data. A number of design considerations have been described for image type documents. Similar concepts have to be developed for all alphanumerical documents and data of radiological interest, e.g., how to access, handle, and display diagnostic reports, request forms, and clinical data.

Responsiveness. As an integral part of the use model, not only the functional requirements have to be defined but also how fast operations will be carried out. For time-dependent, routine actions, e.g., arranging a number of images on the viewing area, the performance features of film-based radiology have to be used as a guideline. This demands that most of the described basic workstation mechanisms be done within a fraction of a second.

6.1.5 Technical Design Considerations

In line with the proposed design methodology, requirements and design considerations for second generation PACS workstations have been discussed so far rather independently of their technical realization. In the following, some technical implementation aspects will be addressed. Of course, a range of quite different design solutions are possible for dedicated workstations in support of different diagnostic tasks. However, generic hardware and software architectures which cover the whole range of applications and which are flexible enough to allow for modifications and extensions appear beneficial and feasible. A generic hardware architecture that is capable of supporting various use models and task-dependent workstation types is sketched in Fig. 6.4. It consists of a multiprocessor system embedded in a dual bus environment. Due to the special requirements for image handling, display, and processing, separate and optimized data paths and image processors are of central importance for PACS. The required workstation components and their dimensions are briefly characterized in the following.

Image Bus. An optimized data path has to be provided for local image data transport between the various hardware processors. According to demands for high responsiveness, throughput requirements in the range of 50–125 Mpixel/s with at least 12 bit/pixel have to be fulfilled. The lower limit of 50 Mpixel/s is already required if a single high-resolution radiograph has to be freely shifted in real time across the viewing area. The upper range requirements arise, for example, for the parallel presentation of several movies of image sequences at 30 frames/s.

Control Bus. A communication path for nonpictorial data is needed for interprocessor links on the control level. Unlike on the picture data level, the emphasis on the control level lies in the flexible exchange of relatively small data packages. A general purpose computer bus seems appropriate (the VME bus appears as a good candidate).

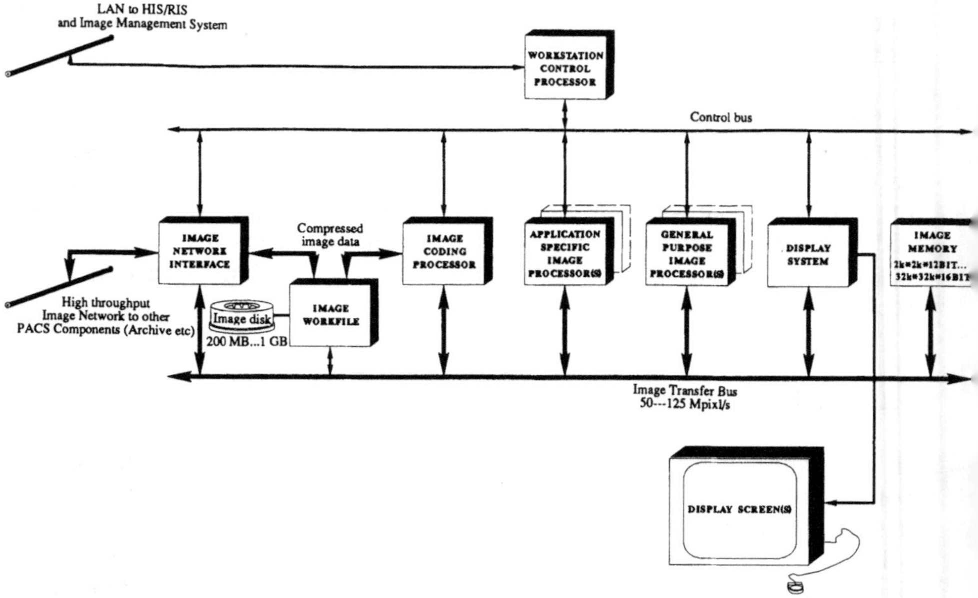

Fig. 6.4. Generic digital image workstation hardware architecture

Display Processor. A high-speed device is needed to map part of the workstations image memory to the viewing area. Typical components of the display processor are: frame buffers that contain all pixels to be mapped to the screen(s); a high-speed address generator to fill the frame buffer; a real-time interpolator; a unit for the overlay of graphical information; a set of look-up tables (LUT) for gray scale mapping; and a processor for viewport management (in case of overlapping documents).

Semiconductor Image Memory. During a worksession, the semiconductor image memory will contain all pictorial objects which are of focal radiological interest. These may be all relevant images of one or several patients which have to be kept in immediate, nondelayed access. For different tasks to be supported by a workstation, the total capacity requirements for the image memory will vary: in low-cost versions for simple viewing tasks, a capacity of $2000 \times 2000 \times 12$ bit may be sufficient. For tasks that involve many high-resolution radiographs and require high image throughput, a capacity in the order of $32 \times 32 \times 16$ bits (allowing 64 high-resolution radiographs to be kept in ultrafast access) is desirable. This, however, also depends on speed and capacity of additional local image disks.

Local Image Disk. A local image workfile has to be designed for all images needed during a worksession. From our observations of film viewing sessions, we can conclude that the workfile has to keep some tens to some hundreds of images (200 MB–1 GB). The required capacity will depend on two other technical design aspects, namely (a) Preloading and (b) hierarchical image coding. For sufficiently fast image access, a relevant selection of images has to be preloaded into the local workfile preceding the user's work session. This translates to rapid usage of images during the work-session (without waiting periods caused by central archive access). The number of images to be preloaded will depend on strategies which are based on knowledge about the diagnostic information requirements (a definite approach to this will be discussed in the second part of this chapter). With respect to hierarchical image coding, lossless image data compression will reduce the overall data volume to be stored. For the sake of efficient usage of disk capacity and for faster image access, images should be held in compressed form also on local disks in workstations. With hierarchical coding techniques, e.g., the S-transform, (Lux 1977; Wendler 1987b) additionally a structured access to images on different levels of spatial resolution becomes possible. As a result, survey information, e.g., pictorial indexes, can be retrieved rapidly, avoiding time and memory consuming transport of the entire documents. Some hierarchical image coding schemes, including the S-transform, have been proposed in a supplement of the ACR/NEMA standard.

Image Coding Processor. The benefits of data compression and data structuring will only be of merit if the decoding process can be done immediately without any increase in retrieval time. Workstation hardware must be open enough to allow high-speed decoding processors to be attached between the image network and the local image transfer bus. For the S-transform coding scheme, a very large scale integration (VLSI) chip set has been designed that supports fast image compression and reconstruction.

Control Processor and Workstation Control Software. A general purpose computer can act as the workstation control system. The software architecture has to reflect quite different functional requirements:

1. Fast and hardware-related software (firmware) is needed to control high-speed image processing operations in real time.
2. For user interface design, software tools are required that allow the rapid and flexible implementation of workstation use models and that support easy extentions and modifications. There is a wide agreement that this part of workstation control software should be based on the object-oriented programming paradigm.
3. For adaptive workstations with co-operative user interfaces, there is a need to integrate knowledge-based systems which act as intelligent consultants at run-time.

In summary, this wide range of requirements indicates the need of a hybrid workstation software environment that allows quite different dedicated and problem-oriented language tools to be integrated. An example for a layered software system of this kind is given in Sect. 6.2.

6.2 Adaptive User Interfaces for PACS Image Workstations

6.2.1 Why Adaptive User Interfaces?

As proposed earlier in this chapter, user-friendliness can generally be approached by a predominantly user-centered design process. User-centered design, however, often results in a compromise that focuses on some kind of "average" user and assumes a number of *general* goals users are interested in. Changing requirements that arise from different kind of users and the diversity of goal oriented tasks and subtasks are rarely considered during system design and almost never at system run-time. Most human–machine interfaces appear to be "static". They function uniformly, regardless of what kind of user is working with a system and what actual task the user is concerned with.

Adaptive user interfaces, in contrast, conceptually take into account that workstation users and their actual tasks–thus their *current* goals and information requirements–are variable at run-time. In radiology, digital image workstations will be used by quite different stereotypic categories of users, e.g., principal or assistant radiologists, physicists, and technicians, with diverging goals, responsibilities, and information requirements. Even within a particular user group, personal preferences and styles are observed, e.g., how to arrange images on the display screen. Analyzing the film-based diagnostic process, various categories of goal-oriented tasks can be distinguished, ranging from simple control actions like image quality check after the acquisition to quite complex image handling and display procedures like preparing a demonstration session for referring clinicians. A variation of information requirements is obvious for different tasks. Furthermore, with the introduction of PACS technologies, initial user requirements are expected to change rapidly. It is assumed that an easy adaptation of user interfaces to developing user and task requirements will be particularly helpful in the initial phase of fully digital information systems in radiology where probably new image handling and viewing procedures will evolve. Adaptive user interfaces appear to be a promising concept for image workstations in second generation PACS.

In the Advance Informatics in Medicine (AIM) exploratory phase, an adaptive, co-operative workstation user interface has been conceived and underlying models of information needs have been acquired and implemented. The remainder of this chapter will discuss these achievements. Before we continue to discuss some of the benefits and drawbacks of adaptive systems, the following definitions of terms shall be given that apply for this chapter:

Diagnostic context. A diagnostic work setting characterized by the current workstation user, diagnostic task, and patient case.

Diagnostic information requirements. All material (documents, facts, data, knowledge) needed in a diagnostic context for successful diagnostic work.

Adaptive workstation user interface. A user interface that changes a distinct part of its functionality at system run-time, if a specific diagnostic context is presumed.

Co-operative workstation user interface. An adaptive workstation user interface that supports users actively in reaching their goals in the diagnostic process by providing relevant information in a given context (on self-initiative or on request). Co-operative actions are based on explicit models of context-dependent diagnostic information requirements. In hospital-integrated PACS, the main motivation for co-operative workstation user interfaces is to simplify and speed-up multimedia document access and presentation. The overall objectives can be summarized as follows:

1. To increase the efficiency of routinely performed work procedures by simplifying and speeding up information access. Unacceptable and unnecessary waiting periods for document retrieval can be avoided by appropriately preloading relevant images. Information requirement models are the basis for preloading mechanisms.
2. To increase the effectiveness and accuracy of the diagnostic work by volunteering needed information (additional information that contributes to solving the problem), and by focusing on relevant information (discarding the vast amount of irrelevant information).
3. To increase the usability and acceptability of digital information systems in radiology by convenient and fast information access and problem-fitting information presentation.

From the user's point of view, co-operative actions should be adequate and supportive, they must not result in "surprising" and disturbing effects. In other words, there is a strong demand that the consistency and predictivity of user interfaces should not be affected by the adaptation mechanisms. An adequately designed static user unterface is an important precondition for a successful adaptive system.

From the workstation designer's point of view, part of the workstation's user interface has to be controlled by explicit, formalized, and computable descriptions (models) of context-dependent diagnostic information requirements. These models will not only guide the design process, but will define distinct parts of the workstation's functionality at run-time. This allows for interactive modifications and extentions of the functionality on a high level of abstraction, for example, expressed by rules. As the models have to be acquired in close collaboration with the user community, a user-centered design concept is mandatory for adaptive interfaces.

6.2.2 State of the Art in Adaptive User Interface Design

The design of adaptive systems is a research discipline in its infancy, although in recent years the interest in various kinds of adaptive user interfaces has substantially increased. Adaptivity appears to be a natural issue in the

Table 6.1. Levels of adaptivity in user interface design

Level	Designation	Description
0	Adapted	Designed system that perfectly fits to its users' needs
0.5	Adaptable	Tailorable (to be adapted by user or system supplier)
1	Adaptive (discriminative)	Discriminates among multiple choices, fixed response per choice
2	Adaptive (self-regulating)	Interprets the environment, learns, evaluates the success of an adaptation strategy
3	Adaptive (self-mediating)	Interprets the environment, builds models and plans
4	Adaptive (self-modifying)	Reasons about purpose, evaluates the evaluation

framework of user-centered design. It is a vital requirement for models that guide the design process to be explicit, formalized, and represented in a computer executable way. Consequently, the discussion of adaptive user interfaces was stimulated quite considerably by the availability of representation techniques offered by knowledge-based systems technology. Basic contributions for a domain-independent design methodology and terminology of adaptive system have been provided, for example, by Browne et al. (1987) and Totterdell et al. (1987). Generally speaking, adaptive user interfaces relate their functioning to the context they work in. To achieve context sensitivity, system actions and reactions have to be based on knowledge about the specific requirements of users and tasks and about the general task domain. These explicit user, task and domain models may be representations of quite a different nature, purpose, and complexity. They may be prespecified, e.g., using a priori knowledge of the medical diagnostic process as derived from interviews or questionaires, or acquired and updated during the users' dialogues. The purpose of adaptation and the degree of adaptivity may be defined in wide limits. A classification of possible levels of adaptivity in system design (Table 6.1) has been proposed by Totterdell et al. (1987):

Among human factors researchers, in the general discussion of the pros and cons of the various kinds of adaptive systems (levels 1–4) a consensus has not yet been reached; for example, there are open questions concerning the difficulty of trading adaptivity against consistency, the effect of recursive human-machine adaptation cycles, or social implications with user models. The investigation of co-operative image workstations described later in this chapter focuses on adaptivity up to level 1, with a clear option to be extended by concepts of automatic model updating through learning mechanisms (level 2). The last two levels mentioned (3 and 4) are certainly not in reach of today's technology, and their desirability for user interfaces in general appears doubtful. A number of adaptive user interfaces have been implemented with knowledge-based tools in the area of office automation (Hein et al. 1987), electonic mail systems (Adhami et al. 1987) or in support of computer operating systems (Alty and McKell 1986). No adaptive user interfaces have been proposed yet for problems in medical care, although their benefits (problem fitting design for heterogeneous user groups and a diversity of tasks, co-operative system behavior) appear to be attractive in this field. A framework for the terminology of user and task models has been proposed by various authors, e.g., Streitz (1988). The content of meaningful user and task models, both for user groups (stereotypes) and individuals, has been investigated for various applications, ranging from computer-aided book recommendation (Rich 1983) to computer-aided learning systems (Benyon et al. 1987). User and task modeling approaches have not yet been reported for workstations in diagnostic radiology. First adaptation scenarios have been discussed by Wendler (1987a, 1989), while benefits of user models have been emphazised by Braudes et al. (1989).

6.2.3 Scenario for Adaptive, Co-operative PACS Workstations

Compared with nonadaptive, static user interfaces, a co-operative workstation needs two additional system components:

1. A formal model of the user's requirements (here: models of information requirements in diagnostic radiology).
2. A strategy by which users can be supported on the basis of this model (the adaptation mechanism).

This section is concerned with the adaptation mechanism. In the course of the hospital integrated PACS (HIPACS) project, the following questions were addressed:

- What is the objective and the scope for adaptation?
- What is the basic theory, how the objectives can be reached?
- What will become visible to the user?
- What are the sources of evidence (data, facts) on which the adaptation process can be based?
- How can the effects of adaptation be measured and evaluated?
- What are the implementation strategies for adaptive systems?

As mentioned earlier, the global objective for co-operative workstation user interfaces was defined to be the active support of document access and presentation in a fully digital PACS. This should simplify and speed up routine work procedures and assist users in problem-solving tasks. The principal adaptation mechanism was designed to volunteer (select, access, and display) needed pieces of information in a given diagnostic context. Thus, the workstation should be seen by its users as being a co-operative dialogue partner that actively (on self-initiative or on request) tries to fulfil the user's current diagnostic information requirements. For practical pur-

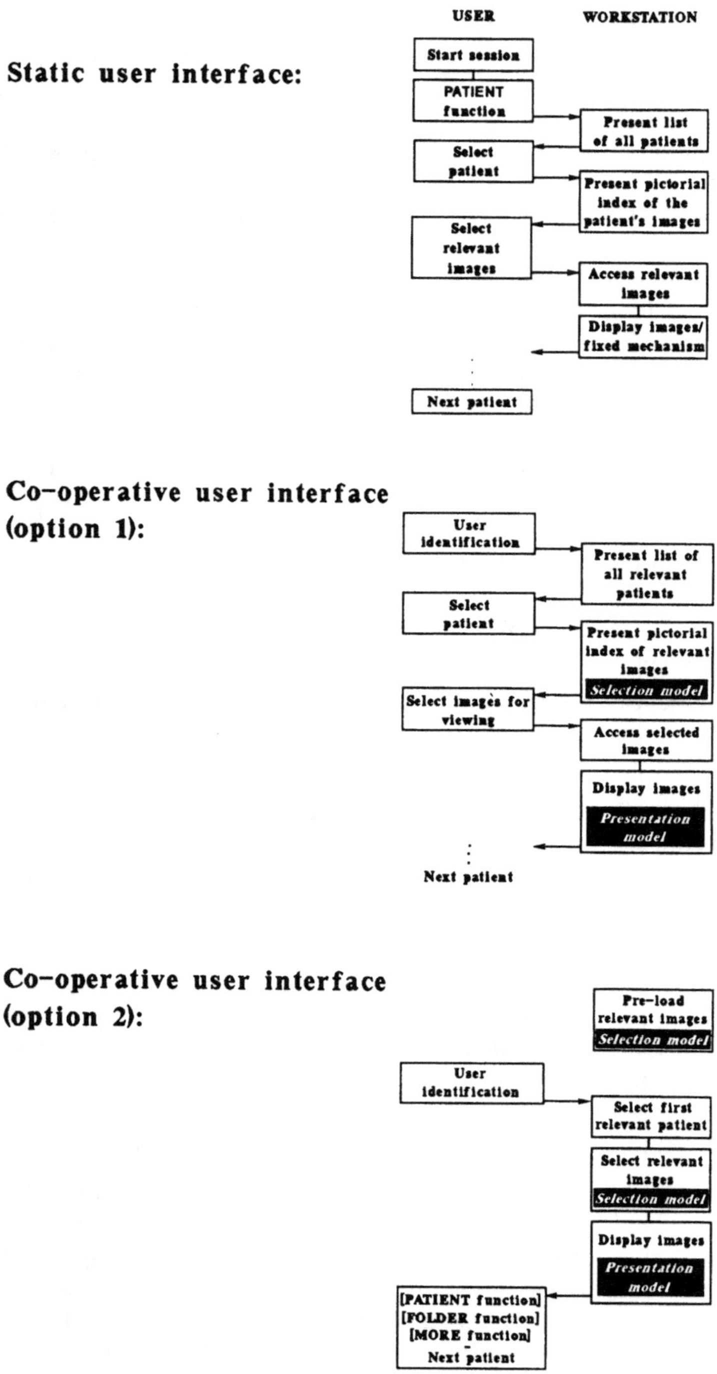

Fig. 6.5. Example of sessions with static and adaptive user interfaces

poses, the scope of the adaptation mechanism was restricted (in the AIM exploratory phase) to the co-operative selection and display arrangement of image-type documents (images and image sequences.)

The effect of possible co-operative actions will be shown by three examples that demonstrate different options for the degree of adaptation. The examples in Fig. 6.5 present a sequence of typical image access and display operations that may occur in a routine reporting session. The actions taken by the user and the workstation are shown separately on both sides on the drawing. The example session consists of (a) session start (user log in procedure and task definition); (b) selection of the first patient from a list of patients; (c) selection of the patient's relevant images from a pictorial index; (d) image access and image arrangement on the display screen; (e) image reading; (f) report dictation; and (g) next patient(s).

Fig. 6.5a gives a possible sequence of actions with a nonadaptive, static user interface. The interaction for selecting images and arranging them on the display screen may be based on direct manipulation techniques with pointing devices. Interfaces like this were proposed and demonstrated early in PACS design (e.g., Wendler et al. 1986). The list of patients and the pictorial index of images show all available information, i.e., all current patients and the complete contents of the patient's image folder. For large folders, paging mechanisms may be used. The arrangement of images on the viewing area follows fixed mechanisms, e.g., images selected from the folder appear in adjacent viewports with reduced size, or in overlapping viewports with the best possible resolution in the middle of the screen. Fig 6.5b gives a possible sequence of actions with a co-operative user interface (option 1). Based on a selection model, only a subset of patient relevant for this radiologist and his/her current task is listed, and only relevant images appear in the pictorial index. As a typical example, from 80 images found in a patient folder only two mandatory images (from the current examination) and four images of additional interest (from previous exams) may be presented. The image arrangement (after selection) is controlled by a presentation model. In option 1, the selection process from lists and pictorial indexes is left to the user.

Fig. 6.5c gives an alternative sequence of co-operative actions that illustrates a far more extended adaptation scenario (option 2). Prior to the user's work session, images expected to be relevant are selected and preloaded into the workstation's fast access memory, During the session, the selection process from lists and pictorial indexes is automated. In principle, this mechanism generates – immediately after user identification – an appropriate presentation of all relevant images for the first relevant patient. Later on, the session may continue by activating a NEXT PATIENT menu field. The selection criteria for preloading have to consider all anticipated tasks and users and will, therefore, generally differ from those used in specific work settings.

Despite these adaptation mechanisms, which are designed to considerably speed up and simplify image access and presentation, the user may at any time decide to perform other tasks if necessary, e.g., look at the complete list of patients or the complete contents of the patient folder, select additional images, and rearrange images on the screen.

6.2.4 Sources of Evidence for the Adaptation Process

The proposed adaptation mechanism can only be realized if sufficient sources of evidence (knowledge, facts, data) for co-operative decision processes are available. Four principal information sources can be identified:

1. *General domain knowledge* about the medical diagnostic process, which includes knowledge about general procedures and concepts found in radiological practice, e.g., information requirements arising from categories of diagnostic work like routine diagnostic, or follow-up diagnostic. Basic knowledge about examination types or anatomical and pathological codes will also be modelled here.
2. *Task and user models*, which define information requirements for specific, predefined diagnostic tasks like reporting, demonstration, or image quality check, and for specific user groups or individuals.
3. *Domain status data*, which describe the properties of all current radiological objects, e.g., all available information on currently existing patients, examinations, images, or reports. For co-operative decision processes, the objects of radiological interest must possess a rich set of descriptions from which conclusions can be derived. A typical set of object descriptions will be described later in this chapter. The properties of object instances are important facts to be used as a basis for co-operative actions.
4. *Interactive data* which are captured from the user's input during the work session. Useful dialogue data such as function calls, or object rearrangements may be gathered and interpreted. The system may also take the initiative itself and enter metadialogues to clarify the user's goals or needs, e.g., for the current task.

The first two knowledge sources in this list describe heuristics about diagnostic information requirements that have been acquired in the course of the HIPACS project in close co-operation with experts from clinical radiology. In the following, the methodology for knowledge acquisition and the resulting models will be described.

6.2.5 Context-Sensitive Models of Diagnostic Information Requirements

6.2.5.1 Methods of Knowledge Acquisition

According to the limited scope of the proposed adaptation mechanisms in the HIPACS project, the following questions had to be answered in order to formulate models of diagnostic information requirements:

1. Which documents (especially images and image sequences) from previous examinations are relevant for the current examination, and which properties (document parameters) define the criteria that make them relevant?
2. How should current and previous images be arranged on the display screen?
3. How can the acquired knowledge of diagnostic information requirements be structured, formalized, and implemented in a computer executable representation system?

A general objective for modelling image selection was to focus, whenever possible, on the goals of the diagnostic process rather than on the features and limitations of currently used tools. Models of diagnostic information requirements were acquired in close co-operation with the two clinical partners in the HIPACS project, the University Hospital of Aachen (Clinic for Diagnostic Radiology) and the University Hospital of Brussels (AZ-VUB, Department of Radiology). For the investigations, the following methodology was used.

Introduction to department organization and data flow. In a number of meetings, a general introduction to the radiological procedures and an explanation of department organization and the image data flow were given in both hospitals by members of the clinical staff. In addition, typical goal-oriented radiological work procedures were defined. The staff involved in radiology was described with respect to their role in the diagnostic process.

Inventory and classification of the documents of radiological interest. A complete list of all routinely used documents, e.g., images, image sequences, reports, and request forms, and document-collections, e.g., various kind of folders, acquisitions, examinations, and studies, was assembled. All document types were described in terms of their typical properties and their relation to other documents. A list of all routinely performed examinations was provided by the University Hospital of Aachen (in total, 386 different types of examinations), and a hierarchical anatomical description was assigned to each examination type. In the course of the project, the assembled information on the documents of radiological interest was directly translated into an object-oriented representation system.

Interviews with radiologists (recorded on audio tape). In the search for heuristics of diagnostic information requirements, interviews with principal radiologists and radiological assistants were made in both hospitals. The participants were encouraged to formulate their answers in terms of rules. In Aachen, the interviews were recorded on audio tape, and the written results of interviews were iterated in various subsequent sessions. After structuring and formalizing the knowledge in a rule-based system, interviews were also used as an initial step to validate the acquired knowledge. Interview questions focused on the relevance of various document types in different work situations. Radiologists were asked to define information requirements that arise for, e.g., a given diagnostic task, clinical question, current examination type, or the patient's actual disease.

Protocols of routine viewing sessions (using questionnaires). Protocols of real viewing sessions were taken at varying work places in the radiology department to detect observable criteria for the selection of relevant images and their display arrangement. To support this, a questionnaire was designed to capture the relevant parameter sets during the work sessions. It appeared to be desirable to protocol completely the currently used (displayed) images and additionally all available documents belonging to a particular patient (even those which existed but were not available due to loss). The image arrangement was also sketched on the questionnaire. During the sessions, radiologists were asked to assess the image arrangement using five categories:

1. Mandatory from the medical point of view
2. Appropriate
3. Clinical standard (may vary among hospitals or departments)
4. Personal style (subjective preference)
5. Pragmatic reasons, e.g., limited space on lightbox

Although this was a promising approach to detect information requirements objectively, it turned out to be quite difficult to fill in the entire questionnaire in synchronism with the radiologists' working speed. Altogether, the reading of 108 examinations was protocoled in reporting sessions at different work places in the department.

Simulated viewing sessions with selected cases. Mainly to validate results of the initial knowledge acquisition, simulated clinical viewing sessions were carried out with well-prepared and completely known patient cases. As an advantage of this method, the entire image material and clinical information of a patient was available, i.e., the complete image folder and all alphanumerical documents. In a simulated environment, it was also possible for the investigator to ask the radiologist for deeper explanations. In the University Hospital of Aachen, a total of ten representative cases were selected and discussed in simulated sessions.

6.2.5.2 Methods for Knowledge Representation

Parallel to the clinical knowledge acquisition activities, efforts were made to structure and formalize the results. Two parallel but interdependent modelling approaches were taken:

- The formal description of all entities found in clinical radiology, e.g., departments, documents, tasks, persons, and data, and their properties and relationships. This can be seen as a descriptive static model of the domain of radiology. Its representation was achieved by means of an *object-oriented* system using a language that supports object-oriented design (OBJECTIVE C).
- The formal description of context-dependent diagnostic information requirements, which was achieved with a *rule-based* representation

system. In this scheme, models are defined by rule sets. The various models were implemented using the expert system shell NEXPERT OBJECT.

Object-Oriented Model of the Entities of Radiological Interest

A complex world of objects was found in both radiology departments investigated that appears to be typical for most hospitals. For the implementation of objects, the principles of object-oriented design were applied. In object-oriented systems, all relevant real-world entities are described as strictly encapsulated units (objects) that communicate with each other via messages. Procedures activated in an object by messages are referred to as methods. The object's methods define the functionality of a static workstation user interface. A comprehensive introduction to the concepts of object-oriented programming is given by Cox (1987). An explanation of its benefits for the design of image workstations in radiology can be found in Grewer et al. (1989).

It is useful to structure objects into class hierarchies. Classes are prototypes for object instances, where instances receive the properties of their class and all super classes (inheritance). Figure 6.6 shows a fraction of the obtained class structure for some documents of radiological interest. Two kinds of relationships between objects are considered in the diagram:

- "IS_A" relations (class structure), indicated by solid lines, e.g., an MR_IMAGE is a kind of IMAGE, an IMAGE is a kind of DOCUMENT.
- "HAS" relations, indicated by dashed lines, e.g., an EXAMINATION consists of (has) a number of acquisitions, an IMAGE SEQUENCE consists of IMAGES. During system operation, "has" relations point to object instances. Only a few example relations are shown in Fig. 6.6.

Most of these object classes possess a rich set of properties. Taking the example of the object class REQUEST_FORM (in traditional radiology this is a paper form used by the referring physician to request a radiological examination), the following typical object properties were found: date of request; patient demographic data, e.g., name, birthday; clinical question; supposed diagnosis; requested examination type; basic disease; actual disease; referring department; and referring physician.

Some relevant properties for other objects are shown in Fig. 6.6. As the property values of object instances represent facts which can be tested in the condition parts of rules, they are of central importance for the formulation of co-operative decision processes.

Rule-Based Models of Diagnostic Information Requirements

The definition of information requirement models will be described in the following using some examples. Participants in interviews were asked to

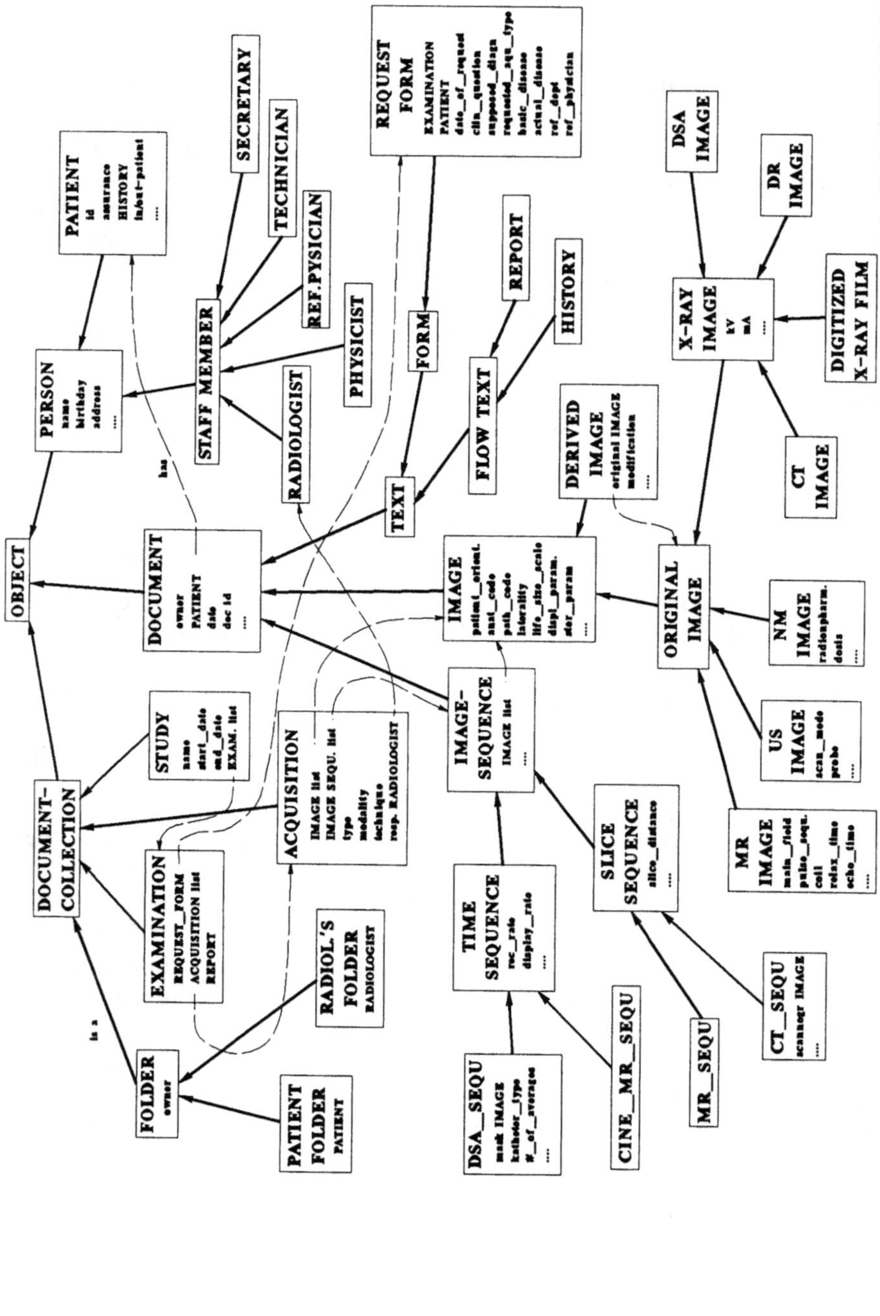

Fig. 6.6. Part of the world of objects found in diagnostic radiology

formulate rule-like sentences for the relevance of images and their display arrangement in the context of different diagnostic tasks and patient cases. A large number of rules and other sentences were recorded on audio tape. Early in knowledge acquisition, it became apparent that the majority of rules focused on a relatively small set of hypotheses. Typical output of the initial knowledge acquisition phase were statements like: "If an examination [in a reporting session] can be classified as 'Routine diagnostic', then only the current images are relevant and images from previous examinations are not. However, induced by the diagnostic findings, previous images may in some cases become relevant. 'Routine diagnostic' then may change to 'Primary diagnostic' . . .". Asked for a definition of the terms used, it turned out that, e.g., "Routine diagnostic" was defined as an event where the clinical question associated with an examination is missing or cannot be clarified by the requested examination type (apparent for thorax examinations with typical clinical questions such as "preparation for treatment" or "blood donation"). Furthermore, it came out that only *thorax* examinations were classified as "routine diagnostic". Ten types of conventional thorax examinations are performed in the department: THOR, in two projections; THBE, in bed; THLI, with patient lying; THPA, posterior–anterior projection; THIE, in expiration; THDL, fluoroscopy; THHA, with patient hanging (padiatrics); THIN, made at the intensive care unit; THKN, bony thorax; KATH, catheter control. Only the first four examination types were designated "routine thorax candidates". From this point, it was feasible to create a number of rules to test the hypothesis "Is routine diagnostic" and, consequently, "No previous images relevant". Part of the rule network for the hypothesis "is routine diagnostic" (belonging to the general model of radiology) is shown in Fig. 6.7. Another example for a rule is given in Fig. 6.8.

Once the decision for a rule-based system had been settled, the main activity was to structure the acquired knowledge and to reformulate and formalize it in terms of valid rules. A set of relevant hypotheses had to be defined with appropriate conditions that could be verified by the system at run-time, using facts (properties of object instances) found in the object world. In creating problem-fitting hypotheses, it turned out that the selection of relevant documents from previous examinations was strongly determined by a construct called "diagnostic category". The diagnostic categories were defined and formulated as rule hypotheses (Table 6.2).

For typical pairs (e.g., diagnostic category: task), the relevance of previous images was defined using the classification scheme "mandatory", "useful", and "of secondary interest". For example, the transcript of the rule for "mandatory" would read as follows:

```
HYPOTHESIS    images_mandatory
IF            task = "pre_examination_viewing"
        AND   diagnostic_category = "succeeding_diagnostic"
        AND   current_exam.type = "MYE" (myelography)
```

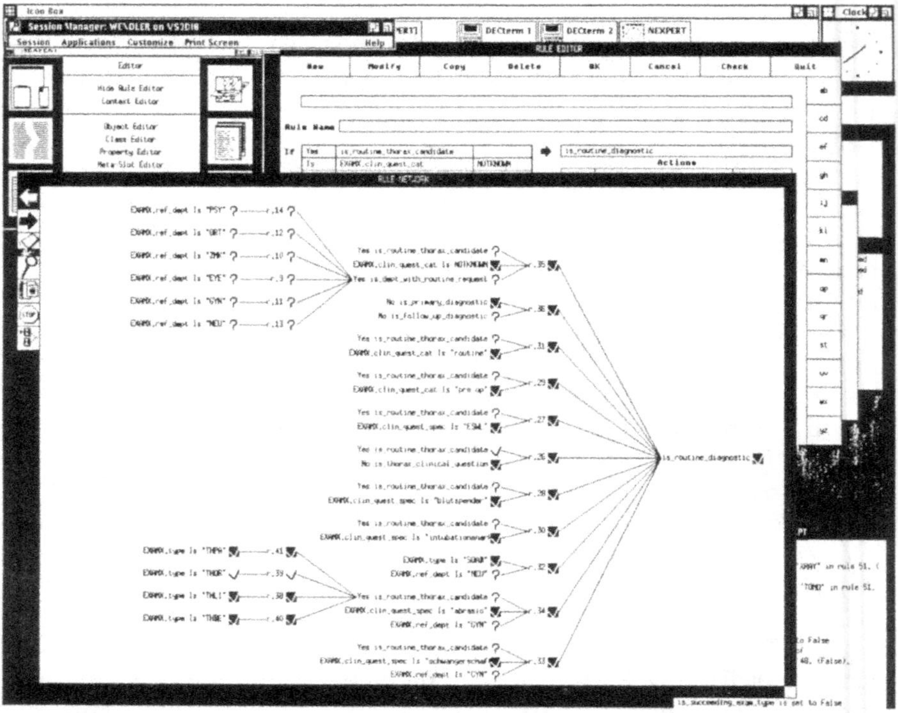

Fig. 6.7. NEXPERT OBJECT rule browsing and editing environment (for hypothesis "is_routine_diagnostic")

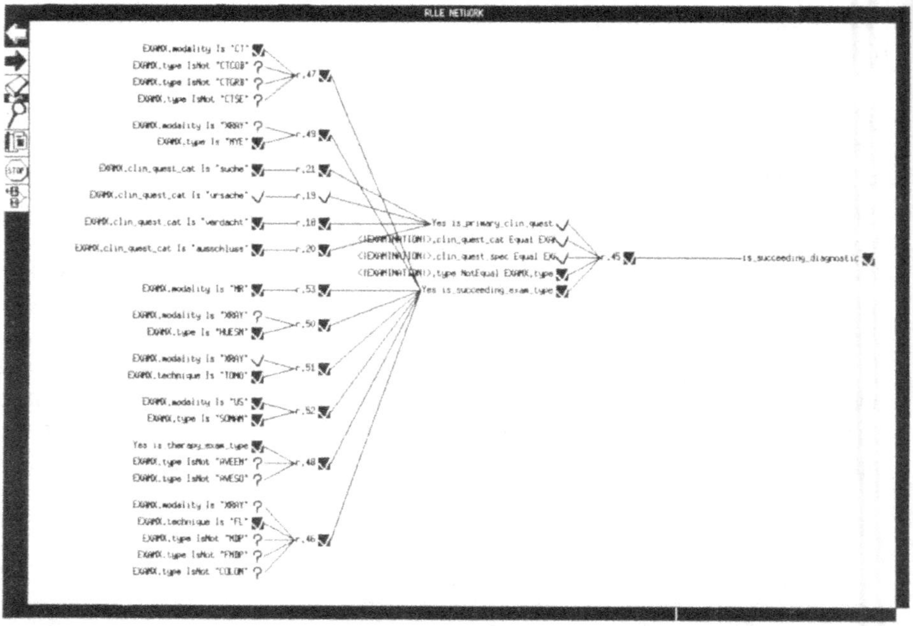

Fig. 6.8. Part of the rule network for the hypothesis "is_succeeding_diagnostic"

Table 6.2. Diagnostic categories and their description

Diagnostic category (rule hypothesis)	Description
Routine diagnostic	Detection of abnormal imaging signs in thorax examinations with nonthoracical clinical questions, mostly in the context of precautions
Primary diagnostic	Image interpretation in the context of primary clinical questions, e.g., reason for . . . , suspicion of . . . , exclusion of . . .
Initial diagnostic	Initial step of primary diagnostic. No radiological history available for the current clinical question
Succeeding diagnostic	Subsequent (2nd to *n*th) step to primary diagnostic (proceeding to more invasive and costly types of examinations). A radiological history exists for the current clinical question
Repeating diagnostic	Primary diagnostic when the same examination type is repeated
Follow-up diagnostic	Control actions in the context of a radiological or clinical patient history
Status control	Follow-up diagnostic that checks for conditions after an event or treatment, e.g., position control of catheter
Comparing follow-up	Follow-up image interpretation that checks for changes by comparison with previous documents, e.g., images before and after treatment, evaluation of the course of a disease

THEN mandatory: exam.type = "LWS" (lumbar spine)
qualifier: "most recent"

This explains that in a pre-examination viewing task, in this case preceding a myelography, the most recently made conventional X-ray images of the lumbar spine in two projections are relevant. These images are known to exist, because myelography is always a diagnostic step following conventional X-ray images of the spine. Using a rule-based representation system, models of context-dependent information requirements can be realized as rule sets, where the appropriate set is activated in a given context. To resolve conflicts, models were assigned priorities, where higher priority numbers overrule lower ones (Table 6.3).

In this priority scheme, preferences of individual users will overrule for example default assumptions defined for a user group or for radiology in general. User models are activated upon user identification, e.g., by log-in procedure. Task models may be activated by declaration, e.g., the user may declare that he is going to start a reporting task by menu selection, or by default assumptions generated by inference processes, e.g., the assumption that this user normally starts reporting at about 2 P.M. Mainly the task and user models contain hypotheses that define the relevance of images. If the models are used as a consultant in a co-operative user interface, the action

Table 6.3. Priority scheme for diagnostic information requirement models

Priority	Model type	Description
1	General model of radiology	Rule set for general information requirements, e.g., the definition of diagnostic categories, and generic object-classes of diagnostic relevance. This rule set will always be activated
2	Task models	Rule sets for task-specific information requirements. One set at a time will be activated if there is evidence for a specific tasks
3	Group user models	Rule sets for user group specific information requirements, e.g., for radiologists. One set at a time will be activated for a specific user of that group
4	Individual user model	Rule sets for specific information requirements of individuals (personal preferences). One set at a time will be activated for the specific individual

Table 6.4. Hypotheses and possible actions

Rule hypothesis	Adaptation mechanism (possible action)
Images mandatory	Images will be preloaded to the workstation's local workfile. On patient selection, these images will be displayed automatically
Images useful	Images will be preloaded, but shown only on the user's request
Images of secondary interest	Images will not be preloaded, but shown as miniature versions in pictorial indexes
Remaining (irrelevant) images	Images will not be preloaded and shown in folder indexes as text strings; they are available only on the user's explicit access request

parts of the rules may contain varying recommendations how to react. Examples for hypotheses and actions are given in Table 6.4.

Information classified as "useful" or "of secondary interest" is, for example, images from previous examinations that share a common anatomical code with the current examination. For this kind of similarity retrieval, a data base was set up that defines "useful" and "interesting" images by means of a hierarchical anatomical key. The example in Table 6.5 illustrates the codification system.

Some common patterns were found that define individual preferences for the display arrangement of images or image series. Typical viewing recommendations for multiple or single images (still reflecting film-based

Table 6.5. Example of the anatomical codification system

Examination	Anatomical key	Subkeys	Related examinations	
THOR thorax	630	620	THKN	bony thorax
		321	BWS	thoracic spine
		308	LWS	upper lumbar spine
		...		

viewing) are, for example, parallel viewing, chronological arrangement (A, B, C . . . left to right/top to bottom); parallel viewing, anatomical arrangement (A, B, C . . . left to right/top to bottom); parallel viewing, paired arrangement (A left of/right of B); concurrent viewing in sequence (A, B, C . . .); image upside down.

This is illustrated by an example of an image arrangement scheme found for two consecutive thorax examinations (current and old exam, each in posterior/anterior and lateral projection): for comparison in follow-up diagnosis the preferred display arrangement for these four images was the following: [(THOR/lat, old) right_of (THOR/pa, old)] right_of [(THOR/pa, current) right_of (THOR/lat, current)]

The rule-based models of diagnostic information requirements were implemented using the expert system shell NEXPERT OBJECT, which offers a convenient graphical user interface for rule editing. Rules can be easily displayed, modified, and extended. The system offers a variety of inference strategies, easy interfacing to the object world implemented in OBJECTIVE C, and the possibility of integrating various data base systems.

6.2.6 Architectures for Implementing Adaptive PACS Workstations

Apparently, workstations with adaptive, co-operative user interfaces must incorporate a variety of knowledge bases, data, and procedures that represent models, facts, and algorithms on quite different levels of abstraction. To handle the complexity of this situation for prototyping, a layered system structure has been designed that separates (from bottom to top) between:

1. Real-time layer. Workstation hardware and low-level (hardware-related) software.
2. Object layer. The object world with a complex structure of object classes, properties and methods.
3. Model layer. The rule-based models of radiological information requirements in the context of tasks, users and patient cases.

A block diagram of the layered workstation architecture is shown in Fig. 6.9. The three layers are briefly characterized in the following.

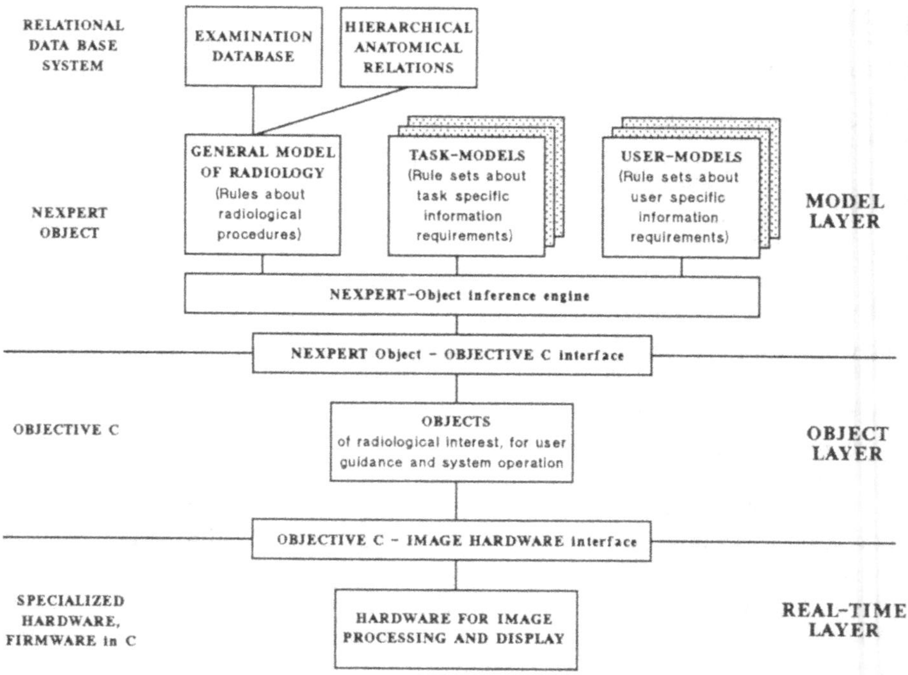

Fig. 6.9. Block diagram of a layered architecture for an adaptive image workstation

6.2.6.1 Real-time Layer

The real-time layer is responsible for fulfilling the conditions of responsiveness defined in the user interface scenario. It particularly has to offer solutions for all speed problems induced by high-resolution image storage, transmission, display, and processing operations. A typical hardware architecture for this problem has already been described in the first part of this chapter (Fig. 6.4).

Besides of special purpose image processing hardware, the real-time layer also includes hardware-related firmware written in C. Although being separated for speed reasons, the hardware and firmware are logically considered to be part of the object layer. They can be looked at as object methods implemented by means of separate high-speed processors.

6.2.6.2 Object Layer

The complex world of objects with their properties, methods, and relationships is represented in the object layer of the system using a language that supports object-oriented design (OBJECTIVE C). Typical objects for medical image workstations fall into a number of categories:

1. Objects of radiological interest, e.g., images, examinations, reports, and folders. These are the most important objects from the user's point of view. The objects of radiological interest have already been discussed in Sect. 6.2.5.2.
2. Objects that support interaction and user guidance, e.g., menu fields and all kinds of graphical objects found in a direct manipulation environment. Most of the workstation's functionality is operated via these objects.
3. System objects that are invisible to the user and help to maintain the proper running of the workstation, e.g., workfiles, memory managers, and network interfaces. The user need not be aware of their methods, properties, or even existence.

6.2.6.3 Model Layer

The model layer represents knowledge about context-dependent diagnostic information requirements and the adaptation mechanism in terms of the described rule sets (implemented with NEXPERT OBJECT). The model layer may act as an intelligent consulting system that serves explicit requests initiated by objects, e.g., the folder object may request a list of relevant images to be presented in a pictorial index. Typical elements of information exchange between object and model layer are shown in Fig. 6.10. The model layer may also act on self-initiative by regularly scanning the properties of available object instances, deriving conclusions, and initiating actions in the object layer.

6.2.7 Discussion and Perspective for Future Work

An adaptive image workstation user interface has been designed that acts as a co-operative dialogue partner, supporting information access and presentation in the complex technical environment of PACS. As a first mechanism for adaptation, the co-operative, context-dependent selection of images and their appropriate display arrangement has been investigated, where the context was defined in terms of different diagnostic tasks, workstation users and clinical patient cases. The realization of adaptive user interfaces is only possible with a deep understanding of the clinical radiological process and the users' goal-oriented tasks in that process. A continuous involvement of end users is mandatory for the design process of such interfaces. As an advantage over nonadaptive interfaces, information requirement models do not only guide implementation, but are also an integral part of the workstation's functionality. The explicitness and formality of models support the convenient and fast revision of design assumptions and facilitate the correction of misconceptions. In summary, the design of adaptive user interfaces is in essence a user-centered design and offers the potential for better user interfaces.

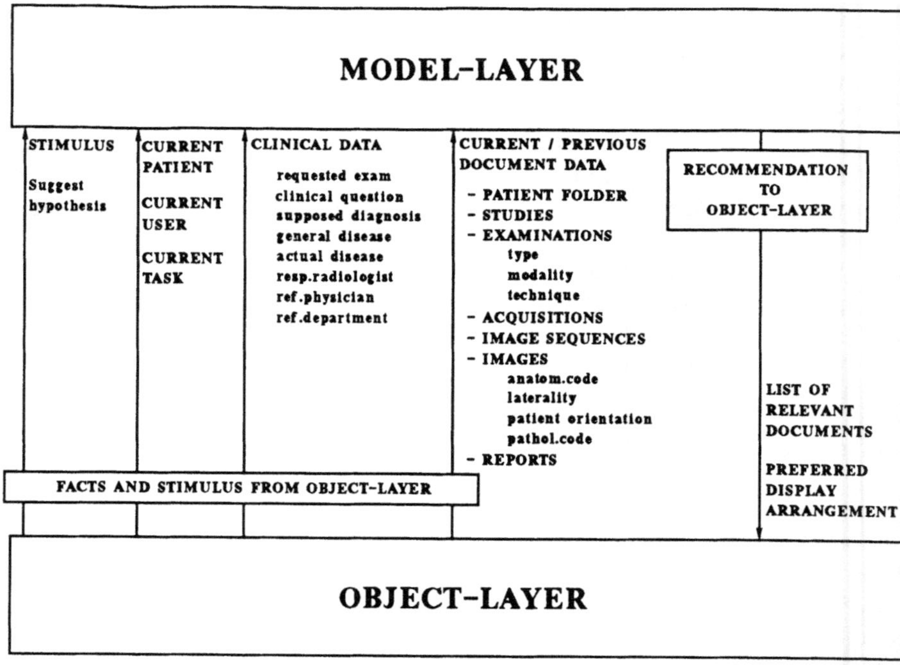

Fig. 6.10. Typical elements of communication between object and model layer

In the course of the HIPACS project, a first attempt has been made to acquire and formalize models of diagnostic information requirements and to implement and integrate these models into a layered architecture of an adaptive image workstation. For demonstration of the adaptation mechanisms in the AIM exploratory phase, all three system layers were realized on a conventional off-the-shelf workstation (VAXstation 3100). The hybrid software architecture and the use of object-oriented and rule-based techniques offered a sound approach for knowledge representation and system integration. The implementation of the real-time layer for a workstation prototype to be evaluated in a clinical environment has started.

The described activities for adaptive user interface design should be regarded as a starting point. The resulting models of diagnostic information requirements acquired so far are certainly incomplete and probably in parts not precise enough. Clear perspectives are indicated for follow-up activities on model validation and evaluation of the adaptation mechanism with adaptive image workstation prototypes in a clinical environment.

6.2.8 Acknowledgement

The acquisition of diagnostic information requirement models and their convertion to an object-oriented and rule-based representation system would have been impossible without the fruitful collaboration between the authors and their clinical partners at the University Hospitals of Aachen and Brussels. We would like to acknowledge the work of all people who contributed to the success of the investigation by explaining radiological procedures, participating in interviews or viewing sessions, and helping to formulate the rule system. In particular, our thanks are due to Dr. Berthold Wein from the Clinic of Diagnostic Radiology in Aachen for his indispensible contributions in generating, structuring, and validating rules and in providing complete and detailed information about the radiological work procedures, examinations, anatomical codes, and numerous other subjects that proved to be relevant for the project. We would also like to thank S. Kaviani who provided a large number of protocols from routine viewing sessions taken at various work places in Aachen. From Brussels we appreciated the helpful input of Renaat van den Broeck, who gave valuable information in the initial knowledge acquisition phase. Finally, we would like to thank Rüdiger Grewer from the RUBI^{3}CON project team for his contributions in object creation and user interface implementation.

References

Adhami E, Browne DP, Mitra SK (1987) Application modelling for the provision of an adaptive interface – a knowledge based approach. In: Bullinger HJ, Shākel B (eds) Human–computer interaction: Interact '87. North Holland, Amsterdam, pp 981–987

Alty JL, McKell P (1986) Application modelling in a user interface management system. In: Harrison MD, Monk AF (eds) People and computers: designing for usability. Cambridge University Press, Cambridge, pp 319–335

Arenson RL (1990) The digital imaging workstation. Radiology 176: 303–315

Beard D, Pizer S, Rogers D, Cromartie R (1987) A prototype single screen PACS console development using human-computer interaction techniques. SPIE (Medical Imaging) 767: 646–653

Benyon D, Innocent P, Murray D (1987) System adaptivity and the modelling of stereotypes. In: Bullinger HJ, Shākel B (eds) Human–computer interaction: Interact '87. North Holland, Amsterdam, pp 245–253

Braudes RE, Mun SK, Sibert J, Schnizlein J, Horii S (1989) Workstation modelling and development: clinical definition of a PACS user interface. SPIE (Medical Imaging III) 1093: 376–386

Browne DP, Trevellyan R, Totterdell P, Norman M (1987) Metrics for the building, evaluation and comprehension of self-regulating adaptive systems. In: Bullinger HJ, Shākel B (eds) Human–computer interaction: Interact '87, North Holland, Amsterdam, pp 1081–1087

Cox BJ (1987) Object-oriented programming – an evolutionary approach. Addison Wesley, Reading, MA

Grewer R, Mönnich KJ, Schmidt J, Svensson H, Wendler T (1985) Design of interactive workstations for the interpretation of medical images in pictorial information systems. In: Lemke HU, Rhodes ML, Jaffe CC, Felix R (eds) Computer assisted radiology CAR '85. Springer, Berlin Heidelberg New York, pp 679–686

Grewer R, Mönnich KJ, Schmidt J, Svensson H, Wendler T (1989) Object-oriented design for medical image workstations. In: Lemke HU, Rhodes ML, Jaffe CC, Felix R (eds) Computer assisted radiology CAR '89. Springer, Berlin Heidelberg New York, pp 780–784

Hein HW, Kellermann G, Thomas C (1987) X-AID: A shell for building highly interactive and adaptive user interfaces. Proceedings of the tenth international joint conference on artificial intelligence. pp 97–99

Kasday LR (1986) Human factors considerations in PACS design. SPIE (Medicine XIV, PACS IV) 626: 581–592
Kowalsky G, Lux P, Meyer-Ebrecht D (1977) The electronic X-ray archive: an integral approach to filing and remote retrieval of computer-generated radiographs. Medicamundi, 22(3): 27
Lux P (1977) A novel set of closed orthogonal functions for picture coding. AEÜ 31(7/8): 267–274
Meyer-Ebrecht D (1980) The management and processing of medical pictures – an architecture for systems and processing devices. IEEE workshop on picture data management and description. August 27–29, 1980, Asilomar, CA, USA p 202
Meyer-Ebrecht D, Wendler T (1983) Concept of the diagnostic image workstation. SPIE (PACS II) 418: 180–188
Monk AF (1984) Fundamentals of human–computer interaction. Academic, New York
Norman DA (1986) Cognitive engineering. In: Norman DA, Draper S (eds) User centered system design. Erlbaum, Hillsdale, NJ, pp 31–61 (New perspectives on human–computer interaction)
O'Malley KG, Giunta JA (1988) The alternator: determination of its fundamental features, as a basis for design of a PACS diagnostic workstation. SPIE (Medical Imaging II) 914: 988–994
PACS I (1981) 1st International Conference on PACS, Newport Beach. SPIE 318
PACS II (1982) 2nd International Conference on PACS, Kansas City. SPIE 418
Pizer SM, Johnston RE, Rogers DC, Beard DV (1987) Effective presentation of medical images on an electronic display station. Radiographics 7(6): 1267–1273
Rich E (1983) Users are individuals: individualizing user models. Int J Man-Machine Stud 18: 199–214
Rogers DC, Johnston RE, Brenton B, Staab EV, Thompson B, Perry JR (1985) Predicting PACS console requirements from radiologist's reading habits, SPIE (PACS III) 536: 88–95
Rubinstein R, Hersh H (1984) The human factor. Digital, Bedford, MA
Shneiderman B (1983) The future of interactive systems and the emergence of direct manipulation. Behav Inf Technology 1(3): 237–256
Streitz NA (1988) Mental models and metaphors: implications for the design of adaptive user-computer interfaces. In: Mandl H, Lesgold A (ed) Learning issues for intelligent tutoring systems. Springer, Berlin Heidelberg New York, pp 164–186
Totterdell PA, Norman MA, Browne DP (1987) Levels of adaptivity in interface design. In: Bullinger HJ, Shākel B (eds) Human–computer interaction: Interact '87. North Holland, Amsterdam, pp 725–721
Wendler T (1985) Human–computer interaction in radiology. In: Lemke HU, Rhodes NL, Jaffe CC, Felix R (eds) Computer assisted radiology CAR '85. Springer, Berlin Heidelberg New York, pp 669–678
Wendler T (1987a) Advanced image display systems in radiology. Documed '87 Elsevier, Amsterdam. (ICS 747), pp 589–597
Wendler T (1987b) Hierarchical image coding. In: ASST '87 6th Aachen symposium on signal theory. Springer, Berlin Heidelberg New York (Informatik Fachberichte, vol 153), pp 217–228
Wendler T (1989) Co-operative human–machine interfaces for medical image workstations: a scenario. In: Lemke HU, Rhodes ML, Jaffe CC, Felix R (eds) Computer assisted radiology CAR '89. Springer, Berlin Heidelberg New York, pp 775–779
Wendler T, Wein B (1991) A rule-based model of diagnostic information requirements for the design of adaptive image workstations. In: Computer assisted radiology CAR '91. Springer, Berlin Heidelberg New York, pp 629–635
Wendler T, Grewer R, Mönnich KJ, Svensson H (1986) Design considerations for multimodality medical image workstations. In: Höhne KH (ed) Pictorial information systems in medicine. Springer, Berlin Heidelberg New York, pp 401–420 (NATO-ASI Series F, Computer and System Sciences, vol 19)

7 Data Bases

7.1 Distributed Multimedia Data Base Systems

D. Bell, D.H.O. Ling, and I.R. Young

Up to the present, picture archiving and communication systems (PACS) have used centralised image stores. It is now widely recognised that there is a need to move towards the idea of a distributed, multimedia filing system if PACS is to become practicable. The trend towards distribution, or decentralisation, of data in organisations has come about because of the need for local autonomy, modularity and extensibility of local systems, robustness of information availability in the event of component breakdown, and efficiency. Former trends which led towards centralisation of processing in the 1960s and 1970s were fuelled by "Grosch's Law", which states that the power of a computer increases as the square of its cost, a law that was clearly repealed in the 1980s. These trends have now been discontinued. So there are now well-recognised reasons, from the point of view of both technology advances and "user pull", for at least considering the possibility of a distributed image archive rather than a centralised one in a PACS.

Clinical users share the need for increased flexibility with users in manufacturing industry and other industries in the service sector such as banks. There is a clear user need, if not yet a demand, for not only accessing image archives which are distributed as described above and may be multimodal, but also integrating (possibly preexisting) relevant textual data in hospital computer files and data bases. The distributed image management functions can clearly be viewed as extensions of the general textual hospital information system (HIS). Such extensions must be based on knowledge of the users' needs and practices, and the system architecture and software must permit the user to "drive" the system evolution. Only by using distribution of information stores can the flexibility and performance of a PACS meet clinical users' needs.

7.1.1 Introduction

Relational data base systems evolved out of a "primordial soup" which came to maturity in the late 1960s. During that decade, there was much talk about integrating systems, where the key idea was to pool many application

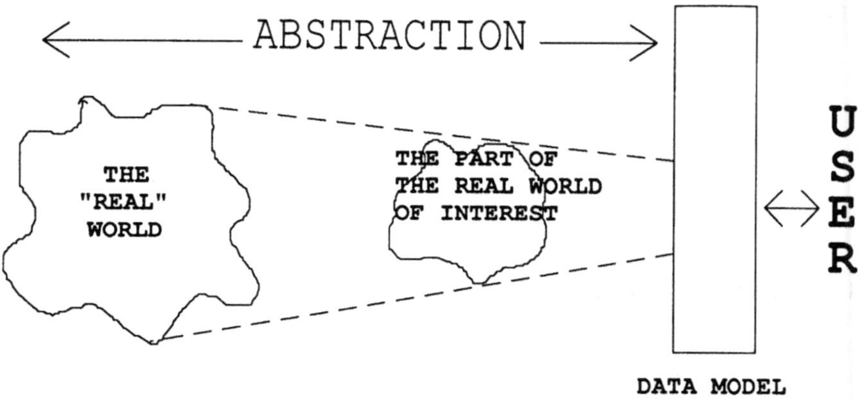

Fig. 7.1. Data model showing user's view of the universe for querying the computer

programs and their associated files to produce an "all-singing-all-dancing" system, to meet, for example, the management information system needs of corporations. A major shift in philosophy, always existing in the background, finally surfaced with the 1967–1968 Apollo space mission. In order to meet the hectic schedule for landing a man on the moon, a very powerful bill of materials package was needed, and it had to have more scope than did packages such as IBM's bill of materials program (BOMP) that were around at the time. This resulted in the development of the embryo information management system (IMS) from IBM, a package which still has considerable presence today.

In many ways this development marked the beginning of the "data base era". IMS supported the concept of a reservoir of data to be shared by the application systems of a corporation or other enterprise. The "sharing" here means that data items are usually stored only once in the reservoir, regardless of how many applications processes accessed them. Clearly this enhanced the consistency and integrity of the data and cut costs due to the redundant storage of data items. The reservoir was managed by a data base management system (DBMS) such as IMS which provided a high-level interface to the data and could be called by application programs. A data model is a logical arrangement of entities in the real world of interest in a particular application, showing their interrelationships and any constraints on the values the variables of the model describing the entities can take. A query language or a data manipulation language is needed to allow users to make queries about the "world" represented in this way (Fig. 7.1).

Although IMS was a DBMS, it was not *relational*. Around the same time as it was being developed, many researchers in informatics were seeking a *data-independent* way of maintaining data in such reservoir. This was aimed at permitting low-level (computer-oriented) changes in the data's organisation and other details to be done transparently, in the sense that these changes did not force programs using the data to be changed. Contrast

PATIENT

PATIENT	DATE OF BIRTH	SEX	DOCTOR
Smith	12/07/59	M	Jones
White	15/08/68	F	Brown
Adams	07/09/32	M	Green
Evans	09/09/86	F	Brown
Kelly	18/03/86	F	Watts

DOCTOR

DOCTOR	HOSPITAL	SPECIALITY
Brown	London	Dermatology
Jones	Leeds	Cardiology
Green	Bath	Geriatrics
Watts	Durham	Paediatrics

Fig. 7.2. The relations patient and doctor. We denote these relations as PATIENT (patient, data of birth, sex, doctor) and DOCTOR (doctor, hospital, speciality)

this with IMS, for example, which has a hierarchical structure (remember the BOMP background), and the corresponding programs accessing data have to include details of the "inverted tree" structures by which the data is represented.

The eventual result of this research was a seminal paper by E. F. Codd of IBM in 1971 (Codd 1970), who proposed a data base structure involving no navigational complexity (such as that inherent in hierarchies). He suggested using intuitively simple two-dimensional tables (relations), very similar to the tables of rows and columns commonly found in bound ledgers and other well-established and well-tried manual record-keeping systems (see Fig. 7.2). An algebra which provided operations for manipulations of the tables corresponding to common data processing operations completed the picture of a relational data base.

It took the rest of the 1970s to get to the stage where commercial products based on Codd's relational data model (ROM) were available for serious information systems. During that time, a clear understanding of the mathematical principles governing relational systems was established, and this added to the basic attraction of the model – its simplicity. This meant that the trend in computational record handling in the 1980s was predominantly relation-oriented. As a means of supporting data-independent access to data stored in the conventional records structures commonly met in accounting and other traditional data processing systems, the relational model has no peers.

However, during the 1980s attention was increasingly turned to applications that have data which are not amenable to storage in conventional fixed-format record structures. Such applications included many engineering design activities such as computer aided design (CAD) and very large scale integrated (VLSI) circuit design and also geographical information systems (GIS), where maps have to be stored. Another conspicuous example are, of course, medical imaging systems. This led to work on more complex data models and DBMS. Moreover, people working in data base research and development also saw great potential in adopting some of the developments of artificial intelligence (AI) techniques. This led to the concept of deductive data bases, which can be thought of as being quite similar to expert systems; in contrast to expert systems, however, the rule collections tend to be small, and the collections of facts governed by the rules tend to be large.

At the same time, the possibility of linking and integrating data bases scattered over many computing facilities, perhaps at geographically distributed sites, became a reality. This led to the development of distributed data base (DDB) systems, where the impression of a single data base can be presented to a *global user*, i.e., one who wants to access a collection of data bases with minimum complications.

Complementing these software and data modelling advances, there have been concurrent improvements and challenges in hardware and system methods. An important hardware (and software) development was the advent of the personal computer (PC). Perhaps even more challenging to people in the information systems industry are the advances that have been made in parallel computing, where configurations of multiple linked computers are vigorously being developed, which can solve problems by splitting the problem up and allocating processing tasks to different processors in order to facilitate the cooperation of distributed, communicating processes.

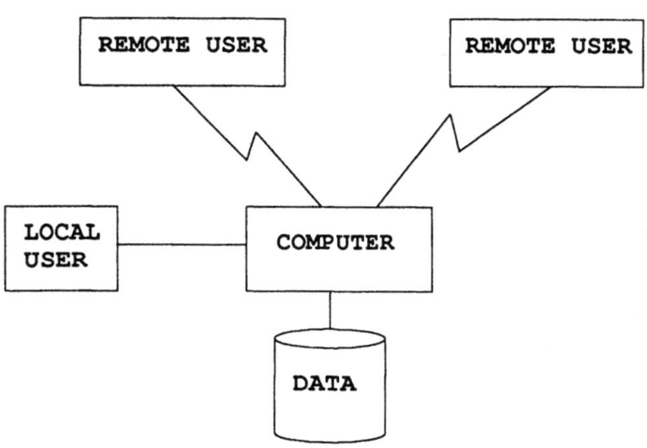

Fig. 7.3. Centralised processing

On the system side, system development methodologies have been appearing, which provide systematic neoformal methods of developing data bases and even complete application systems.

Another concept which has more recently captured the attention of many data base researchers is that of the object-oriented paradigm. One of the directions in which programming languages have advanced has been in accordance with this way of looking at things. Essentially, this approach to data modelling provides a change of orientation, away from fact-based data collections systems such as relational DBMS, to an object-based perception. So, for example, the behaviour of a real-world object of interest can be represented as a procedure and stored in a data base along with the data itself. This has the advantage of taking some application program code – that describing the behaviour under consideration – from the application program and putting it into the base, where it intuitively belongs.

The concepts and developments introduced in this very brief historical account will become clearer as we proceed through the next four sections.

7.1.2 Starting Point

7.1.2.1 Distributed Data Bases

Introduction

During the early 1970s, a DBMS and its data were often stored in one central computer and were shared among different groups of users running different applications. Terminals were linked directly into the central computer containing the DBMS and its reservoir of data (Fig. 7.3). Terminals which were local (i.e., close) to the central computer were normally physically connected to it via an RS232 wire and terminals; those far away from the computer, remote users, were linked via telephone lines. This centralised approach to data base processing was cost effective then, as it served a variety of users for both local and remote access and using various applications, and brought economies of scale.

However, as both the volume of data stored in the reservoir and the number of users increases, the central computer system becomes a bottleneck because it has to handle many activities of data processing. Firstly, it is responsible for communication processing (acting as a front end to the DBMS) for the remote users. Secondly, it handles data base processing tasks which are not complex but involve time-consuming and repetitive computer input/output operations. Finally, other general routine usage of the operating system must be carried out on the processor. As the system degrades, the waiting time for the remote users becomes intolerable. With advances of computer technology such as the provision of faster communication networks and efficient computer architectures coupled with reasonable costs of hardware, it is now possible to accommodate a wider

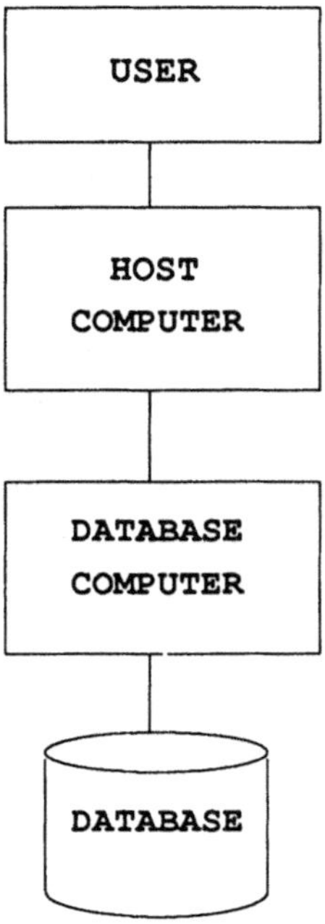

Fig. 7.4. Data base computer

range of user applications with different levels of complexity. Today, there are four existing alternatives to the centralised data base approach: DDB, data base computers, microcomputer data bases, and parallel data base computers.

The DDB approach seeks to integrate all participating computing facilities, which are all connected via some communication network, into one homogeneous software system. Among other things, this provides location transparency, i.e., users need not know on which computer a given item of data resides, and services queries in a uniform manner. This approach is attractive because it is based on the "bottom up" approach and provides ease of incorporating new computing nodes into the network.

Data base computers are conventional (Von Neumann) computing machines specifically dedicated for data base processing (Fig. 7.4). Normally there is a front end processor used for handling data communications. The main advantage of having a data base computer is that the data base machine is solely used for data base processing, freeing the other processors to handle only the remaining general processing. This increases the efficiency of data base processing and levels of security, too.

Microcomputer data bases are usually small data bases set up for the industrial needs of some restricted locality. Microcomputers or PCs have proved to be valuable assets in many organisations or enterprises today. One can get off-the-shelf data base or file management packages for this type of computing facilities at reasonable cost. This approach is justifiable because the running costs, say, for two PCs operating at two sites may be substantially less than the centralised approach when both sites require intensive data processing. However, for the purposes of our present classification they are not linked together.

Parallel data base computers, perhaps based on commodity components such as the transputers (small, powerful computers which can be linked for parallelism) are attractive because they can speed up data processing, and the components can be slotted into the back of a PC. There is still a considerable amount of research required to realise their potential for efficiency and make them user-friendly. We shall restrict the discussion in the remainder of this subsection to issues involved in DDB.

Distributed Data Base Systems

A distributed DBMS is a software system which handles data shared among a community of users, while ensuring the integrity of the data in dispersed reservoirs and providing security against unauthorised access. It provides transparency of the location of data so that users can access data from any site in the network without being aware of the geographical location of the data and details of the participating DBMS.

DDB development can be identified as falling into two different phases. During the 1970s, the development of the system R* by IBM and SDD-1 by the Computer Corporation America (CCA) marked the first generation of DDB systems. They were designed to handle a single integrated data base which was distributed over a number of geographically dispersed nodes or sites. There were no local users in such DDB systems – all users used the DDB to access data, even if they were local. These systems have several advantages over the centralised approach. Firstly, they increase the system availability in that when one or more computer nodes are down, users of the active node(s) will not be affected. Secondly, they improve performance by storing data closer to the appropriate users, and thirdly, information transmitted across the data communication channels between computer nodes is minimised. One of the main problems with DDB systems designed in this early phase is that every participating node must have identical computing software and hardware. There are referred to as homogeneous systems.

The second generation of DDB systems has been developed since 1980 to overcome the limitations of first-generation DDB systems, coupled with the desire of organisations who wish to integrate existing data bases which may have differences in character and features. The multi-data base technique was proposed as a DDB system in order to permit heterogeneity of the underlying DBMS and computers. Indeed, underlying DBMS may continue to function individually as before, supporting local users even though they are involved in the DDB. This provides the advantage of local autonomy (Fig. 7.5). At each of the local nodes, the data base administrator (DBA), who manages his local DBMS, will have the right to decide which portion of the data in his local reservoir to contribute to the reservoir of the global DDB system.

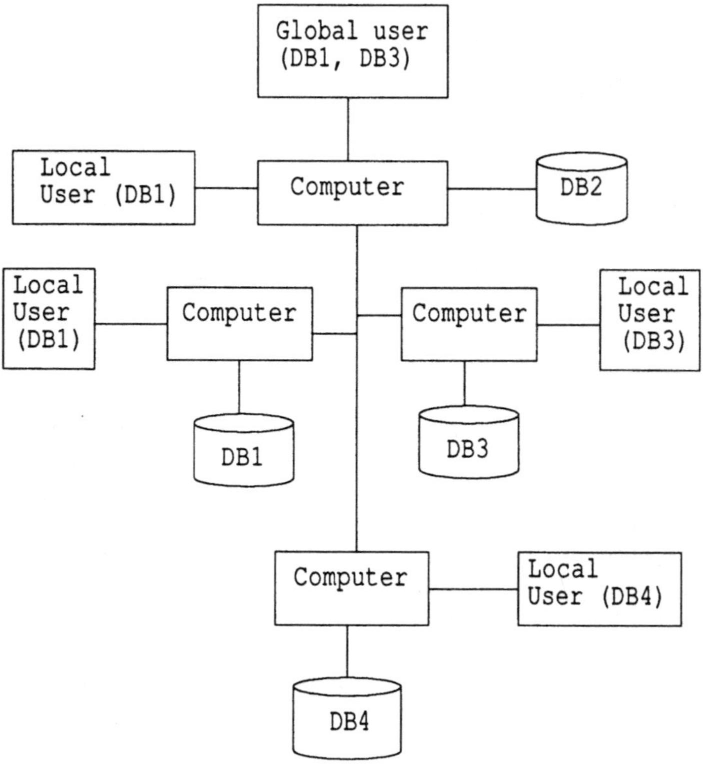

Fig. 7.5. Local and global data base users (*DB*, data base)

Issues in DDB

The architecture of the multi-data base approach is attractive because it reflects the nature of organisations well. For example, in a typical HIS, different departments may have different budget allocations for purchasing their computing equipment, which may be specialised for use, and different kinds of policies among them. Eventually, different departments would be equipped with different kinds of computer hardware and software, and often these departments are not physically close together. The philosophy of the multi-data base approach is that it should be able to incorporate any preexisting node into the DDB system with minimal human interaction. The multi-data base schema (i.e., data description layout) architecture is relational and has evolved from the three-level ANSI/SPARC data base architecture (Fig. 7.6). The main advantage of using the concept of levels schemes (see below) is the data independence – the way a user perceives the data is different from the way they are represented in the physical storage.

There are four schema levels in a multi-data base system: external, global, participation, and internal schemas. The global schema contains

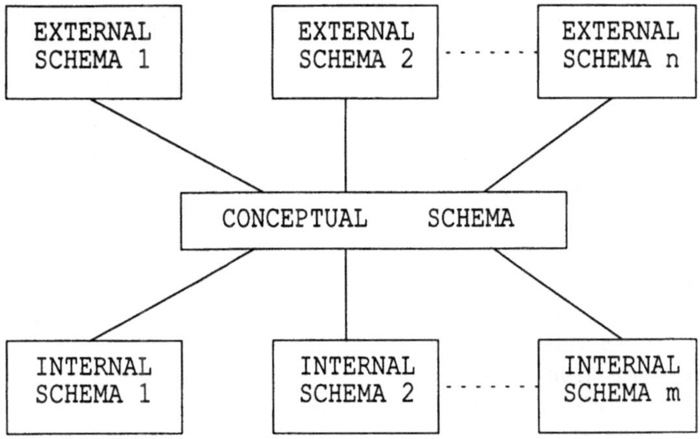

Fig. 7.6. ANSI/SPARC data base architecture

descriptions of the entire underlying data base of the DDB system together with other information used for query processing. To date, most DDB systems are based on the relational concept, and, therefore, their global schemas are described in tabular form. External schemas are collections of subsets of the global schema as presented to the end users. Therefore, different users may use different external schemas. Internal schemas describe their local site schemas. In a heterogeneous DDB system, internal schemas may be collections of representations of inverted trees (from the CODASYL or IMS DBMS), tables (from the relational DBMS) or even flat files. Participation schemas convert the underlying local internal schemas into relational form. An alternative to using the single integrated global schema is the use of qualification procedures to retrieve its underlying data bases. This approach is referred to as the federated approach.

Distributed query processing is a fairly complex process, especially in a relationally based DDB system where users only specify the results they wish to obtain and leave the system to decide upon efficient ways of processing them. Efficiency in processing in this context means very short user waiting time at minimal processing costs. A possible solution for minimising user waiting times in a DDB system is to broadcast user queries to every (relevant and irrelevant) node in the network to exploit parallelism which may speed up the processing time. Upon receiving the query, each node will begin to process the request; irrelevant nodes (nodes which do not contain data required by the query) will soon discard the request, and only relevant nodes will send their results back to the requesting node. On the other hand, a solution for minimising total processing costs, which include local processing and communication costs, is to eliminate as many messages transferred between nodes as possible, both in terms of volume and number of messages, because communication costs incurred could be more than local processing costs. Here a DDB system has to meet two conflicting goals – minimum time and minimum costs. Often, a compromise solution is sought for practical reasons, whereby the system develops some pragmatic query optimisation technique, based on quick estimates for formulating some "near optimal" strategy to reduce data transfer between nodes.

The query processing strategy provides a schedule for servicing queries at appropriate nodes in a given order. In general, this strategy attempts to restrict the data that are being shipped to another node for further processing (Fig. 7.7). Furthermore, certain data base operations could result in increasing data volume and, therefore, need to be performed as late as possible during the query processing stage in the system. A good query optimisation technique is clearly needed to meet the requirements of the two conflicting goals mentioned above.

Coupled to this heavy reliance on the query optimisation technique for improved performance, DDB data base design is another important fact to consider. Some DDB systems such as Distributed INGRES allow a logical table to be physically split up for efficiency purposes according to frequency of demand. Here one can split the logical table either vertically or horizontally or both. It is also possible to replicate data over several computer nodes, although maintaining data to be consistent over the entire network can be complicated in this case.

When data are replicated over several nodes, making changes on a value at a site would require the system to propagate this change to be made at other sites containing such replicated data. Complications arise when one or more of these nodes is suddenly down of when many users are trying to make changes to a given data element at the same time. A range of "soft" solutions have been developed for these problems.

The Current State of Play

With technological advances in the area of data communications networking, it it hoped soon data transmission between physically separated node will be a much less of a system bottleneck than present. Further it is hoped that it will not incur high an overhead cost. Already for some time local area networks (LAN) have been used for supporting distributed DBMS (DDBMS) such as the Polypheme, Multi-star and EDDS systems. In future use can be made of fibre optics and satellite communications, which will further decrease communication costs. Distributed query processing strategies would need to be slightly altered but they are certainly still very much needed in DDBMSs.

The move towards heterogeneous DDBs, whose nodes are preexisting, would imply the need for standardisation in areas such as formats for communicating queries and data between nodes. Some efforts are being made to achieve this, for example many recent relational systems support structured query language (SQL) as an interface between the local system and other DBMS, but more standardisation remains to be done.

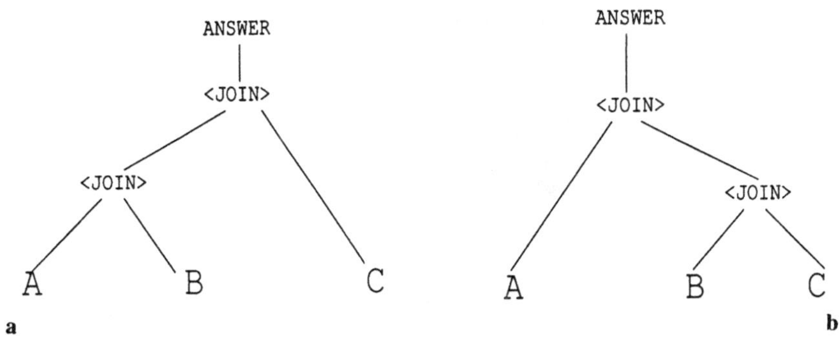

Fig. 7.7a,b. Query processing strategies. If *A*, *B*, and *C* are relations at different sites, strategy **a** – where *A* and *B* are first combined at one site and shipped to another before being combined with *C* – might require less transportation of data than the alternative strategy **b**

The incorporation of intelligent knowledge-based systems (IKBS) techniques into DDB systems, and extensions of the DDB architecture to include statistical data and voice, free text, and images, present challenging future research areas of interest in the evolution of the centralised data base to a DDB.

Already DBMS have been used to store different kind of data – multimedia data, e.g., voice, text, images and graphics. A future possible trend would be in investigating appropriate data types and operations to homogenise multimedia data over a multimedia DDB network to provide better services to the end users. Recently, research into multimedia issues have been actively explored. Multimedia data management would certainly require DDB research and technology as part of its support component/system. The multimedia issues will be discussed in Sect. 7.1.3.

7.1.2.2 Image Data Bases

Image Storage and Retrieval

In the 1980s, it became possible to develop image storage and retrieval systems. The developments which underpin this advance came from a wide variety of sources, including both hardware and software advances. Mass storage devices, image processing devices, specialised peripherals, communications systems, and satellite sensors provide the hardware scenario for image management systems, and on the software front, as we have seen, there have been great enhancements to the functionality of DBMS and DDBMS, and the advent of multimedia DBMS has opened up exciting possibilities. This section takes the form of a survey of the literature describing research, development, and application of image database management

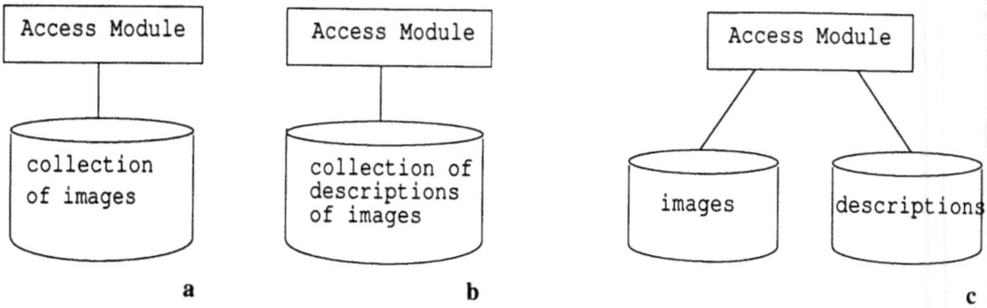

Fig. 7.8a–c. Three different types of data base. **a** Of data base. **b** About data base. **c** With data base

systems, and considers briefly their interrelationships with multimedia data base systems and distributed information systems. One of the most enlightening articles on image data bases was written by Boursier (Boursier 1985). The paper gives a good feel for the issues and progress being made in about 1984. We include much of the material in that paper as a starting point for the survey presented here and update it. Our headings for this subsection are: representation, interrogation, harmonisation, and performance. While we cannot hope to be exhaustive in our survey, we do hope that this treatment will give a good appreciation of the current state of the art in this area.

It is important to distinguish between the concepts of data bases of, about, and with images (Sloan and Lipman 1982). We refer to these three classes as OF data bases, ABOUT data bases, and WITH data bases, respectively (Fig. 7.8). OF data bases are defined as simple collections of images, i.e., a collection of slides or digitised images. ABOUT data bases treat the images as the entities of interest in the Universe of Discourse and are classical symbolic data bases. WITH data bases are perhaps the most interesting class. Experience has taught that image-related information should really be separated into two classes – one consisting of data which are closely coupled to the images, and the other being the data items which are segregated into a conventional data base so we have a database with images. These are described as WITH data bases by Sloan.

Representation

The abstract data type (ADT) approach has been recommended by several authors for data modelling for engineering and CAD-oriented databases. Extending the RDM has been a popular approach. For example, the well-known INGRES has been extended to include several of the features presented in the section headed object oriented data bases (see below), and complex objects and features to support conversational transactions have been added to IBM's prototype System R. Other researchers have also taken the ADT approach to image processing. In Chassignet (1985) an "iconographic kernel" is superimposed on the relational data model to remove the limitation imposed by its flatness. Molecular object is a concept which generalises that of relational object to allow arbitrarily complex objects to be represented. Versions of a design object have a common interface, but different implementations and, expressed as molecular objects, they are accompanied by interface and implementation descriptions. Basic modelling concepts and user operations can be identified for the capture of object semantics in terms of molecular objects, and for their manipulation. Related approaches have been taken to the specification and modelling of CAD component information used during design.

Semantically meaningful data types are also the focus of attention in Lohman et al. (1983). The application in this case is that of remotely sensing geographical information, but the approach can be extended to other scientific applications. The special needs of these applications for data management are discussed, for example, the automatic, real-time collection of large volumes of data by spacecraft, with respect to the regular nature of the data collected by a particular sensor; the fact that continuous data domains are prevalent in contrast to the discrete objects usually dealt with in commercial applications; the need to integrate data from relatively unrelated sources; and the combination of stability of data with dynamism of their structure. There are clearly substantial overlaps between the needs of these applications and those of medical imaging data bases. The authors describe a prototype data base that uses a relational data base management system (RDBMS) to link oceanographic data and metadata from remote and in situ sources. At a more theoretical level, work is proceeding in the object-oriented and AI fields which is closely related to the issues being considered here.

Interrogation

Extensions to relational algebra have been proposed which would facilitate the manipulation of pictorial information. Extensions to the well-known relational language query by example (QBE) called query by pictorial example (QPE) have also been suggested. QPE is the user interface for the IMAID image data base system, which combines an image understanding system with an RDBMS, and this is also the approach adopted in the ELF model. A related approach, which can be described as a deductive image data base approach, is described by Fox and Walker (1989).

An extension of the SQL language is described by Assman et al. (1984) called image SQL (ISQL) language. This language has been implemented in a prototype radiological picture information system, and the paper illustrates the properties of the language by a number of examples. A hierarchical menu management arrangement for the processing and retrieval of image data, which are represented as heterogeneous data structures – vectors, rasters, point, arc, mesh, table, and video – under a common administration system, is described by Nagata and Oonishi (1985). Some of the capability is illustrated using geographical data.

Harmonisation and Integration

When reviewing images, a user often relies on display-oriented functions such as grey mapping, zoom, and scroll. If the image collections are dispersed around the nodes of a communications network, the functions must still be invoked, preferably with as much ease as if they were local. A system architecture which supports a large number of display subsystems is clearly required, each with its own memory, and its own processing capability. When an image has been transferred to a local system, the local node is decoupled from the rest of the network, and acts as an independent system. If capability greater than that supplied locally is required, the node must be recoupled to the global system.

In the distributed medical image data bases described in the literature, the harmonisation is accomplished locally and is the responsibility of the local user. To allow different manufacturers' equipment to be linked requires a standard interface which can be used as a common and stable link between the stations. Standard product interface for this have been presented by Alzner et al. (1984).

Simple file handling systems for images which aim to "harmonise" heterogeneous image collections are also available. Limited prototype implementations of these in a PACS environment have been carried out which allow the user to access files by patient name, name of doctor or study type.

A system for harmonising heterogeneous data collections is presented by Abul-Huda et al. (1988). Its designers take an approach to the harmonisation problem based on the multi-data base approach (Bell et al. 1987a,b) to the heterogeneity problem in structured record-based data bases described earlier. A software superstructure is placed over the (possibly distributed) data collections, managed by diverse systems, and this ensures that the heterogeneity and distributed nature of the data is hidden from the user to a large extent. This system permits the integration of pictorial data with voice and text data. The REMINDS system is a further example of a system which provides harmonisation – in this case between images and text only.

Performance

As data bases grow they make heavy demands on storage capacity. Terabyte (10^{12} bytes of data) systems are likely to be needed in future large image data bases. A system aimed at trying to provide the required specialised mass storage devices based on a Hitachi 301 digital optical disk device has been developed. The result was a system which proved invaluable for managing large image databases, i.e., for Radiology applications.

A key problem in designing these systems is to provide the required levels of performance. The real-time digital disk (RTDD) is a system which acquires and displays images at about 30 frames per second, and also provides a range of functions for image processing and enhancing that add to its attractiveness.

During the last few years, optical mass storage technology has matured to the stage where various standards have been developed for organising different types of information on CD-ROM. In comparison with alternative mass storage systems, this technology has special features such as slow access to data. An example of the mechanical differences between optical and magnetic disks is the fact that when the read head is in a given position, it can read information from neighbouring tracks, as well as that on which it is currently positioned, using mirrors with a low inertia. Access methods and data placement methods can take advantage of these features to compensate for the poor performance of the devices in other respects. Developments in other systems for storage are not transferable directly to optical systems. There exists a large volume of literature on optical mass storage systems. No work has yet been carried out on the clustering/placement aspects of physical data base design for CD-ROM, and research is called for in this area. The fact that optical media are currently often WORM-based means that special care has to be taken with the placement of data, which must clearly take into account the likely growth rates of data, and also the fact that access patterns may change during the systems operational lifetime.

Data in a data base are stored physically according to some organisation method on the storage cells of a computer facility. The physical access method, on which any given organisation is based, specifies some relationship between the cells. To meet a request for data an ordered collection of cells has to be visited, and then a physical access path formed. Choosing a physical access method for images is currently an important area of research in data bases.

Image data are not well represented using point locations. An example of a query is to search for all objects meeting a given criterion and falling within a particular distance (in three dimensions) from another given object – classical single-dimensional indexing structures for data bases are not suitable for this type of application, nor is the use of exact matching using hashing supplemented by access structures suitable for such *range* queries. Furthermore, B trees and indexed sequential access method (ISAM) indexes, which are commonly used in conventional data-bases, are inappropriate in three-dimensional space. Examples of the structures which have been proposed to solve the problem are quad trees, K-D trees, K-D-B trees, gird files, bang files, and R trees. The latter is a height-balance tree like a B tree. The leaves of the tree hold pointers, i.e., disk addresses, to data objects. The idea is to keep the number of nodes of the tree to be visited in a search to a minimum. Insertions and deletions are carried out gracefully. All the entries are in pairs; in the leaves, the pairs consist of an identifier and an n-dimensional rectangle bonding the object of interest, while elsewhere they consist of an identifier and a pointer to a child. Searches are carried out in a similar way to those for the ubiquitous B tree, but more than one subtree may have to be searched from a particular node. This method has been found to be efficient in a series of performance tests. Moreover, it is considered to be amenable to adoption by relational DBMS which use conventional methods.

Other data base management functions such as query optimisation (see Bell et al. 1989) will also have a special character in image systems. It will not be the order in which joins of relations are executed that will have the greatest effect on the response time of a given query execution, but the indexing and data movement operations, which are perhaps simpler, but hard to alter. Buffer management is another example of such a function.

7.1.3 Multimedia Data Bases

7.1.3.1 Multimedia Computing

Multimedia computing was one of the buzzwords in computing circles in the late 1980s, and many computing industry watchers predict it will be a major trend in the 1990s. It covers a number of areas, because the pertinent information is contained in journals and conference papers, for example, in a variety of domains – both in computer science itself and in the literature of computing applications such as in geophysics, education, and medicine.

In this section we will consider the issues in the area under a number of headings, which we believe permit a systematic approach to be taken to the subject. Essentially we are presenting an appraisal of the status quo in this area at the end of the 1980s.

7.1.3.2 Objectives

There have been a wide variety of recent contributions to the growing body of literature pertaining to an extensive range of data storage and manipulation issues. The literature in the area of multimedia data base systems (MMDBS) is to be found in many apparently disparate subject areas such as office automation systems, medical information systems and various other application-oriented areas as well as in a wide spectrum of (hard and soft) computing fields such as workstation design and semantics data modelling.

We limit our attention here to those aspects of the overall subject which are most pertinent to the hospital integrated PACS (HIPACS) project. We give good reasons for our choices or aspects and choose between using descriptive appraisal and more tightly informative discussion for each system. The items of most significance are emphasised, of course.

Our ultimate goal of an assessment such as this is to ensure that developers of future MMDBS take into account all relevant previous work and avoid duplication of this work.

7.1.3.3 Multimedia Data Base Systems

MMDBS can be considered as a natural evolution of DDBS. The main aim of an MMDBS is to provide integrated representation and manipulation of heterogeneous data on multiple media. A distributed dimension to such systems is clearly desirable in many application areas such as in medical information networks and in open or distance learning systems (Forsdick et al. 1984; Christodoulakis et al. 1986). As indicated earlier, we consider a data base to be a store of information used as a buffer between the suppliers of information and its users, so we can see that the stored information is used essentially for communication purposes and that in daily life it takes many forms in addition to those encountered in bound ledgers, and other record-based devices. So voice data, image and picture data, free text data, and even video data should ideally be contained in the reservoir or data base. In addition, this information has to be moved between suppliers and users to be of any use.

The historical introduction to this chapter indicates that the stage has now been reached when generalised MMDBS capable of being applied to many diverse applications can be contemplated. Users of information have continually asked for richer varieties of data to be stored in their reservoirs, and this gives a "user-pull" to stimulate development of MMDBS. There has also been a "technology-push", for example, optical storage devices which are ideal for storing large nonvolatile chunks of information, such as images, and improvement in input/output peripherals have complemented the development outlined in Sect. 7.1.1.

We can define a MMDBS as a data base system that integrates data bases which are represented using a variety of media in a variety of styles such as pictures and images, tape recordings, films and, of course, conventional computers' mass storage devices. Several survey papers on this topic have been produced (see Bell and Abul-Huda 1987; Christodoulakis 1987). Issues to be addressed are: data modelling, e.g., is the relational system any use in this case, or do we need object oriented systems in order to get generalised commercial MMDBS?; storage management subsystems, e.g., how do we cluster objects which are needed at the same time, and what sort of physical access methods do we use?; and, of course, system architectures to support this approach to information processing.

There are three main approaches to handling multimedia data. The bottom-up technique seeks to adapt existing DBMS to handle data on several types of media, e.g., the extended relation approach of POSTGRES. A top-down approach can be taken by developing a new MMDBMS, perhaps based on object-oriented principles integrating the multimedia data; this has been proposed by the Microelectronics and Communications Technology Corporation in the United States. The third alternative, which is much less general, is to develop a specific MMDBMS tailored for a given application environment. An excellent example of this is the Doomsday project in the United Kingdom, but this indicates the shortcoming of this

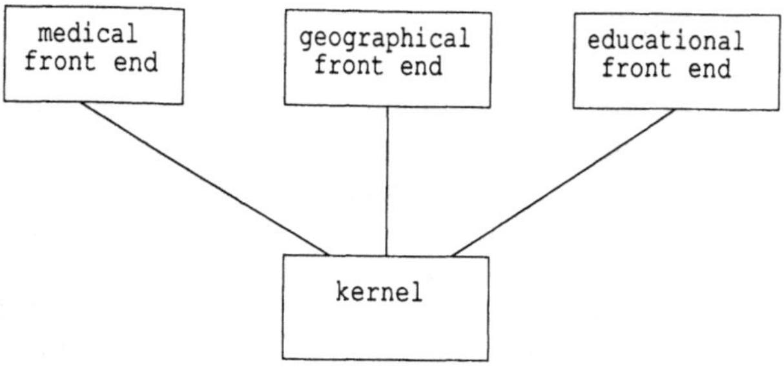

Fig. 7.9. Application-specific interface to a kernel

approach, because the system cannot be applied to other applications and domains.

7.1.3.4 Representation Issues

As indicated earlier, many of the current prototypes and system proposals which use the bottom-up approach are based on the RDM. Some, however, are based on network and functional data models which are more object-oriented than the RDM (see Sect. 7.1.1). Possible extensions to the RDM for a MMDBMS that have been suggested include:

1. Supporting variable string length to accommodate free text as attribute values (this was an early suggestion for the POSTGRES system);
2. Supporting ADT, e.g., allowing nonconventional data types such as office folders, polygons and even procedures;
3. Non-first-normal-form (NF^2), i.e., the basic structure used is not just "flat" tables or relations; the relations can appear as values in the columns of the tables. A major trend in this area is towards extensible DBMS, where a *kernel* DBMS is used to underpin application-specific interfaces to the real world, or front-ends (Fig. 7.9).

The object-oriented model has been acknowledged by some leading researchers as the most appropriate data model for handling multimedia data. However, this fact is not yet established. Advocates of the object-oriented model claim several advantages over the existing DBMS-based models such as the RDM. These include:

1. The data base can be perceived as a collection of abstract objects, each with its own identifier;
2. Semantic relationships among objects can be represented clearly and explicitly;
3. Encapsulation of the behaviour and the state of objects are stored in the data base.

We will discuss object-oriented data bases in a later section.

7.1.3.5 Presentation

Making use of multimedia data requires an efficient, flexible and user-friendly user interface. Various techniques for presenting the multimedia data have been proposed. Among these are the use of a presentation manager which could allow a user to choose and specify a final output in a very idiosyncratic manner; windowing facilities where an output screen or screens can be subdivided to show, for example, multiple objects/subobjects at one time; and special media presentation devices.

7.1.3.6 Interrogation

The user interface language (UIL) depends entirely on the data model and DBMS that the MMDBMS is built upon. Early proposals were to extend to the relational SQL query language. From the object-oriented view point, there have been many suggestions; one example is an object-oriented programming system called Oz for office information applications. An object-oriented programming language Smalltalk-80 is used for the GEMSTONE object-oriented DBMS. In a multimedia filling system called MUSE, the UIL is based on windows and menu facilities.

7.1.3.7 Harmonisation and Integration

Harmonisation and integration are perhaps the most challenging problems encountered when developing a MMDBMS. The problems of integrating and harmonising multiple data on various different media which are specific to the application environment have not been adequately explored.

Examples of integration approaches are (a) integrating structured-text, free-text, image and voice media in a command and control workstation (CCWS) multimedia mail system, and (b) integrating structured text, free text, and image and voice media in the DIAMOND system. Further examples are the two experimental mixed-object data base systems (MODES1 and MODES2), aimed at handling mixed object data such as text, images, graphics and voice. MODES1 is relation-based and MODES2 is based on the functional data model. The integrating of text and images is treated in Sect. 7.3.

7.1.3.8 Performance

Performance is one of the key issues in MMDBMS because of the large search space when the huge data volumes are stored. Various searching techniques have been proposed and developed to improve the performance of the systems. These include new methods of compressing data, of providing look-up indexes to locate data, ensuring that there is a good chance that the information needed is in the user's workstations even before they wish to access it (buffering), making deductions, and searching the data.

7.1.4 An Architecture for MMIP

In this section, we outline a pragmatic but general relation-based, layered architecture for a distributed image and text data system which is an evolution from the current data base technology. For example, we use the base schema of architecture of MDBS as a foundation for this. An example is given from a medical environment of the schemas existing at each layer of the architecture. A hierarchical chart of the functions in a medical image data access module (MIDAM) is given.

The main reason for basing our architecture on the RDM is that relational systems, e.g., INGRES, ORACLE, and DB2, have been commercially available for some time, and the RDM has been successfully used in different real world applications. Furthermore, issues concerning data independence, data integrity, data sharing, minimal redundancy and security in textual data systems are dealt with well in a conventional DBMS. These issues are relevant to image data as well as the textual data.

The three-level scheme for data base system architecture was proposed by the ANSI technical committee X3 group, which aimed to standardise and harmonise the interfaces between different levels of data base system components. It also enhances implementation and integration. A straightforward evolution of the ANSI/X3/SPARC architecture that accommodates different data media and a distributed dimension is shown in Fig. 7.10.

A local schema representing logical data, which can be either explicit or implicit as defined below, stored in the underlying system, may exist in every site-specific and medium-specific local system. It consists of the description of all the information stored on the local media expressed in the local description language, e.g., using the RDM. We say that the logical data in the local schema are explicit when the schema extensions provide actual data *values* to be presented in response to a query. In some cases the local schema may not be explicit. For example, a local user may be presented with a "representative symbol" or "pointer" as a the result of a query against a given schema, e.g., an image key as the pointer to retrieve the actual image. Alternatively, the local user may have no logical schema but the user knows what to retrieve, e.g., for content accessible retrieval.

Associated with each local schema is a local participation schema which describes the subset of data that the local system wishes to contribute to the distributed multimedia system. A local subsidiary schema (not shown) might also be required to be coupled with each local schema for resolving any incompatible data/information. The global conceptual schema represents the entire, collective MMDBS. This schema describes every object, entity, and relationship of the underlying data on various media. The external media

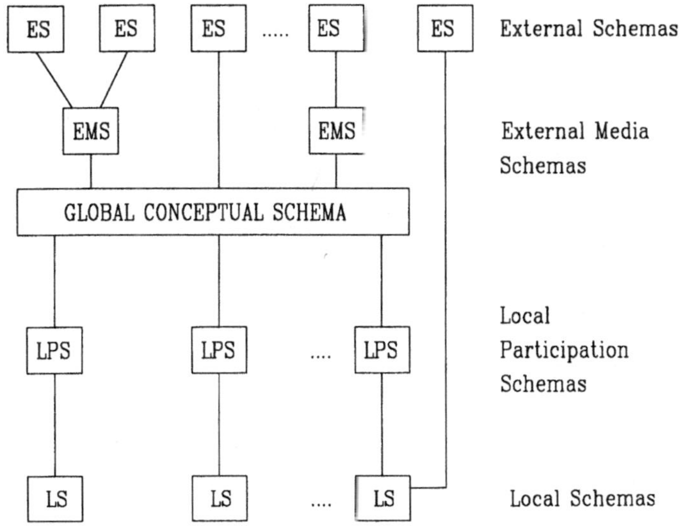

Fig. 7.10. Schema architecture

schema (EMS) may be required to describe the mapping functions between the global conceptual schema and the external schemas for a single medium. An external schema (ES) represents a view for each individual end user or designated group of end users. A view of a single medium could be expressed in different conventional query languages, and the view could be over the EMS.

Alternatively, the ES could be a multimedia view of the global conceptual schema. Special consideration is required for the case of the content accessible retrieval mentioned above. Schema levels (components) within the architecture should be independent of each other as far as possible. For example, altering the data object of an ES should not affect any other, underlying schemas. By standardising interfaces between each component, it is possible to include/exclude a local schema into/from the multimedia system with relative ease of implementation.

A second, and in some cases a pragmatic, contender for distributed MMDBS architecture would eliminate the global conceptual schema and use a qualification procedure to refer to local (specific media) data bases, as in the federated approach mentioned in an earlier section. In order to obtain a better understanding of this (idealised) architecture, we shall go through the system component architecture for the case where there are only two sites (global and local), using a query trace. We use a direct analogy with the structured DDB query trace, so that all the possible components of the trace can be identified even if they are not important for a particular medium (such as image). This architecture in simplified form is shown in Fig. 7.11.

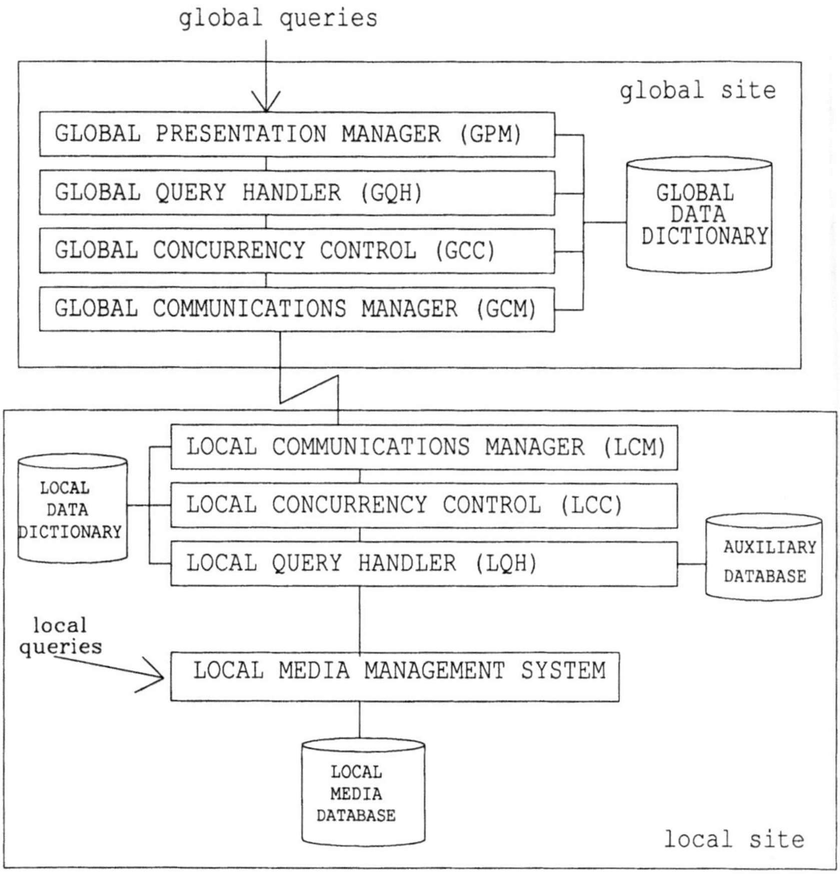

Fig. 7.11. System component architecture

Suppose a consultant, considered as a global user, would like to conduct a research study concerning the degree of knee cap fractures of recorded patients. At his workstation, he poses a global query to the system. This may be done at a very high interface level, in which case a data base query over a special "research" ES or global schema is produced by an interface module. Here the global representation manager (GRM) parses and validates the query, and then passes it to the global query handler (GQH). The GQH further decomposes, optimises and verifies the query. Note that these functions are not identical with those in purely relational systems. The output from the GQH is a query tree/graph, which represents the original global query. The concurrency control modules (both global and local) are used when a global update of transaction is initiated. This may not be an important function in this particular application domain, but may be replaced by a different form of transaction control. The communication manager (both global and local) is responsible for routing the query/result file package from one site to another designated site via the communication network. When the query file package arrives at the local site, the local query handler (LQH) may further optimise the subquery according to the specific media of the management system. In our system, the response to a query for images, and perhaps text in some cases, although text can be stored directly as relations, is a relation which gives a representative symbol or pointer for access to an image file, possibly via an image data base system.

Intermediate results generated from the local sites are then passed back to the LQH. Any local incompatibilities will also be resolved here using the information stored in the auxiliary data base. The semiformed result is then transferred to the global site for further processing. The final result(s) will be presented to the users by the GPM. The GPM has to be equipped with windowing facilities, an SQL-like query language, and also object-oriented features so that users could either use an image on the screen to retrieve a "similar" type of images, or select image retrieval based on an object hierarchy.

As our architecture is based on the relational model, associations between the physical and logical images are via pointers; the system provides a relational directory to the image store and the text store. This is the key distinguishing feature of our approach. Both the image and text can be retrieved by content; the image can be retrieved via the image key, and the text can be retrieved via the abstract terms. As mentioned above, text can be handled well by the conventional DBMS functions. The Starburst system, developed by IBM, also treats image data as a complex object attribute in this way. The long field manager is proposed to manipulate object data up to 100 MB.

It is possible to construct a hierarchical chart which depicts the functionality of this system. The higher level modules in he chart are explained in the following:

Common System Services deals with communication and synchronisation, process control, condition handling, memory management and conversion functions.

Global Data Dictionary provides a permanent description of the global definition of the distributed image data base. It contains a global part and local part.

Local Storage Manager provides temporary storage, queue handling, and query handling facilities.

Communication Network Manager interfaces and handles the communications with the data network, e.g., TCP/IP, ACR/NEMA.

Query Language Processor performs all the data access and manipulation functions necessary for the execution of a query.

Prefetching/Fetching controls transfer of data to local sites in preparation for examination.

User Interface Server handles the communication between MIDAM system software and the user terminal.

Process Control Monitor initialises, and controls MIDAM run-time environment.

Transaction Processor manages the execution of MIDAM transactions.

This layered architecture is sufficiently general to integrate data of any medium across computer networks. However systems built according to this idealised architecture will not give favourable response times. For example, as noted earlier, during the reporting session in the radiology example, a response time of more than 5 s is unacceptable. Therefore, a "prefetching" strategy has been proposed which predicts the sets of most relevant images (stored in the image data base) for the given examination/reporting, and then transfers them to the image server (fast buffer store) that is next to the viewing workstation.

The image data base has a large storage capacity, but is slow in retrieval (Fig. 7.12). Therefore, selecting the relevant image from the image data base and then transporting it over the network to the desired workstation would take a long time. In the prefetching scenario on the other hand, some heuristic/rule is used to select the relevant images from the slow huge store to the image server (fast but limited in storage) prior to the start of the examination. The problem of selecting images which are relevant and have to be moved to the image server depends on the type of examination to be carried out. In its simplest form, this is similar to the buffer management problem in computer operating systems. It is possible that the image server is close to several workstations, and each workstation demands sets of images simultaneously.

Clearly the site/medium independence properties of this architecture makes it suitable for integrating nontext data with conventional systems, such as HISs.

7.1.5 Linking HIS and Image Data Bases Using These Architectures

There are essentially two practical issues to be considered in the application of multimedia information processing systems to a PACS environment. Firstly, there is the issue of integrating PACS modalities, e.g., radiography, computed tomography to allow efficient and effective handling of diverse digitised images. This is a problem involving distributed image handling, since the images may be generated and stored at multiple locations. Secondly, there is the issue of how such a PACS system might be integrated in the HIS. This addresses the problem of integrating single-media data from many sites as well as integrating multimedia data.

Both issues may be resolved using the multimedia data base approach described in the previous section. This approach allows integration of both distributed single-media data, e.g., structured text or image, and of multimedia data, e.g., structured text *with* using an extension of the multi-data base approach used in the handling of distributed structured text data bases. Firstly, an simplified model of an HIS and PACS system is presented

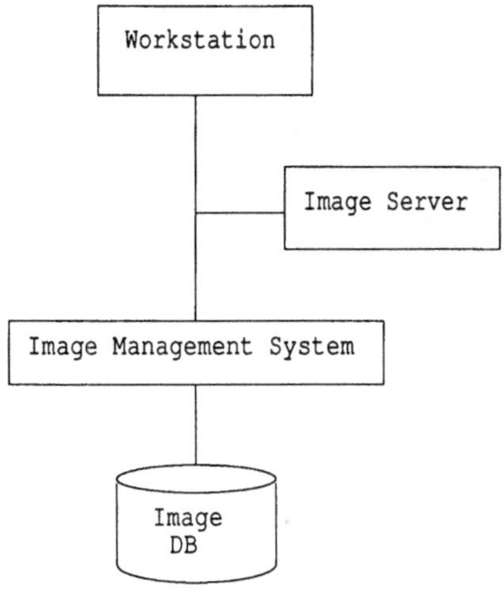

Fig. 7.12. Image management and processing schema

using a set of relations which constitute the EMS. In this simple scenario, the part of the HIS global schema is made up of information on consultation sessions at a hospital in which X-rays are taken. The set of relations is then as follows:

1. Patient (*Hosp_no*, Pat_forename, Pat_surname, Birthdate, Address)
2. Appointment (*App_No*, App_date, App_location, Hosp_no)
3. Doctor (*Dr_no*, Dr_name, Dr_phone)
4. Consultation (*App_no*, *Dr_no*, X-ray_no)
5. X-ray (*X-ray_no*, X-ray_type, X-ray date, X-ray_ptr)

The first four relations are in the form of structured text and the fifth is part of an image database of x_rays (a limited amount to structured text must be stored with images to facilitate image handling). These relations are physically stored at three different sites and are thus defined in three different participation schemas:

1. Site A – local participation schema.
   Patient (*Hosp_no*, Pat_forename, Pat_surname, Birthdate, Address)
2. Site B – local participation schema.
   Appointment (*App_No*, App_date, App_location, Hosp_no)
   Doctor (*Dr_no*, Dr_name, Dr_phone)
   Consultation (*App_no*, *Dr_no*, X-ray_no)
3. Site C – local participation schema.
   X-ray (*X-ray_no*, X-ray_type, X-ray date, X-ray_ptr)

Since the participation schema defines how much of the local data participates in the global system, the local schema may also be composed of nonparticipating information. For instance, at site A there may also be information on patients' general practitioners, i.e., "Patient (*Hosp_no*,

Pat_forename, Pat_surname, Birthdate, Address, GP_no)" and "GP (*GP_no*, GP_surname, GP_address, GP_phone)." Having defined the data in the global schema, participation schemas and local schemas it is appropriate to consider the applications that may be defined over the global schema. These can be split into three classes depending on whether single media or multimedia data are involved. The processing of a typical multimedia query is outlined at every stage of the system using the module architecture diagram (Fig. 7.10).

7.1.5.1 Single Media Applications

In single media applications, the relations involved are defined in the ES. In these cases, an EMS will also be accessed. This may be to enforce security in that one application does not necessarily need to see data from other relations. The EMS is thus a subset or view of the global schema, e.g., for the above system an example of an external media schemas could be:

- Patient (*Hosp_no*, Pat_forename, Pat_surname, Birthdate, Address)
- Appointment (*App_No*, App_date, App_location, Hosp_no)
- Consultation (*App_no*, *Dr_no*, X-ray_no)

Thus a single media external schema may involve relations of only one medium type distributed over multiple sites. For example if information is required about patients and their appointments an external schema would be:

- Patient (*Hosp_no*, Pat_forename, Pat_surname, Birthdate, Address)
- Appointment (*App_No*, App_date, App_location, Hosp_no)

Since this application is single medium a typical query such as "list all the patients and their appointment times for location A2 on 27th October 1990" will involve use of the external text schema.

7.1.5.2 Multimedia Applications

In multimedia applications an EMS is not used since information is required from more than one medium. An example of an application using this approach would involve information about patients and their X-rays:

- Patient (*Hosp_no*, Pat_forename, Pat_surname, Birthdate, Address)
- Appointment (*App_No*, App_date, App_location, Hosp_no)
- Consultation (*App_no*, *Dr_no*, X-ray_no)
- X-ray (*X-ray_no*, X-ray_type, X-ray date, X-ray_ptr)

A typical example of a multimedia query might be "Get the hospital numbers, patient names and previous X-rays for the last 5 years for all those patients with appointments at location A2 on 27th October 1990." This query is an example of information which must be prefetched prior to a particular clinic. The ES will first be checked to see if the data may be accessed, and then the global schema will show the mapping between the media objects. After the query is parsed and validated by the GRM, it is passed to the GQH, where it is decomposed into a number of subqueries. At this stage, optimisation of the query takes places. Access to the global schema held in the global data dictionary allows the query to be decomposed into a number of subqueries according to medium and site:

1. Subquery 1 to site A
   Patient (*Hosp_No*, Pat_forename, Pat_surname)
2. Subquery 2 to site B
   Appointment (*App_No*, App_date = "27/10/90", App_location = "A2")
   Consultation (*App_No*, X-ray_No)
3. Subquery to site C
   X-ray (*X-ray_no*, X-ray_date > "27/10/85", X-ray_ptr)

These subqueries are sent to the local sites by the global communication manager. At each local site, the data base holds the local participation schema and local schema in the local data dictionary. The local participation schema checks to see whether the data in the subquery are permitted for use by the global system and also gives the mapping rules between global and local representation, e.g., from relational to network model for structured text data bases. The local schema gives the mapping between relations at the local site.

The results of the subqueries are passed back to the global site where they are concatenated according to the query tree which has been constructed for the outgoing subqueries. This allows the results to be properly related. The results can then be stored for viewing by the presentation manager or for sending to a remote workstation at the clinic site.

7.1.5.3 Local Queries

Local queries are not posed over the global schema, but represent queries that a local user may make on a single site, single media data base. They are thus posed over the local schema only. A typical query such as: "Get a list of all patients whose general practitioner is called Dr. Wilson," would, therefore, bypass the global system and be posed only over the local schema for site A as previously defined. The information required may involve relations not participating in the global schema. The single media query thus corresponds to the PACS scenario, where different image types at multiple locations require limited integration, and the multimedia query corresponds to the HIS/PACS link that is required for the integration of medical images with HIS data.

7.1.6 Open Issues of Working Systems

There are several areas in which research is necessary before a system represented by the MIDAM architecture above can become an practical reality. We have pointed out the problems under the headings representation, interrogation, representation, integration, and performance. Each of these issues has an impact on individual modules of the component architecture given in Fig. 7.11 and we are convinced that they are essential if the model is to be used for HIPACS applications.

7.2 Distributed Image Archival*

C. Schilling, B. Wein, and D. Meyer-Ebrecht

7.2.1 Introduction

Medical imaging has been important for the diagnostic process since the advent of X-rays. Its importance is growing even more due to new medical imaging techniques such as magnetic resonance imaging (MRI) computed tomography (CT), and digital subtraction anglography (DSA), which give precise additional information about the patient's diseases. Therefore, the total number of images produced by image sources in various medical examination types is increasing more and more. An average hospital currently generates about half a million images per year. The information content of these images is in the order of several terabyte. Particular conceptual and technical attention must, therefore, be paid to archiving digital data, as well as taking into account the data management aspect discussed in Sect. 7.1.

A basic problem with film archives is that it takes too much time to retrieve images. The time needed to retrieve an image which was archived only a short time ago can be up to 1 h. It may even be up to 1 day for older images. Another problem with film archives is the loss of images that occurs because only one original image exists, and this original has to be handed out on request. Moreover, a significant percentage of films never find their way back to the archive. Finally, films are not an appropriate storage medium for images produced by digital modalities, because an essential part of the primary information content is lost.

Stimulated by evident progress in computer technology and application, e.g., the high-density storage of images on optical disks that was demonstrated first in the early 1970s, or the scenario of the "paperless office" which was also under discussion as early as the 1970s, there has been an enthusiastic hope for more than 15 years that *digital* archival of the

* This research was supported by the Commission of the European Communities under Project A 1008. We would also like to thank the Department for Radiology of the University Hospital Aachen for their excellent collaboration.

medical images could solve all these problems. Although the necessary technologies have reached an appropriate state of maturity since then, full-scale digital image archives have not yet been implemented, and we are far from having satisfactory "off-the-shelf" solutions. Obviously, the simultaneously occurring requirements for vast quantity data storage and high-speed access, in addition to a complex interlinking between images and other types of health care information have hampered progress on this key part of a full-scale picture archiving and communication system (PACS).

Recent investigations into the current situation of hospitals and their radiologic departments concerning image production, image transports and the behavior of the user, e.g., the radiologist performing a reporting session at the lightbox, brought more insight into detail problems. Armed with that knowledge, an attempt was made to match carefully the properties of the available technologies with the user's requirements, rather than attacking the problem with "brute force", to make acceptable compromises, and to conceive a generic solution which offered the ease and flexibility to adapt systems in size and structure to the diversity of different hospital organizations.

7.2.2 Analysis of the Current Situation

In the following we will describe investigations about current work organizations of radiologic departments and the resulting image storage and retrieval actions versus time, aiming at deriving, e.g., figures of equivalent digital data volumes and data flow rates and distributions of load versus time. The investigations were carried out at the University Hospital Aachen. We will complement this by a survey of the state of the art in digital mass storage technology. With regard to the limitations of storage media, the critical issues for the conceptual design of digital image archives will be pointed out.

7.2.2.1 Image Data Production, Retrieval, and Flow

In order to get quantitative data about the total numbers of examinations and the distribution over different examination types, we first analyzed the examination data which were supplied by an existing radiologic information system (RIS). We then observed the ten most important work places for image evaluation at the reporting rooms of the investigated radiology department. Altogether we observed 404 examinations in which 1566 images were used. We did not regard the old images which had been transported to the reporting rooms, but were not used for the ongoing examination. In order to access the hospital-wide overall image data flow, we assumed that each image used by the radiologist must also be retrieved at least once more by the referring department.

Table 7.1 shows the tremendous amount of image data which must be handled by he image archive, the image network, and the image work-

Table 7.1. Image production at the University Hospital Aachen (January 1989 until June 1989)

Type	Matrix	Bit/Pixel	MB/Image	Images/year	GB/year
X-ray	≈2908[2a]	10	≈10.57[a]	227 000	2400
DSA	512^2	8	0.26	22 000	6
CT	512^2	12	0.39	160 000	22
Nuclear medicine	128^2	6	0.01	ND	ND
MRI	256^2	12	0.1	ND	ND
Ultrasound	256^2	6	0.20	75 000	4

[a] An equivalent average pixel matrix and data volume has been calculated based on the film sizes and spatial resolution of the different types of X-rays
DSA, digital subtraction angiography; *CT*, computed tomography; *MRI*, magnetic resonance imaging; *ND*, no data

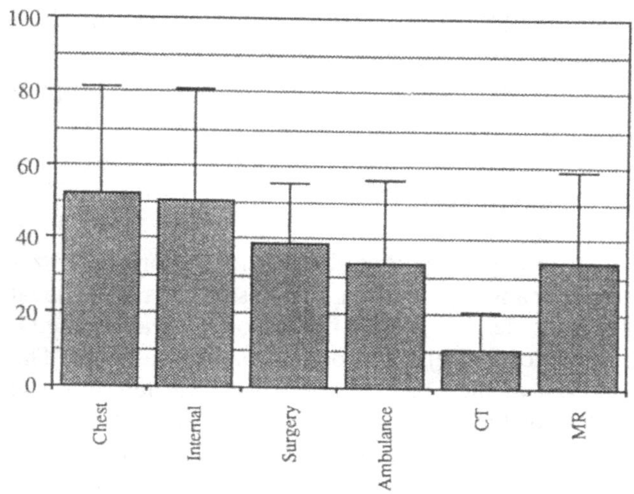

Fig. 7.13. Equivalent volume of image data per patient at different types of reporting places (mean volume and standard deviation)

stations. We found that chest X-rays contribute to the total image data volume by about 65%. A typical chest X-ray film is approximately 35 × 43 cm, its spatial resolution is about 5 lines per millimeter, and the contrast range is about 1–1000. Therefore, the equivalent digital data volume is up to 20 MB (3600 × 4300 pixel at 10/8 B per pixel). During the reporting sessions at a chest reporting place, two to four chest X-rays (average 2.83) are used per patient, which are equivalent to 56 Megabyte per patient (see Fig. 7.13).

All images which are needed during the treatment period of all current patients must be accessible at tolerable response times, i.e., within a couple of seconds. However, Fig. 7.14 illustrates that 87% of all reviewed images

→

Fig. 7.14a–c. Age of images used during reporting sessions (age 0: new images). **a** Long-term average at ten reporting places. **b** short term, average at ten reporting places. **c** short term distribution at one chest reporting place

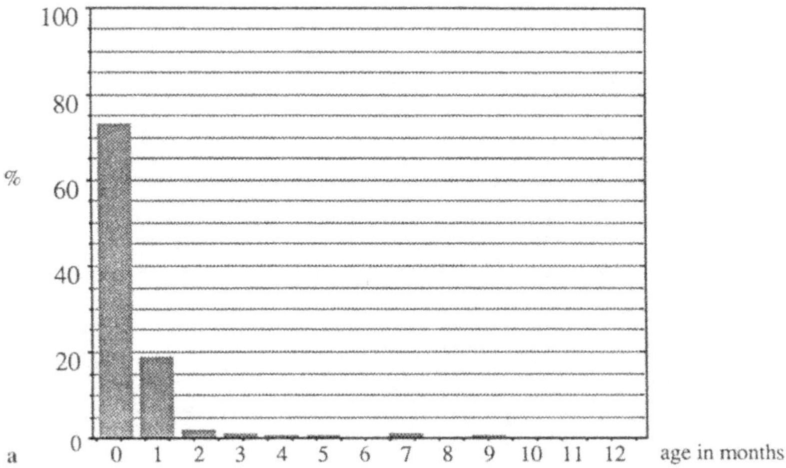
100
80
60
40
20
0
%
0 1 2 3 4 5 6 7 8 9 10 11 12
age in months

a

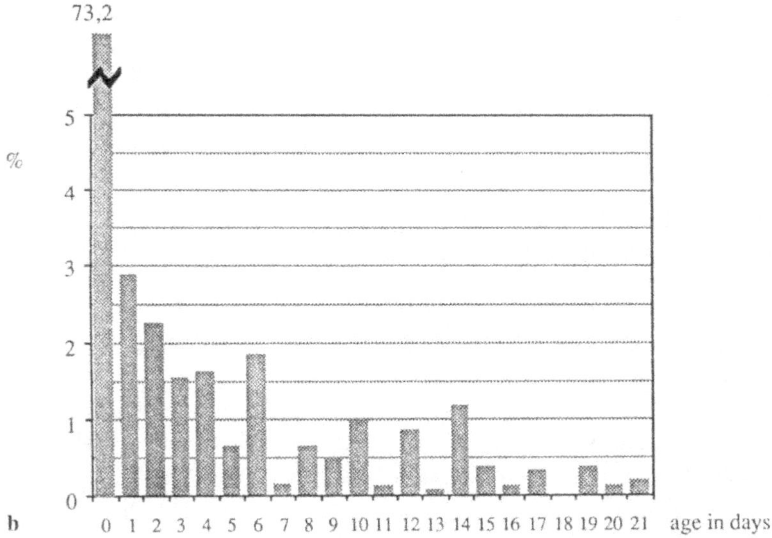
73,2
5
4
3
2
1
0
%
0 1 2 3 4 5 6 7 8 9 10 11 12 13 14 15 16 17 18 19 20 21
age in days

b

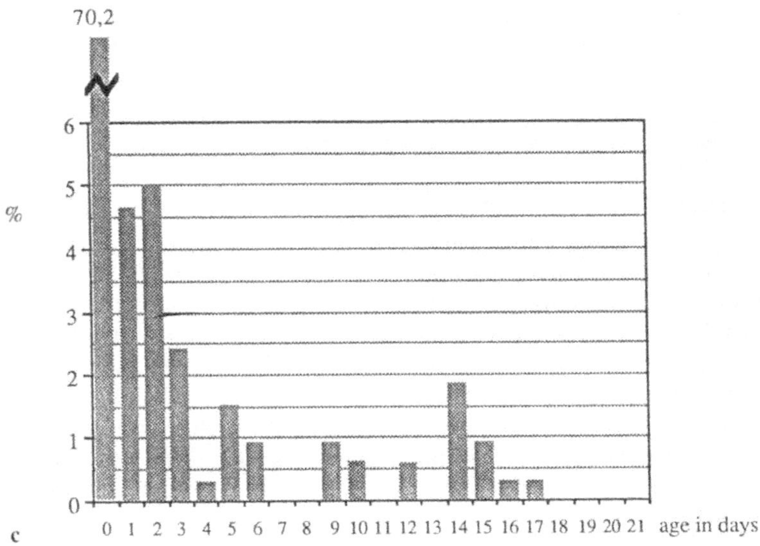
70,2
6
5
4
3
2
1
0
%
0 1 2 3 4 5 6 7 8 9 10 11 12 13 14 15 16 17 18 19 20 21
age in days

c

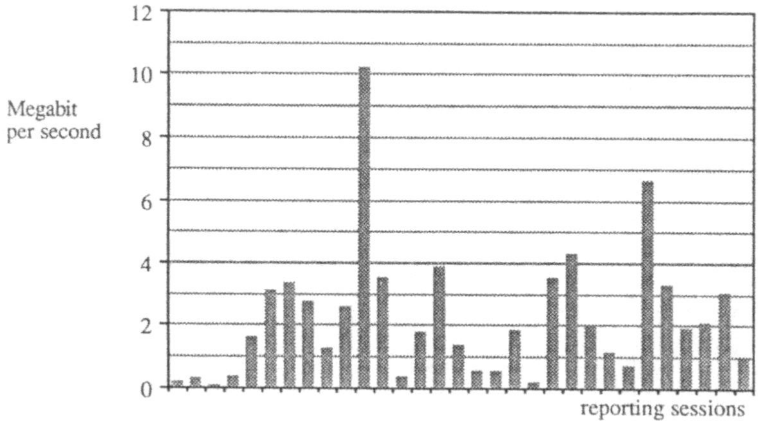

Fig. 7.15. Mean equivalent image data flow calculated from 31 individual reporting sessions. Equivalent data volume of the Complete set of images used during one reporting session devided by session's duration

are no older than 14 days. Images which are older than 14 days are retrieved much less frequently. At the University Hospital Aachen, for example, where there are 1500 beds and the daily image production is about 6.5 GB, 14 days of image production equals a data volume of about only 90 GB. These results give some indications for the organization of image stores, and we will use these below.

In Fig. 7.15, it is shown that typical radiological reporting sessions require a mean continuous data flow rate of approximately 4 Mbit/s. From this, it can be estimated that a hospital like the University Hospital Aachen, which runs 12 image reporting places, needs an image archive that offers a continuous throughput of at least 100 Mbit/s for image retrieval at routine workload (two retrievals per image at 12 workplaces at 4 Mbit/s per reporting session). The required data rate can be much higher in the worst case.

7.2.2.2 Storage Technologies: State of the Art

For a *digital* archival, the images must be stored on nonvolatile media. A suitable state of the art technology for nonvolatile digital image storage is the write once read multiple (WORM) technology. A WORM disk consists of a metallic layer which is protected on both sides by glass plates. The write process is performed by a laser beam which changes the optical reflective properties of the surface of the metallic layer. The information can be read by measuring the reflection of the surface. Due to the physically irreversible write process, data which have been written onto such a disk are, to a large extent, protected against electromagnetic waves, temperature influence, and

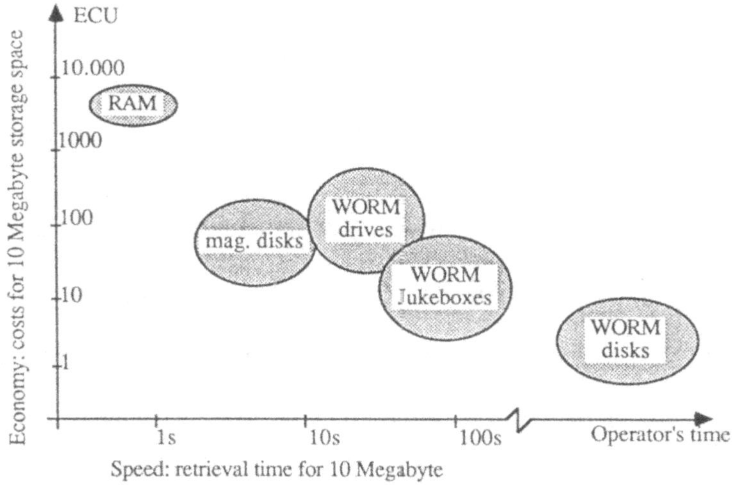

Fig. 7.16. Economy versus retrieval speed of available storage media

mechanic shock. WORM disks are designed to save data for at least 30 years.

WORM disks are available in 5.25 and 12 diameter, with a storage capacity of 0.4–1 or 2–7 GByte per double sided disk, respectively. Due to the high density of recording, the relative costs (price/Megabyte) are extremely low for the medium. WORM drives, however, are still much more expensive than magnetic disk drives of a comparable capacity. Moreover, access speed and data transfer rates are about a factor of 10 below those of magnetic disk drives. On the other hand, WORM disk drives may be combined with automatic disk-changer modules ("jukebox"), which can contain about 100 WORM disks in automatic access. Disks can be changed within approximately half a minute.

WORM disks are the favorite media for image archival storage due to their storage density, economy, and nonvolatility, but their transfer speed is far too low for routine image retrieval. In contrast, magnetic disks offer the required speed, but cannot be used for long-term storage because of the volatility of stored data and the excessive storage costs. In Fig. 7.16, the relations of the storage costs versus the retrieval time are given for the different storage technologies.

7.2.2.3 Conclusion

At first glance, digital image archival poses the problem of a safe and reliable long-term storage for a terrific amount of data with reasonably fast access *and* at reasonably low costs – an apparently contradictory requirement! Looking closer at the mechanism of radiologic departments and the user's work, we can see several possibilities of reducing the problem:

1. Islands of operations, inside which the amount of image data is much smaller than the total, could be isolated and equipped with separated storage modules.
2. The total volume of images could be partitioned into a small amount of recent images, which are frequently retrieved, and a much larger amount of old images, which are retrieved only in rare cases, i.e., fast media with a low capacity could favorably be combined with big, but slow storage media.
3. Existing resources for data management could be appropriately extended or modified to perform a "smart" management of image retrieval and image data flow, e.g., to apply so-called prefetching strategies.

A combined use of measures to circumvent the physical, technological, and economic bottlenecks – distribution of resources, hierarchies of storage media, sophisticated management and internetworking with heterogeneous services – makes image archival a tremendously complex task. Moreover, we have to attack the problem of dynamic growth. There is only one countermeasure to make that complexity manageable: a carefully designed concept of the mechanisms which control the allocation of images and, the information flow between the distributed resources, and which let the clients keep control of the diversity of servers and services.

7.2.3 A Generic Concept for Distributed Digital Image Archives

Let us first define the *clients* and the *servers* in a PACS. Basically, the clients are the users, i.e., the radiologists and other medical personnel. In the terminology of the computer network community, clients are also all those systems which are operated by users. Hence in a PACS, clients are image modalities such as CT, MRI, or film digitizing stations and image workstations. Servers are the modalities which deliver services at the request of a client. In a PACS, these are image stores, patient data base systems, radiologic organization systems, and hospital administration systems (these services are delivered by RIS and hospital information systems HIS), film hard copy printer stations, and, possibly, resources for remote image processing.

Image archival and retrieval can be subdivided into three basic services, which we will call SEND_image, FIND_image, and GET_image, adapting the terminology of the ACR/NEMA protocol proposal.

1. *SEND_image*. A server which is equipped with nonvolatile archival storage media after transfer of the image takes over the responsibility for its availability over a period of at least 10 years.
2. *FIND_image*. When a user wants to retrieve specific images, information such as the patient's name and kind of examination is normally

available. So, in order to get the desired images at the end, a query must be sent to an appropriate server, which is then supposed to search for all images corresponding to the search criteria. Possibly, the user will be asked to make a selection, add more precise information about the roots of the desired images, or change the search criteria. The query process will then become a kind of dialogue.

3. *GET_image*. The selected images are immediately to be transmitted from the image stores to the workstation.

The amounts of data which have to be moved for these three services differ significantly. Only SEND_image and GET_image require a physical transfer of images. FIND_image, however, requires a search in text files: a typical function of conventional data bases. SEND_image and GET_image effect the one-way transfer of typically several megabytes of image data, whereas FIND_image effects the movement of only some kilobytes of alphanumerical data, but normally two-way. Conventional data bases perform the FIND-image service on textual data, but they are by no means designed for a fast access to image data. Because of these significant differences, the FIND_image service and the SEND_image/GET_image services should be performed by separated servers which are each appropriately optimized. Servers for the latter services must be equipped with storage capacity up to the desired terabytes, though it must be possible to move images extremely fast between its stores and network ports. In the following, such a server will be called an image storage module (ISM). The other server, in the following called image management module (IMM), can be a conventional data base or a subfunction of a RIS or HIS. The performance of both the IMM and ISM services can be enhanced considerably by distributing the load and/or

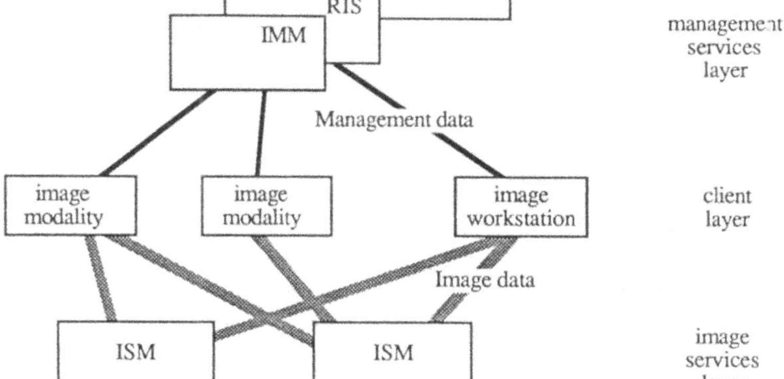

Fig. 7.17. Decomposition of a hospital-integrated PACS (*HIS*, hospital information system; *RIS*, radiology information system; *IMM*, image management module; *ISM*, image storage module)

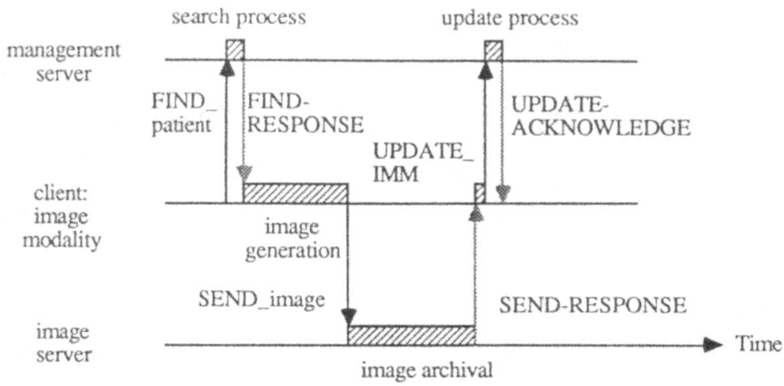

Fig. 7.18. A protocol for image generation in a decomposed hospital integrated PACS

the functions. For this purpose, several of both types of modules are meant to cooperate. Then, at any time the performance or functionality of the whole system could be increased by installing additional modules of the required type into the PACS.

7.2.3.1 Networking the Clients and Servers

The complexity of a PACS, which is due to heterogeneous functionalities of its components, can effectively be reduced by a clean decomposition of interactions. As a first step we define a *client layer* and two *server layers*: the management services layer, which contains all services that use alphanumerical data like the RIS, HIS, and IMM, and the image services layer, which contains all services that exclusively perform image data handling or processing (Fig. 7.17). This type of decomposition also supports the use of high-speed networks which are particularly dedicated to image data transport such as described in Chap. 5.1.5. Based on this model we define the communication protocol which distinguishes only four types of interactions between clients and servers (one forward and backward to each of the two service layers) and avoids direct interactions between servers.

To start with an image generation and the subsequent image archival process, the client (in this case an imaging modality) first requires a query type interaction to the RIS or HIS to get information about the patient to be examined (Fig. 7.18). After its generation, the image is sent to an ISM (SEND_image). As long as the image has not been stored on a long-term storage medium, the image source must keep the image on a local store for safety reasons. After the image archival has been completed, the ISM sends a response to the client which contains information about the final location of the image. At last the client has to update the RIS or IMM (UPDATE-IMM). After that the image is accessible to all clients. An image retrieval is performed as shown in Fig. 7.19. The client starts with a query to the RIS or

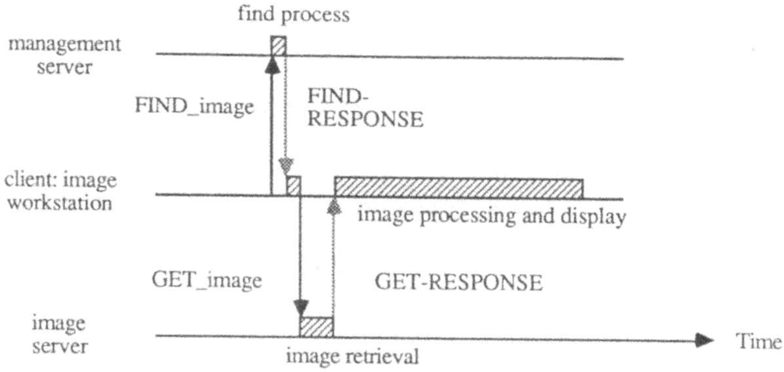

Fig. 7.19. Protocol for image retrieval

IMM (FIND_image). The RIS or IMM returns the unique image identification and, in addition, the information at which ISM the image can be found. The client then sends a retrieve command (GET_image) to the designated ISM, which will return the desired image.

7.2.3.2 A Hierarchical Storage System Meets the Conflicting Speed and Capacity Requirements

So far we have not talked about the internal structure of the ISMs. We have to match the properties of bulk memories – quick but small *or* big but slow – which the archival storage requirements, i.e., big *and* quick! A solution for an acceptable compromise is indicated by the results of the evaluation of the *hierarchical store*, which makes best use of the advantages of fast, volatile storage technologies (solid-state RAM and magnetic disks), and the advantages of the slow nonvolatile WORM technology. For example, at the University Hospital Aachen, the image archive could be equipped with 100 GB of fast buffer store (magnetic disks), WORM jukeboxes with a capacity of 2 TB (about 1 year's image production) and manually operated WORM magazines with a capacity of at least 20 TB (10 years image production).

Such a storage hierarchy needs a smart management which copies the images to be retrieved with high probability into the fast buffer store. In a first straightforward approach, the management strategy is simply based on the statistical correlation between access probability and age of images. Each image which is received by the image archive is copied into the buffer store as well as into the longterm WORM store. The buffer store is operated as a first in first out (FIFO) store, which means that storage space for new images is allocated by subsequently deleting old images. Also, those old images which have been retrieved for comparison are kept on the buffer store level after their retrieval, because the probability for further retrievals

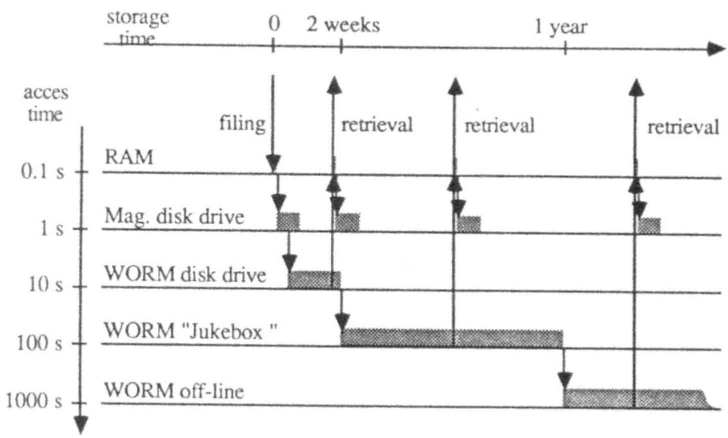

Fig. 7.20. Image flow through the hierarchy of stores

is now the same as that of the related new images. Each further retrieval of an image residing on the buffer store level will pop the logical entry of that image back to the top of the FIFO store. The image storage and retrieval mechanism is illustrated in Fig. 7.20. A special advantage of this type of store management strategy is that it does not need any additional information for the control of the store beside the image itself.

The performance of the storage management can, however, be further improved by prefetching old images which are likely to be retrieved before long. The prefetching strategy uses patient information which normally can be supplied by RIS or HIS systems. In general, as long as a patient stays in the hospital, all her/his images are very likely to be retrieved. It will, therefore, improve the speed of retrieval if all images which belong to this patient are simply copied into the buffer store before they are requested for the first time. More sophisticated prefetching strategies are discussed in Chap. 5.3.

The prefetching mechanism can be added to the store management described above. When a patient is registered in the hospital, information about all old images of this patient will be requested from the IMMs. A PREFETCH_image command is then sent to the ISM. Inside the ISM, all addressed images will be copied into the buffer store in the same way as it is performed after the GET_image command. In fact, the only difference between a PREFETCH_image and a GET_image service is that for the former no transport of the images via the network is performed.

7.2.3.3 Parallel Processing Makes Image Storage Modules Fast

A parallel operation of ISM distributes the retrieval load and increases the chance of getting an immediate response. However, are current computer

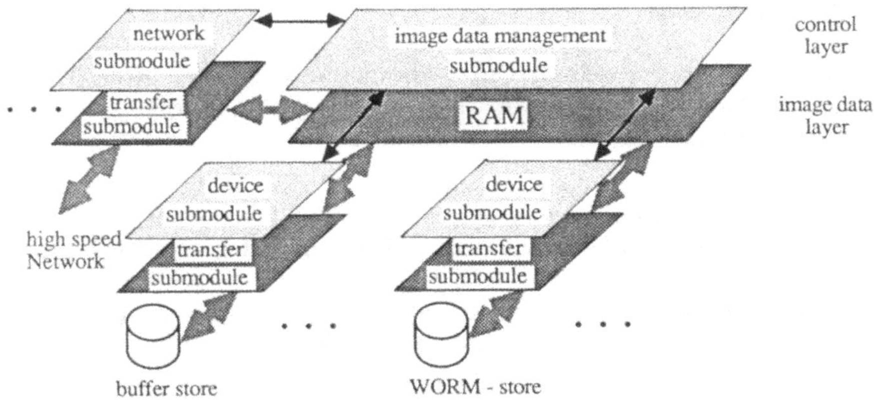

Fig. 7.21. A parallel-oriented image storage architecture

systems fast enough to perform even a single retrieval at a sufficient speed? A data throughput of the desired 100 Mbit/s (see above) can be achieved via state of the art computer buses, but the image to be retrieved has to be moved several times over the one and only bus – WORM to RAM, RAM to disk, RAM to input/output (I/O) port – and filing activities and management processes are still to be interleaved. In order to get image after image at the desired 100 Mbit/s, the processes inside the ISM must be performed in parallel. This needs distributed hardware and a sufficiently powerful internal communication structure. A recent prototype design employs *device submodules*, each of which is responsible for the complete administration and control of one physical storage unit. Network submodules take care of the communication via the image network (Fig. 7.21). An image management submodule coordinates all activities within the ISM. Now the GET_image and the SEND_image service are split up into several tasks which the submodules can execute in parallel. So, for example, GET_image consists of a first task SEARCH_image, to find out which of the storage device submodules can supply the required image, and at least two "TRANSFER_image" tasks. SEARCH_image can be executed simultaneously by all storage device submodules. After its completion, the image management submodule triggers the appropriate storage device submodule to transfer the image into the random access memory (RAM). After this task has been finished, the storage device submodule can immediately continue with other tasks. At the same time, one of the network submodules is selected to transfer the image through the network to the requesting client.

Fast multiprocessor architectures, which are, for example, designed for high-performance image processors, would be an appropriate hardware basis for this type of archive concept. So far, the concept has been implemented software-wise on a VME bus computer using a given multitasking operating system. Though on a reduced speed level, advantages in the performance of the system are gained by a reduction of overheads due to the decomposition described above.

7.2.3.4 Conclusion

Several benefits are achieved by decomposing the image archival service into the IMM and ISM layers, which may in return each be composed of distributed server modules. These benefits are:

1. *Migration*: Additional ISMs or IMMs can be added subsequently in accordance with a growing load or increasing functionality.
2. *Open system philosophy*. ISM or IMM of different vendors can be adapted more easily.
3. *Fault tolerance*. If one server module fails, this will only affect part of the whole system. Other modules can take over the load or at least deliver the required services at a reduced level.
4. *Flexibility*. Many hospitals are already equipped with some kind of HIS or RIS systems. These could possibly be extended by a FIND-image service. Such an integrated IMM also avoids the duplication of data bases (see also Chap. 5.3.2).
5. *Acceleration of image retrieval*. Distributed ISM operate in parallel and hence speed up the access to images.
6. *Image data transport economy*. Since ISM can be installed at those locations where their images are required, data paths can be disentangled and the network load can be minimized.

7.3 Image Indexing by Content*

P. Kofakis and S. Orphanoudakis

7.3.1 Introduction

Many diagnostic imaging modalities are currently available and routinely used to support clinical decision making by providing the physician with anatomical and physiological information. It is possible to extend the capabilities of diagnostic medical imaging techniques by developing medical image data base (MIDB) systems, which support the storage, retrieval, presentation, and interpretation of multimodality medical images. In this section, we present issues related to the design and implementation of an MIDB system which supports image indexing by content. The presentation is focused primarily on the justification of design choices, an illustration of the major features of such a system, and the definition of requirements for its implementation. In this work, image data are viewed as a component of

* This research was supported in part by the Commission of the European Communities under project AIM-1008. We would like to thank the members of the PRIMIS group (AZ-VUB Brussels) and the Department of Diagnostic Imaging, Yale University School of Medicine, for providing most of the midical images. We also like to thank Y. Kavaklis, S. Kostomanolakis, D. Lagouvardos, and E. Petrakis for valuable contributions in this project.

a multimedia document, i.e., a structured collection of image, text, and attribute data. Pictures cannot be described efficiently by words (textual or formated data), and this necessitates the development of indexing techniques for the efficient retrieval of images in picture archiving and communication systems (PACS). An image data base (IDB) system will be presented which also supports image retrieval by (textual and image) content and can be considered as a tool that is used over an existing PACS rather than a separate system. We are not concerned here with physical storage problems such as the encoding of image pixel values (image format), compression techniques, or the short- and long-term storage of raw data on magnetic or optical devices. We are only concerned with issues specific to image indexing by content. These are:

1. How to describe the content of images?
2. How to use such descriptions efficiently for the indexing and retrieval of images?
3. What (graphic) tools and user interfaces are appropriate for IDB systems?

The main objective of the work presented in this section is the development of a system that permits the quick and intelligent access of images, based on their content, from a large set of:

- Reference images for diagnostic and educational purposes (data bank)
- Images archived in a PACS IDB

It is expected that such a system will also provide valuable clinical decision support and will increase the efficiency of diagnostic image interpretations. Specifically, if a physician encounters a difficult case and needs supporting evidence to make a diagnosis, the proposed system will allow him to consult similar images associated with a confirmed diagnosis.

Medical information systems and PACS are among the fastest growing application areas which integrate local area networks, advanced workstations, and image processing systems. Sophisticated IDBs with flexible user interfaces are important components of an integrated PACS. The simplest way to index images is to use textual attributes or keywords that are organized in a tabular manner and used for the indexing of raw images. These keywords and text can be handled by conventional data base management systems (DBMS). Figure 7.22 shows the indexing of images using textual attributes. The physical image identifiers can be used as an input to a PACS query. A new approach is to use *image content + text* (textual support) to store and retrieve images. A schematic diagram of a pictorial information system is shown in Fig. 7.23.

Recently, there has been much interest in various kinds of DBMS for nontextual information. The data base community has expressed this interest by proposing the development of multimedia data bases, spatial data bases, object-oriented data bases, and various marriages between data base and artificial intelligence (AI) techniques. In the computer vision com-

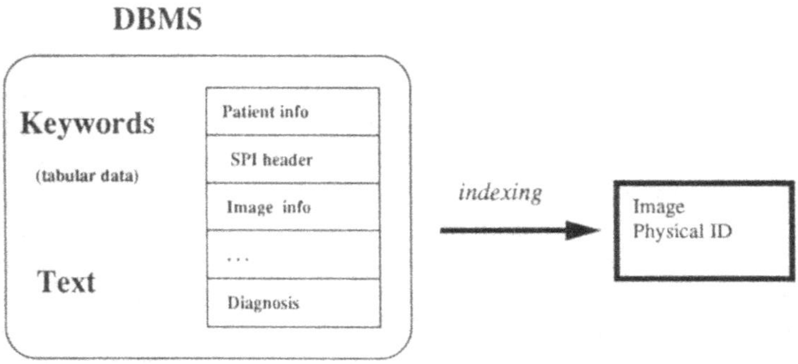

Fig. 7.22. Textual attribute (keyword) retrieval

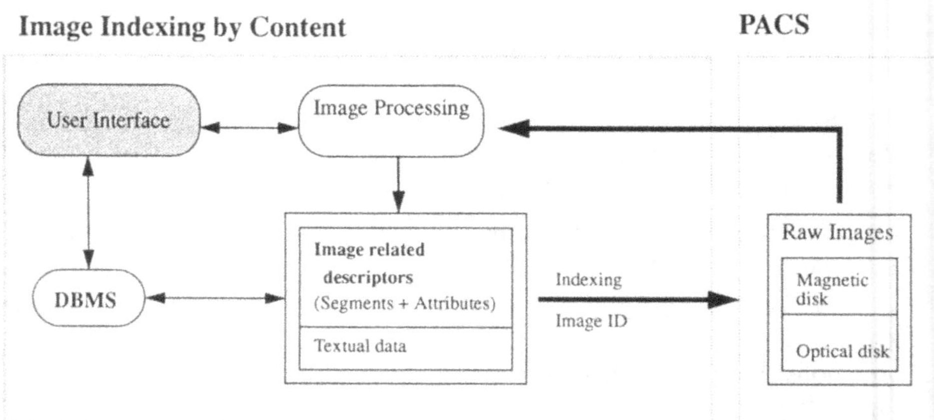

Fig. 7.23. Image database system block diagram

munity, interest has focused primarily on the design of IDBs and efficient retrieval of iconic information by content. This iconic information is often used as a component of various query processing strategies. Both the data base and computer vision communities have a lot to offer toward the formulation of good design proposals. The data base community is evolving from the relational paradigm to the object-oriented paradigm. Systems currently proposed by the data base community for the management of nontextual information are based on object-oriented techniques. A pictorial data base or IDB is a collection of sharable pictorial data encoded in various forms (Chang 1989). The problem of efficient and flexible retrieval and manipulation of vast amounts of pictorial information is very important and requires careful consideration. IDBs are useful as subsystems of advanced information systems such as PACS, or as stand-alone systems, depending on the requirements of specific applications. With the exception of some applications in the area of spatial data bases, data base designers have not concentrated on designing efficient access methods for IDBs, nor have they considered efficient image interpretation as part of their approach. These tasks have been left to the computer vision community. The type of information to be managed can be classified broadly into four categories:

- The images themselves
- Image-related data (registration information, format descriptors, patient name, modality and image file header information such as that of ACR/NEMA)
- Information extracted from images
- Image attributes (textual data such as diagnosis related text)

7.3.1.1 Existing Image Data Base Systems

Chang et al. (1988) have described a prototype IDB system based on spatial reasoning, visualization, and traditional IDB operations. The data structure used, based upon two-dimensional strings, provides an efficient means for iconic indexing and spatial reasoning. However, the two-dimensional strings representation is not always suitable for the description of gray-scale images. The encoding of information, based on the enclosing rectangles of segments in a picture, is rather nonspecific.

In Chang et al. (1977), an approach to designing an integrated data base system for tabular data, graphical data, and image data is described. It is based on a generalization of the relational approach to data base design. The main idea is to represent pictorial information by physical (raw image data) and logical images. A logical picture can be regarded as a description of the real image and is defined as a collection of picture objects. The logical picture can thus be stored in a relational data base and manipulated using a relational data base manipulation language. Once a logical picture has been identified for retrieval, the corresponding physical picture can be retrieved from the image store.

Orenstein and Manola (1988) have developed an IDB based on an object-oriented data base system and the architectural concept of extensibility, which permits specific extensions to the data model. Joseph and Cardenas (1988) use a high-level query language for pictorial applications, which is designed to reside as a major software layer above a robust, commercially available, DBMS.

To date, much effort has been put into making image processing operations "friendlier" to the user. Tanaka and Ichikawa (1988) propose several visually oriented user-friendly facilities, including semantic panning and zooming, overlaying, and retrieval of elements in a specific region on the basis of their relevance. The data structure used includes logical and physical hierarchies for the management of relationships.

7.3.2 Image Representation

7.3.2.1 General Considerations

Methods of image analysis have been used in other domains such as robot vision, remote sensing, and medical imaging to describe and model images. The content of a particular image is determined based on the correspondence between the derived image description and some appropriate model(s) of an image class (Binford 1982; Chin and Dyer 1986). Such methods can be implemented at the array (pixel) level, the region (segmentation) level, and the relational (semantic, syntactic, or structural) level. So far, most of the methods which have been developed are knowledge based, i.e., making use of application- and domain-specific knowledge, and are not particularly well suited for retrieval by content and IDB work. This is primarily due to problems with computational efficiency, uncertainty, and knowledge representation. Methods specific to IDB applications have been developed (Chang et al. 1987), but their usefulness is strongly restricted by their limited expressive power and applicability. Nevertheless, for certain aplications within well-specified domains, it is possible to find techniques of image analysis, modeling, and interpretation which can be used to process images efficiently. Such applications can be found in radiology and microscopy, which yield two-dimensional images of good quality and high contrast. In such cases, the problems mentioned earlier are simplified, image models are easier to construct, accurate image segmentation is easier to achieve, and picture descriptions are simpler to derive. The completeness of any representation ultimately depends on the complexity of the specific image.

In an IDB application, efficient and robust techniques are needed in order to meet speed requirements and to minimize storage space. The resulting descriptions must be compact, and invariant under scaling, rotation, and translation of the image. Furthermore, they must facilitate matching operations and allow the representation of image content at various levels of abstraction. The last requirement stems from the need to reduce the search space during retrievals, by organizing the storage of images into classes with similar characteristics.

Computer vision has been investigated extensively over the last 20 years. During this period, it evolved from image processing to AI, while passing through pattern recognition and syntactic modeling. Vision is most important, mainly because it can get a considerable amount of information from the environment (Ballard and Brown 1982). However, making a vision system demands a considerable amount of work for each specific application.

Computer vision assumes there are several levels of descriptions between the raw image data and their semantic interpretation. First, primitive features are extracted from the image such as regions of different color or texture, edges, or zero crossings. This kind of processing, which is sometimes called "low-level" processing, is not always straightforward, but has reached a certain level of maturity. Examples of low-level tasks are:

Edge detection. Edge detection attempts to find lines or local changes in image features. Edges contain much information that is complementary to regions.

Region segmentation. The basic idea is to segment images into regions according to low-level features such as texture or color. Local or global criteria may be used for this task.

Texture analysis. Texture has been analyzed using syntactic models, models based on statistical features (such as entropy or correlation), functions of distance, and local energy analysis.

7.3.2.2 Automatic Segmentation

Low-level image processing can be model-driven. We know a priori, from the header of an image, which class the image belongs to at a high level of abstraction. Information contained in the description of this class can be used to set default parameters, rules, or procedures so that preliminary image processing is fairly robust for this class of images. Once some easily detectable constructs of the image content have been identified, we can iterate using information contained in the description of classes at the lower level of abstraction and selectively execute some of the image processing procedures (automatically or interactively) with parameters and procedures set to a more discriminating level.

In order to describe the content of an image for storage and retrieval purposes, we *do not need as fine a description* as for interpretation or diagnostic purposes where we need many details. Thus, a description that can adequately describe the important entities of the picture can be used. After noise filtering and operations such as histogram equalization and normalization, images are reduced to segment boundaries, and these are then approximated by linear segments. Chains of edge pixels can be extracted by any suitable method; in this work, Canny's edge detector, as modified by Deriche (1987) was used. The image is first convolved with an optimal filter yielding x- and y-gradient images. Then, local maxima of the gradient magnitude in the gradient direction are extracted and linked to form chains of edge points. During the linking phase, hysteresis thresholding is applied to remove spurious edge points. Finally, a chain-generating algorithm is applied in order to obtain the edge map data (Giraudon 1987). The algorithm requires a single pass over the image, and the result is a minimal set of chains. Every chain is a set of pixel coordinates, with information about junctions with other chains.

Each chain of edge points is approximated by a set of linear segments. Several techniques can be used, the simplest one being *polygonal approximation* by successive splits (Ballard and Brown 1982). Only the x,y coordinates of the linear segments are stored. This representation is used to extract some morphological and relational features of image segments and to compute a set of geometrical features for each segment.

7.3.2.3 *Interactive Image Analysis*

As mentioned earlier, to perform retrievals in terms of image content, some image processing and analysis techniques must first be applied to images to extract appropriate representations. Image analysis can also be performed interactively under the supervision of an expert. In the IDB application, the performance of individual image analysis algorithms is not our primary concern. Instead, we are interested in providing the user with an environment which supports the direct manipulation of image data for interactive, flexible, and globally robust image analysis as needed for image storage and retrieval by content. In many other highly interactive systems that are based upon the principles of *direct manipulation* and graphical control, it is desirable to manipulate data directly, rather than issuing commands to the system, by exploiting the interactive communications facilities afforded by the display system. Anything displayed on the screen is active, and pointing at a specific location of a picture should activate a specific set of processing or display actions.

The need for an interactive image analysis environment arises from the fact that image analysis methods are not always robust. It is often difficult to

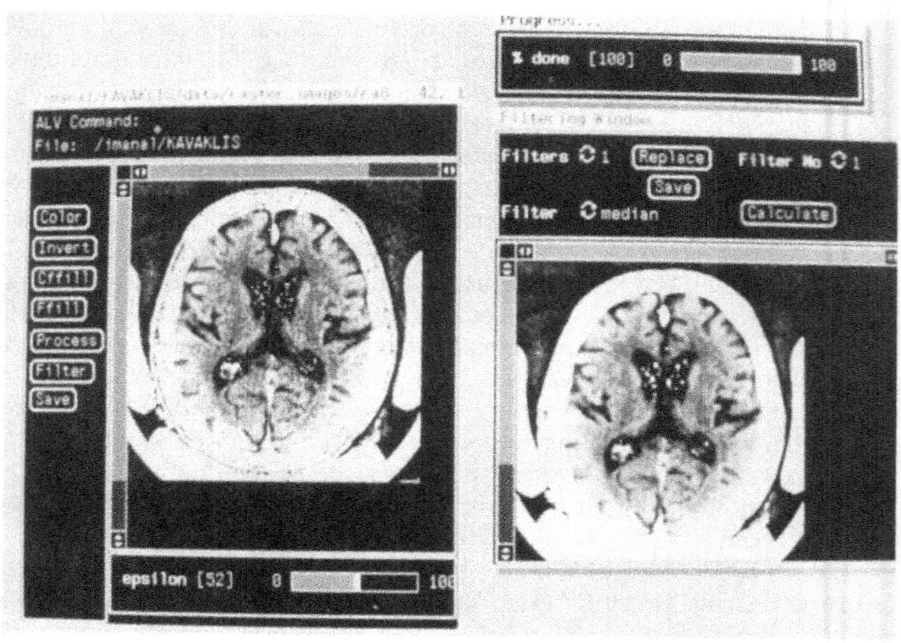

Fig. 7.24. The interactive image analysis window

automatically detect interesting regions (e.g., tumors) or accurately segment parts of the image that represent soft tissues. Thus, we can automatically extract the "easy" or reference contours and manually add other interesting or ambiguous contours. Abnormal/pathological regions can then be defined interactively. To edit the results of automatic image segmentation or to define other regions of interest, the physician must be provided with a variety of tools which are easy to use. For example, the physician can draw a curve which is an initial estimate of the contour of the region of interest, and this crude estimate can automatically converge toward the correct boundary (Kass et al. 1987). A fluid-fill-like tool can also be used to choose regions of interest: The user can click with the mouse at a point in a region of interest. This point is the seed for a region-growing process that defines the region of interest. A slider and panel can be used for the setup of parameters, depending on the type of image to be processed (see Fig. 7.24). Image processing can also be performed in selected parts of the image (included in a contour). In our particular implementation, an integration of many different image processing libraries was achieved in a way transparent to the user. Our system can also support a variety of image file formats.

Image Manipulation

In addition to image processing operations, image manipulation operations can be used to perform certain transformations on the image designed to provide different views. Apart from trivial operations such as panning, shifting, rotation, windowing, zooming, color transformation, and projection, the system should support, for example, the registration (manual or automatic) of images from many modalities or the dynamic display of image sequences.

A language or an interactive tool is also needed to enable the user to define his environment (e.g., windows, type of images, or colors) and the type and sequence of operations for each image. The system should also invoke and guide the different modules (programs) and keep track of the processing of images in order to avoid storing redundant data.

Direct Manipulation

As in many other highly interactive systems, we wish to manipulate data directly, rather than issuing commands to the system, by exploiting the communications facilities of the display. As mentioned earlier, anything displayed on the screen is active, and pointing at a specific location of a picture activates a specific set of actions.

7.3.2.4 Two-Dimensional Representation Requirements

Among all possible features, one must select those that are most discriminating for the application of interest. Another important issue has to do with the semantic level of knowledge that is to be represented. Real world images are mainly three-dimensional. In our case, we have two-dimensional images of relatively good quality (low noise and good contrast). An approach to image representation is suitable for a medical IDB if it satisfies the following requirements:

- Is general enough to be adaptable to new applications.
- Captures the important details that describe the image content, but also small details that may contain useful information.
- Is compact to minimize storage space.
- Is computationally efficient to support real-time processing of large amounts of incoming image data.
- Is immune to noise.
- Is immune to small geometrical distortions.
- Is not dependent on how the object is situated, i.e., it is intrinsic to the object and invariant to two-dimensional transformations.
- Facilitates matching operations (simple and fast matching algorithms).
- Allows easy implementation in specific DBMS environments.
- Is sufficiently discriminating for the application of interest. Redundancy should be minimized.

7.3.2.5 Two-Dimensional Representations: Feature Selection

Features such as regions and edges and their spatial relations are combined to generate object descriptions. Because they represent higher level primitives that correspond to physically meaningful properties of the image, they are less sensitive to variations than the original pixel values. Two-dimensional representations can be divided into several classes, depending on whether they are based on: (a) global features, (b) relational features, (c) graph-based representations, or a combination of these.

Global features can be geometric, statistical or textural (such as average gray or texture values) (Chin and Dyer 1986). A set of such features can be thought of as an n-dimensional feature vector. These features are easy to extract. This type of method is usually associated with the classical feature-space classification scheme (statistical pattern recognition). Matching involves statistical pattern recognition methods. Alternatively, global features can be specified in some transform domain. Examples of such features are the Fourier descriptors, the Hough transform (Duda and Hart 1972), and descriptions of object curvature (Asada and Brady 1986). Examples of local features include line segments and corners. These features can be organized in a highly structured manner such as an ordered list and used to construct abstract models.

Examples of *relational* features include a variety of distance and relative orientation measurements interrelating substructures and regions of an object. To handle occlusions and distortions of shape, an image can be described in terms of local properties (local features) of subparts of the objects/regions contained in the image.

Among the representations that have been used in vision, much attention has been paid to *graph-based* representations (e.g., attributed graphs, semantic nets, and frames). Objects can be represented structurally by graphs. In this representation, geometrical relations between different parts of the image are represented by a graph in which each node represents a part of the image and is labeled with a list of properties. Arcs represent relational features linking pairs of nodes and are labeled with lists of relation values (e.g., distance or adjacency). Attributes can take values on a continuous interval. Labeled links can be replaced by nodes to yield a graph with labeled nodes. Links may be either directed or undirected. Directed links correspond to asymmetric relations, while undirected links correspond to symmetric relations. Although such structures do not solve the problem of representing image content in general, we find many advantages in using them for IDB work. These are the following:

- They represent image content explicitly at the desired level of abstraction.
- They can be considered as generic. Graph representations have been used in a wide range of applications.
- They are powerful and compact.
- Graph theory and AI research offer solutions to problems relevant to the manipulation (representation, matching) of such structures.

Among possible drawbacks, the more important are:

- The matching of graph structures is in general a difficult combinatorial problem.
- The storage and indexing of graphs in conventional data bases in tabular form cannot be done efficiently.
- Graphs may not be analogical representations. Small variations in images may result in unpredictable variations in their graph representation.

Three central issues arise for the specific application:

1. What features should be extracted from an image in order to adequately describe physical properties and their spatial relations in a scene?
2. What constitutes an adequate representation of these features and their relationships for characterizing a semantically meaningful class of objects, that is, in what form should features be combined so that this description is appropriate for describing all objects?
3. How is correspondence or matching between image features to be determined?
4. What kind of knowledge is to be represented?

Our problem is analogous to the problem of object recognition and localization in computer vision where we have to find the: *position* (e.g., translation, rotation, or scaling factor) and *identity* of the object(s) of interest.

Corrections for Geometric Distortions of the Image

In general, the images can also be subject to rigid body transformations such as rotation (patient orientation), translation, scaling and shearing (perspective projection). We do not consider nonlinear distortions, which are often due to the image acquisition process. In order to compensate for these rigid body transformations, we must transform each image to a frame of reference that is common to all images in the data base. The affine transformation that transforms the original image to a "normalized" description can easily be identified using a reference contour for a specific image. This contour is the body boundary in the case of axial tomograms. In the case of sagittal or coronal images, instead of a reference contour which is rather hard to define, we have to define at least four characteristic points of the image which are specific for each class of images. These points are known by the system and are indicated on the reference image. The normalized description constitutes the new IDB representation of the picture and will be used for the retrieval of images based on pictorial content. Spatial relationships between segments are not needed because the spatial reasoning is done in absolute coordinates regardless of distortions, translations, and rotations of our image. This reduces dramatically the combinatorial complexity of the matching process, while the representation without relationships is more suitable for machine learning algorithms, as explained in Sect. 7.3.7.1.

In our system, regions (closed contours) and edges (open contours) with their characteristic features/attributes are combined to generate image descriptions (Fig. 7.25). Selected features that can be used to represent the content of an image (slots of instances of segmented objects) for IDB applications are:

1. Segments and their attributes. The x,y coordinates of the polygonal approximation of segments are stored. This segment representation is

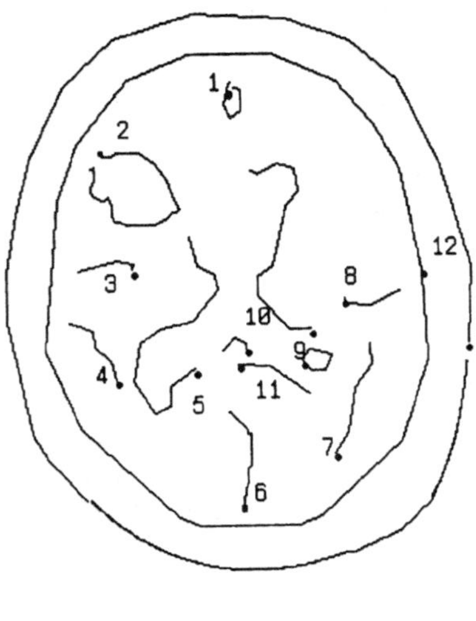

Fig. 7.25. Segment based representation of image content

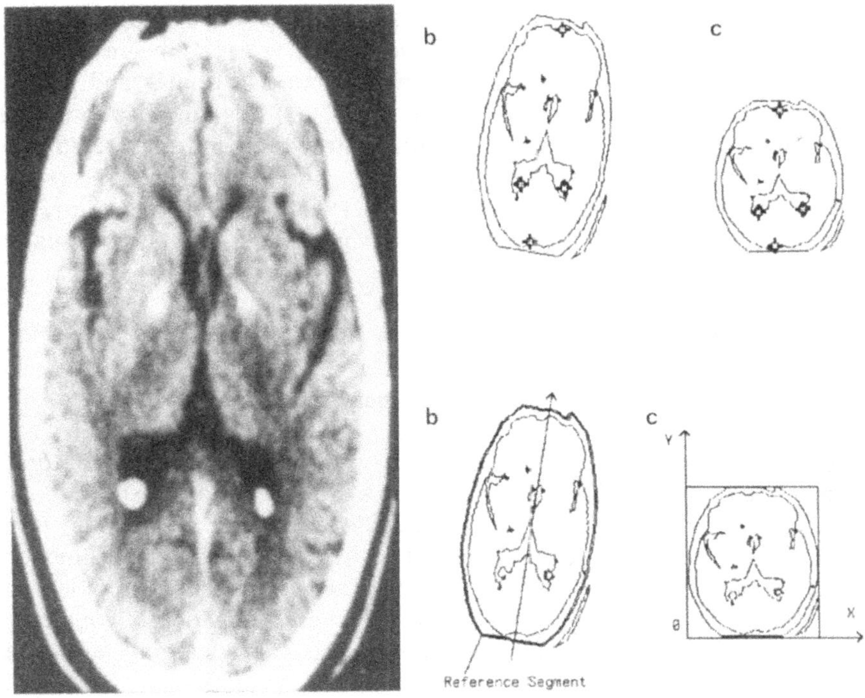

a

Fig. 7.26. **a** Example image. **b** Segments of example image. **c** Internal representation

used to extract some morphological and relational features of segments contained in the image, and to compute a set of geometrical features for each segment. For each object these are: x_{min}, x_{max}, y_{min}, y_{max}; area; perimeter; position; orientation (moments); shape factor; covering with its enclosing rectangle; compactness; elongation; Fourier descriptors (for closed segments); texture class; gray value; color; gradient; mean intensity and standard deviation; area of 1st, 2nd, 3rd, 4th quadrant; and contour length of 1st, 2nd, 3rd, 4th quadrant.

2. Parts of segments and their attributes. Segments are reduced to points: linear segment midpoints, skeleton endpoints, high curvature points, and other characteristic points together with a list of attributes such as length, orientation, position, gray value, and gradient.
3. Relationships. Only the inclusion relationship among objects is used. Given a normalized representation, spatial relationships such as relative orientation, minimum distance, and relative position are not needed explicitly.

Images consist of parts (segments) and their properties that in turn are made up of subparts with their own properties. Thus an image can be described as a hierarchical structure using classes of segments that contain other classes of segments at a lower level of abstraction. The multilevel description of the image has the advantage of modularity and incremental construction of the system. This means that we can begin from a flat structure and incrementally add more and more attributes and features at different levels of abstraction. It is obvious that this kind of representation of image content uses complex internal structures and may require larger numbers of (possibly substructured) properties. Figure 7.26 shows: (a) an example image; (b) the segments of the example image and the reference segment or reference points; and (c) the internal normalized representation.

7.3.3 The Object-Oriented Approach

7.3.3.1 General Description of a Relational DBMS-Based IDB

The different components of an IDB system (i.e., image descriptors, raw image data, image processing procedures that are used to extract the image descriptors, display procedures, the DBMS, and the storage and retrieval rules) are usually loosely coupled. That is, there is a clear distinction between data and the procedures that operate on this data. An older version of our system (Orphanoudakis et al. 1989) used this loosely coupled paradigm (Fig. 7.27). Raw images were processed by an image processing

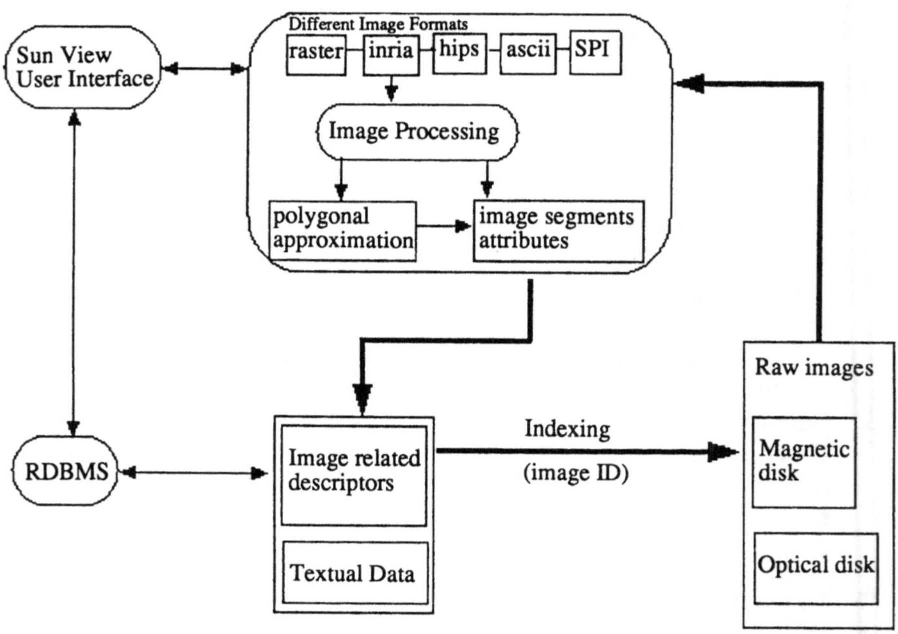

Fig. 7.27. Block diagram of a RDBMS-based IDB system

module and image descriptors were obtained. The descriptors were medium level descriptors, i.e., segments, their attributes, and their relationships. These image descriptors were handled by a relational DBMS (RDBMS) and used for the indexing of images. Queries were formulated using a structured query language (SQL) and could be assisted by an expert system on top of a RDBMS in order to define domain-specific retrieval strategies (matching).

The data base was interfaced with an image processing and interpretation system for coding images prior to storage and the extraction of appropriate image descriptions. Images together with their descriptions and other document components were stored in a document base, which consisted of two parts:

1. The *physical data base*, in which the raw image data is stored, and
2. The *logical data base*, which consisted of three basic tables, in which only the discriminating features were stored. The first table described the image as a whole; the second table held information for segments within each image; the third table described relationships between any two segments in each image. All queries addressed the logical data base. Queries were executed using a command-oriented query language (e.g., SQL).

7.3.3.2 Limitations of RDBMS

RDBMS allow many relationships, but they are completely syntactic, based on operations like joins of entries in the data base. We need the ability to deal with many relationships, and it is not easy to model such relationships in an RDBMS. The aggregation hierarchy is not supported directly by the data base system. Nodes at each level of the hierarchy represent an abstraction of all the nodes below. This abstraction provides for the integration of diverse types of information. The flexibility offered by a hierarchical structure is essential for the storage and manipulation of complex images which may be represented by hierarchical structures of considerable depth where subtrees may be shared by other pictures. The relational model does not support this type of structure directly. RDBMS allow very little flexibility for evolution of their schema, i.e., the schema is static. Furthermore, RDBMS support a limited number of data types. One cannot define complex objects that include edges and regions as well as recursive descriptions of such objects based on their structure. It is also difficult to define a set of basic objects (e.g., edges, curves, regions, arrays, and quad trees), and combinations of these basic objects. Finally data and procedures (user interface, display, image processing, retrieval and rules) are loosely coupled.

In the rest of this section, we present an object-oriented approach which enables the integration of the various components of an IDB system. In an object-oriented IDB system, data, the image analysis module, the data base, the user interface, and the display modules are tightly coupled and considered as a single module.

7.3.3.3 Object-Oriented Systems

The object-oriented approach is particularly attractive for the design and implementation of an IDB. It provides mechanisms for capturing the semantic content of an image in a highly modular and hierarchical manner at various levels of abstraction by making use of abstract data types (ADT) and the principle of encapsulation. It also provides a framework for representing both image content and operations in a uniform way, while the property of inheritance can be used to reduce the amount of stored data. As the problem of designing an object-oriented data base (OODB) is highly application dependent, the user can define his or her own data types and classes and design a query language that is best suited to the specific application, without the limitations of the strict formalism of a query language that is not intended to serve such an application (i.e., SQL).

Object-oriented systems have received considerable attention in the past few years for several reasons. The primary focus of such systems is to provide powerful concepts for applications development and programming, e.g., modularity, encapsulation, inheritance, overriding, protocols and polymorphism (Banchillon 1988). Conventional data base systems are effective in handling files containing fixed-length fields and provide a range of facilities such as interfaces for both end users and applications programmers as well as management facilities to enforce security, reliability, and integrity (Bell et al. 1989). However, such systems have a number of shortcomings, primarily due to inadequate support for the semantic and functional properties of real-world objects. Current data models are thus unable to support the semantic richness of the conceptual model of the real-world. DBMS also cannot store and handle rules, except for limited integrity constraints, and thus are unable to fully support the functional properties of data. The OODB model has several advantages over conventional DBMS models. Specifically, it combines the advantages of:

1. Knowledge based systems, which support complex and dynamic structures of objects in the virtual memory, abstraction and inheritance mechanisms, procedural objects, inferencing and deduction capabilities, and constraint mechanisms; and
2. Data base systems, which support permanent data in the long-term storage, recovery from crash, resiliency of data, concurrent access, consistency checking, and query capabilities.

Furthermore, the concepts used in an object-oriented environment can drastically accelerate the prototyping of a complex system. In contrast, conventional data base systems emphasize data independence by separating the world into two independent parts, namely the data and the procedures operating on them. Thus, we have to split our application into persistent, uninterpreted data and programs that manipulate and share them. Object-oriented systems emphasize object independence, by encapsulating individual objects, and a design composed entirely of objects, only some of which are persistent.

The basic criteria for the choice of an object-oriented approach (Kofakis et al. 1990) to the design of an IDB system are: (a) The use of an environment and a representation/data model that would enable the integration of the different components of the system; (b) the efficient manipulation of the data base schema (classes); (c) enabling new and complex data types that can represent the composition of and the complex relationships among image segments; (d) the need for an extensible and flexible system; and (e) the need to facilitate rapid prototyping. The final goal is the design and implementation of a highly interactive system.

7.3.3.4 Object-Oriented Concepts/Capabilities

The most significant concepts and capabilities of object-oriented systems for the specific application, are described in the following.

Data abstraction. The most important concept in the object-oriented-approach is data abstraction. By this we mean that we are interested in the behavior of an object, rather than its representation. Furthermore, the programmer is not restricted to a fixed set of types, but is free to add new types as required and define objects of various degrees of complexity. An object packages data and the operations that apply to it. Changes to the representation of an object or the implementation of its operations can be made without affecting users of the object, so long as the externally visible behavior of the operations is unchanged.

Abstraction supports the incremental design (possibly top-down and bottom-up) of composite objects (Nguyen and Rieu 1988). This allows the instantiation of objects with partially known descriptions and the incremental design of large objects (complex images containing many kinds of objects). A set of basic objects (e.g., edges, curves, regions, arrays, and quad trees) are defined and then combined to construct more complex objects. A region can be defined as a complex object consisting of other regions or curves. When a representation is chosen, the object inherits from its superclasses all procedures and relevant messages and can immediately be manipulated by other objects of the system. The message passing mechanism can be used for control of the system.

Extensibility. Objects can be easily modified or specialized. New classes of objects can inherit structure and procedures from old ones in a controlled way.

Encapsulation. Data and procedures (called methods) are packaged together in a single, autonomous structure called an object. Data and operations are modeled at the same time. For each object, there is an interface and an implementation part. The interface is the only part of the object visible on the outside and includes the specification of the operations that are allowed on the object. The implementation part includes a data part that describes the structure and the properties of the object and an operation part which consists of the code which implements the various operations on the object. Encapsulation of data with procedures significantly reduces the complexity of large systems by minimizing the interaction between objects.

Independence (object identity). Every object has a unique identity, independent of its value, which characterizes it. Two objects can be identical only if they are the same object. They are equal (not identical) if they have the same value.

Schema evolution. Traditional data bases allow very little flexibility for evolution of their schema (classes). Relational systems sometimes permit adding attributes. However, dropping attributes or moving them to other relations is seldom permitted, i.e., the schema is static.

Schema change operations fall into three categories:

- Changing class definitions, i.e., instance variables or methods.
- Modifying the class lattice by changing the relationships between classes.
- Adding or deleting classes in the lattice.

Types and classes (classification). If every object is to carry its own attribute names and methods, the amount of information to be specified and stored may become unmanageably large. For this reason, "similar" objects are grouped together into a class. Objects that belong to a class are called instances. The concept of class hierarchy reduces information redundancy. A class can have more than one superclass (generalization). These features enable the construction of a hierarchical data base in a similar way to the anatomical hierarchy of the human body.

A type describes a set of objects that have the same characteristics. The notion of type in an object-oriented system corresponds to an ADT. The use of types increases programmer productivity and ensures program correctness. A class consists of a set of objects which have similar characteristics. Unlike types, classes are used only for the efficient creation and manipulation of the objects belonging to the same class. Types are used at compilation time, while classes are used at run time. There are similarities between types and classes. In some systems, there is no distinction between them.

Data bases traditionally have very few classes with large numbers of instances per class. Classification in (relational) data bases serves mainly to provide means for the efficient management of large amounts of data by differentiation between entities by attribute contents. Classification in an object-oriented system supports instantiation, encapsulation, and class inheritance.

Inheritance. A class inherits properties and methods from other classes (single or multiple inheritance). Furthermore, the inheritance mechanism makes it possible for applications to define new classes and have them inherit properties (data and operations) from existing classes. This makes the application easily extensible. Inheritance is a powerful and useful concept in object-oriented programming. It allows objects at different levels in a hierarchy to share data and operations. Data and operations to be shared are put in a level at which the largest number of objects can inherit them. The property of inheritance can be used to reduce the amount of stored data. Furthermore, dynamic inheritance permits the automatic propagation of schema changes on the object instances.

Passive/active objects. Conventional data bases have always viewed data objects as being passive. Active objects can be considered as processes, each with its own script of actions waiting to be activated. One of the most interesting aspects of OODBs is that the objects can be viewed as active agents. They can respond to requests (messages) from other objects, but they can also trigger themselves (e.g., constraint checking when a value is entered).

Navigation. OODBs can support point-to-point navigation between instances in the data base. Thus, it is easy to access objects with many instance-to-instance relationships when they are stored in a data base. This can help queries and the access of objects (e.g., browsing, iterative queries).

Virtual objects. A virtual object looks and acts like any other object, but is just a filter. A simple example is a virtual image (G_GRAD), which is the smoothed gradient of an existing image and is used in the interactive contour detection. Virtual objects can also be operators like gradients, median filtering, and other filter operators without creating intermediate images. Although there is a speed disadvantage, there is a tremendous advantage in terms of space efficiency. Virtual objects are also very important in a display system where minor modifications of existing objects are desired to tune the appearance of the display. Here, virtual images could be used as filters between images coded in different formats that are not directly displayable on the screen. Virtual objects can also provide an excellent interface to various types of display hardware, for example, display of an 8-bit image on a monochrome monitor. Virtual curves and regions can also be created, for example, the zoomed part of a contour or the polygonal approximation of a contour could be virtual objects.

Dynamic classification. Mechanisms for the propagation of changes performed on the schema are referred to as dynamic classification. Once schema modifications are performed, their impact on relevant classes are characterized. For each modified class, necessary changes on relevant classes are defined and checked. Should all these changes be correct with respect to the model and the semantic rules (background knowledge), the corresponding sets of instances are modified. This means that modifications can be propagated on whole sets of instances belonging to relevant classes as atomic operations. Changing a constraint in a class implies that instances of this specific class may also become instances of another class. For example, if we assume that the perimeter constraints on various contour subclasses are as follows: SMALL, ≤ 20; MEDIUM, 21–99; LARGE, 100–200; VERY_LARGE, >200, then changing the perimeter constraint in the VERY_LARGE class from 200 to 180 implies that some instances of LARGE will also be instances of VERY_LARGE.

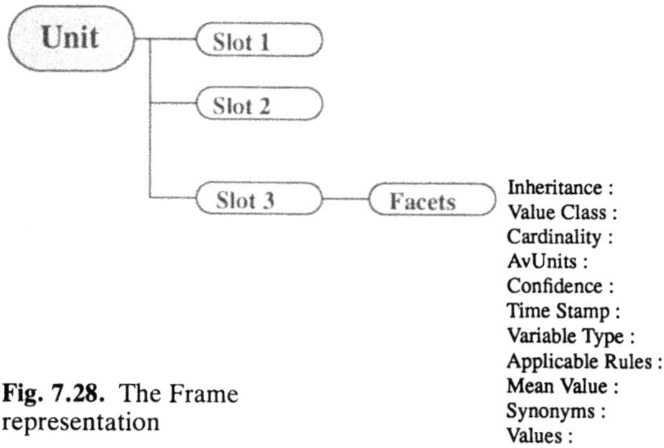

Fig. 7.28. The Frame representation

7.3.3.5 Data Representation

The data representation model used in our work is the Frame model, which is one of the essential knowledge representation techniques used in AI (Mitschang 1988). The primitive element is called unit. Each unit has a name and consists of a number of slots, which in turn consist of a list of aspects called facets. Slots are used for describing the unit they belong to (attributes). Facets are needed for proper specification of the slot and its value. Thus units are formed by an aggregation of slots and facets. A unit can be a class-object or a member-object. Relations (links) relate member-objects to class-objects. As data structures, frames benefit from slot access procedures and value inheritance. The frame is a control mechanism as well as a data representation. The slots may have constraints of their own (e.g., cardinality or value class) or constraints that reference other slot instances or other objects implemented in the form of active values or rules. Figure 7.28 shows the Frame representation.

The slots can also contain information about the organization of the data base (Kleck and Murphy 1990), for example, *hosts* (the names and addresses of hosts in the network), *names* (the name of each image), *image location* (the host and directory where an image is stored), *image size*, and *image format* (how an image is stored such as SPI, ACR/NEMA, or binary).

7.3.3.6 Integration of Background Knowledge

The system should allow the integration of background knowledge (knowledge about the specific domain) such as constraints, assertions that describe a class, and procedures and production rules that change and manipulate the schema (e.g., if attrM = X, then it belongs to class N).

Knowledge is encapsulated in *if–then* rules which interact with the body of data. Rules are also considered as objects. Because of the large number

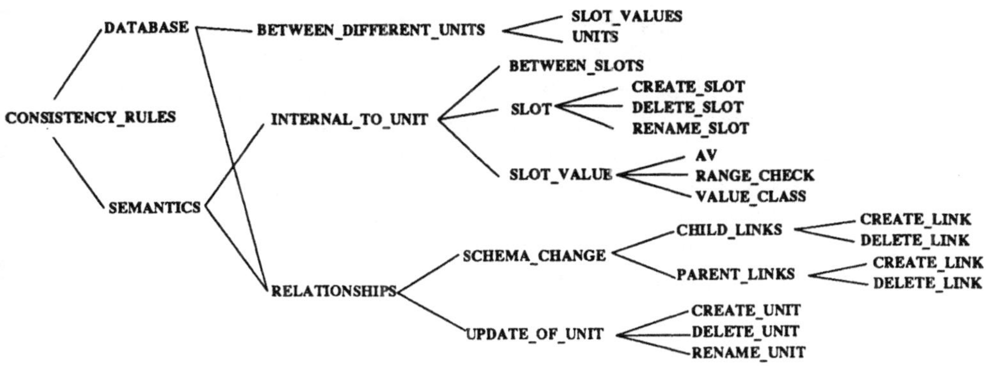

Fig. 7.29. Organization of rules for checking consistency

of rules, additional control has been added by structuring the rule base into classes, and attaching methods to specific classes of the system via the APPLICABLE.RULES slot. Using rules, we can build several models and express knowledge for a specific class of images.

One of the basic functions of the knowledge is to check the consistency of our data. This class of rules applies spatial and contextual constraints. Slot values are checked to determine whether they satisfy constraints with respect to slot values in the same object and slot values of other objects. For example, we can update or modify values of slots for the segments of a specific image. The rules can also check the consistency of the data base schema and be used for constraint propagation or dynamic classification (data base schema evolution). After the activation of consistency rules, links are updated, and objects are moved or deleted, for example. Figure 7.29 shows the organization of rules for checking consistency. Active values are pieces of code which are executed when a specific change in data (slot value) takes place. We can use this code to check for consistency, to update something else in the data base, or simply for debugging purposes. The combination of active values and rules can facilitate the construction of the system's knowledge base. We can attach an active value to specific data, and, when these data change, the necessary rules are triggered so that the state of our knowledge is always consistent.

Strategies are control structures that are implemented in the form of rules and encode knowledge about which methods to apply and in what order. There are also rules for the initialization of the input arguments and testing of the results. Strategies can also be used to optimize the image processing for a specific class of images. Advanced image analysis systems use knowledge-based approaches in order to integrate image processing procedures. The OCAPI system (Thonnat and Clement 1989) is a tool for the semantic integration of existing image processing programs. An expert system built with OCAPI selects sequences of programs, runs them and optimizes the results. The reasoning can be summarized in: (a) the selection of substeps and subgoals, (b) the selection of operators, (c) initialization of the input arguments, (d) effective execution of the programs, (e) a test of the results, and (f) a new execution of programs with different parameters.

Retrieval rules for a specific image class encode knowledge of how to reduce the complexity of a query description, which parameters to use for the search (range), which query evaluation methods to use, and what possible readjustment of parameters is needed for iterative search. The use of prior knowledge helps us eliminate many search paths, so that response time during retrievals will be shorter.

7.3.4 Image Retrieval

7.3.4.1 Matching Considerations

In order to retrieve images based on their content, one must find solutions to the problem of correspondence between a query image and a set of images in the data base. Although it is possible to use very simple attributes that are easy to compare (simple similarity metrics) (Ballard and Brown 1982) or very efficient matching techniques (Ayache 1986) working at the edge segments level, one is still faced with a combinatorial explosion in the case of large image data bases (100 000–1 000 000 images). Thus, in our system, matching is performed at two levels.

7.3.4.2 Medium-Level Matching

Medium level matching can be considered as a filtering step that eliminates many of the possible candidates. The medium-level attributes of image segments are used to prune all irrelevant candidate images for a given class by using large width range queries. The images that pass this step will be candidates for the low-level matching step. We must note that we store in the data base the full description of an image (all segments and all attributes), but only a few are used for a specific retrieval. Retrieval strategies can reduce the complexity of a query graph.

In order to reduce the complexity of the matching process, a query reduction is needed. The query reduction implies that, if we try to find matches for images belonging to a specific class, we are not going to use the "reference" segments that are characteristic of the class and may be present in most of the images in the class, but only the set of segments that are instances of the UNKNOWN class. Thus, the general description of a class stored in the hierarchy in the form of decision trees can be used for the definition of retrieval strategies based on "differential" similarity (Fig. 7.30). Decision trees (Duda and Hart 1973) are popular for their efficiency. In a decision tree, every leaf node carries the name of the class, and every internal node selects a feature (attribute) to be tested. The classification

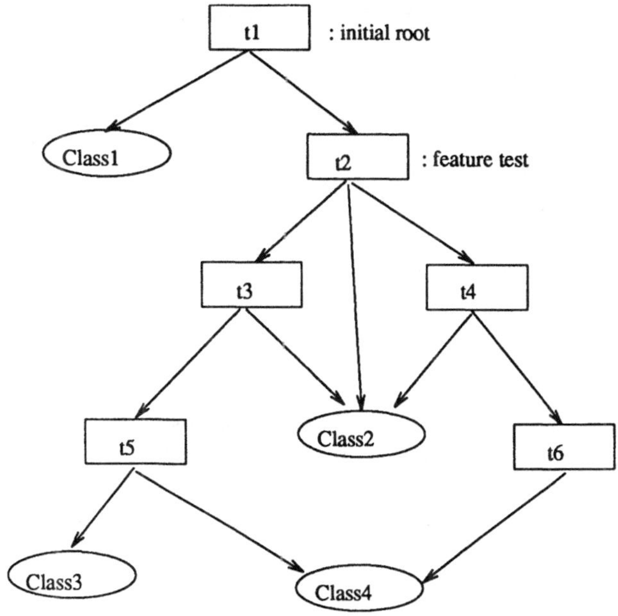

Fig. 7.30. Classification procedure using a decision tree

procedure begins by making the root of the decision tree the current node. The procedure then enters a loop in which the current node determines which feature should be tested and the resulting feature value dictates which child node should become the current node. The loop is exited when the region is assigned to the category associated with the leaf node. The advantage of a decision tree is that it requires only a few of the features to be computed. Some segment features that are costly to calculate need not to be computed in advance. The function that computes a specific feature can be implemented as a method and activated when it is needed. The method knows if the value has not yet been computed, calculates it, and returns the appropriate value which can also be stored in case it is requested again. Thus, computing unnecessary feature values is avoided. Machine learning algorithms can be used for the automatic generation of decision trees. For example, the CN2 algorithm (Clark and Niblett 1989) uses a set of training examples to induce an ordered list of classification rules of the form "*if* {*complex expression*} *then predict* {*class*}".

A measure of similarity is usually defined as a proximity measure in a multidimensional space spanned by selected object attributes. Vectors of values of these attributes for individual objects serve as descriptions of these objects. Each object description corresponds to a point in this multidimensional space. The similarity between objects can then be defined as a reciprocal function of the distance between the corresponding points in the description space. Consider two objects X and Y which are described with features X_i, Y_i $(1 \leqslant i \leqslant n)$. Thus, object X is mathematically represented by the vector $(X_1, X_2, \ldots, X_n)$ and object Y is represented by the vector $(Y_1, Y_2, \ldots, Y_n)$.

The Euclidean distance (D^2) or the Attribute Dissimilarity between these objects can be defined as:

$$\sum_{i=1}^{i=N} (X_i - Y_i)^2$$

Another similarity measure is the Canberra metric which is defined as:

$$\frac{1}{N} \sum_{i=1}^{i=N} \frac{|X_i - Y_i|}{X_i - Y_i}$$

In our system similarity is expressed as a weighted sum of differences of specific attributes. Appropriate thresholds are used to define the required degree of similarity.

$$COST = \sum_{i=1}^{i=QS} W_{1i} AttributesDissimilarity + \sum_{j=1}^{j=MS} W_{2j},$$

where the first sum is evaluated for all the query segments and the second sum is evaluated for all the missing segments.

The weights W_{1i}, W_{2j} define how relevant an attribute is and the importance (focus of attention) of a specific segment in a given query. In general, a significant weight is associated with segments that belong to the UNKNOWN class (pathology). At the end of the medium-level matching, only the segments that satisfy the condition $COST \leqslant threshold$ are retained.

The use of an image representation that does not use explicitly relationships between segments reduces dramatically the complexity of the matching process. The complexity is $O(I\,S)$ where I is the number of candidate images and S is the number of segments used for the retrieval (usually 1–3 segments). The matching process can also be parallelized, i.e., the search space can be partitioned and assigned to multiple processors.

The object-oriented model is associated with an interactive user-friendly environment. The model itself encourages and simplifies the concept of pointing at an object to find out the allowable operations on it and then select a desired operation. A number of different modes of access are:

- Access to an object through its class.
- Access through the aggregation hierarchy (e.g., requests for descendants).
- Access through relationships (relationships can be used to move from one object to another).
- Access through specific features of intrinsic data (e.g., search for specific patterns).
- Combinations of the above.

7.3.4.3 Low-Level Matching

Low-level matching is performed using the midpoints and other characteristic parameters of linear segments constituting the polygonal approximations to all image segments used in the query, e.g., skeleton end-points (Boissonat and Kofakis 1985) or high curvature points (Asada and Brady 1986). The characteristic parameters used are: the x,y coordinates of the midpoint, the orientation, the length, and the gradient value across the segment. Thus, the input is a list of points in a multidimensional (*k*-D) space. The use of spatial access methods is very fast and easy to implement when the dimension of the space (number of attributes) is not very large. The matching algorithm used is similar to geometric hashing algorithms (Lamdan and Wolfson 1988) that use hash tables and voting. The main difference is that we do not use hashing, which imposes quantization of the key (the set of real numbers is reduced to a finite subset) and a limitation on the number of entries in the hash table (if there are too many entries with the same key due to unequal distribution of the entries); we prefer to use indexing and range search.

In the preprocessing step, we create an indexing scheme for all the segments (in normalized form) of all images in the data base. The data base contains the full description of all images (all the segments present in the image and all their attributes).

LOW-LEVEL MATCHING ALGORITHM:
Initialize search parameters (define size of search area).
Set "votes" for all images to zero.
For all linear segments (multidimensional points) in the list:
do

- *Find all "similar" linear segments in the database (k-nearest neighbors in a (k-d) space).*
- *For each similar segment found in the database increment the "vote"* for the respective image.

done
Sort Images with respect to "vote".
The image with the largest vote is the most "similar".

In the current implementation of our system, the voting is purely binary: for the segments that are similar, the vote of the respective image is incremented by one. This has proved to be very fast to implement as well as robust. In order to increase the robustness of the voting procedure, the vote increment can be a function of the segment's characteristics and the distance from the query segment, i.e., $V_c = f$ (segment characteristics, similarity distance). Thus large segments are more robust and will contribute a larger vote than small ones.

If the results of the query do not satisfy some constraints (e.g., vote > threshold, quotient of vote of best match and succeeding retrieved images > threshold), we adjust the search parameters and start the low-level matching step again. In order to increase robustness, we can use several polygonal approximations for the query segments with different line-fitting tolerances (maximum permissible error), because there is not always a unique polygonal approximation for a curve. In order to adjust the search parameters, analysis and modeling of errors is necessary. The advantage of the above method is that we can change the low-level representation of the image (i.e., use high curvature points) without having to change the underlying storage and access mechanisms.

The matching process can be parallelized. Each segment can vote in parallel with other segments, and/or the search space can be partitioned and assigned to multiple nodes/processors. The system can be distributed in the sense that all query formulation and class selection mechanisms can be independent *client* processes that run at different workstations which preprocess the query formulation and then pass this query request to a *global control* module which in turn passes this request to the different *servers* that handle the fragments of the search space. This global control module is responsible for global communication and the concurrency control of the system. It is also responsible for collecting the responses of the different servers and passing the results back to the client.

The matching procedure can be used for multimodality image matching. Although in general this may require very sophisticated transformations, it is possible to obtain matches between computed tomography (CT), magnetic resonance imaging (MRI), and other tomographic images. Suppose we have two sequences of images, obtained with CT and MRI, and we want to match images in one sequence to images in the other sequence. All the images are transformed to a normalized IDB representation. The best one-to-one correspondence can be calculated (matching between the two sets), and an overlay of the two modalities can be displayed.

7.3.4.4 Methods for Spatial (Point) Data Access

As indicated by Preparata and Shamos (1985), range searching problems are similar in some sense to the point-location problems. Normally we have a collection of records (in our case linear segments of all images in the data base) which are represented by an ordered d-tuple of "keys" (points in a d-dimensional space), and several queries are possible on such a file. A range query specifies a domain in that d-dimensional space, and the result is a list of points that are contained in the query domain.

In order to handle spatial data efficiently, data base systems need indexing mechanisms that will help retrieve data items quickly. Classical, one-dimensional indexing methods are not appropriate for multidimensional data. Methods such as B trees and indexed sequential access method (ISAM) indexes do not work efficiently because the search space is multidimensional. Particularly hash tables and similar techniques are not useful because a range search is required. Spatial data access methods provide means for accessing objects that are n-dimensional points (objects of zero size). Most of them optimize retrievals for points that are enclosed in a specific search region. Recently, many methods for handling point and object data have been proposed. R trees are multilevel tree structures designed to handle n-dimensional objects. K-D-B trees are another type of multilevel balanced tree structure designed to handle n-dimensional points. R+ trees combine the features of K-D-B trees and R trees. Like R trees, R+ trees use enclosing rectangles (in two dimensions) to partition the search space at each successive tree level. The local split decision (LSD) tree can support spatial access to multidimensional point and nonpoint objects. A performance study of real implementations of these methods can be found in Greene (1989).

In order to access and retrieve the points which are enclosed in a specific search region the equivalent query is:

if{
$(x_{low1} \leqslant X \leqslant x_{high1})$
and . . .
and $(x_{lowi} \leqslant X \leqslant x_{highi})$
}

A good design methodology is to use a conventional DBMS that can support addition, deletion, and update functionalities and use different indexing (access) methods. In our system, the POSTGRES DBMS is used to store the low-level description of images and support the low-level matching. POSTGRES (Stonebraker 1986; Rowe and Stonebraker 1987) is an extensible DBMS that provides the relational model with general mechanisms that can be used to simulate a variety of semantic data modeling constructs. The mechanisms include: (a) ADT, (b) data of type procedure (active data), and (c) rules. These mechanisms can be used to support complex objects or to implement a shared object hierarchy for an object-oriented data model. In POSTGRES, a collection of POSTGRES commands can be defined as a procedure and stored in a relation. The procedure can then be executed with user supplied parameters. POSTGRES supports user defined access methods. The abstraction for the access methods is a collection of 13 functions, such as *am_build*, *am_insert*, and *am_retrieve*. These functions can be called directly by a user program. This enables us to short circuit many of the database services that would cause a considerable overhead.

7.3.5 Description of the System Model

7.3.5.1 Logical Organization

The data base is organized hierarchically using the object-oriented paradigm (Kofakis et al. 1990), with only large-grained or a high level of abstraction

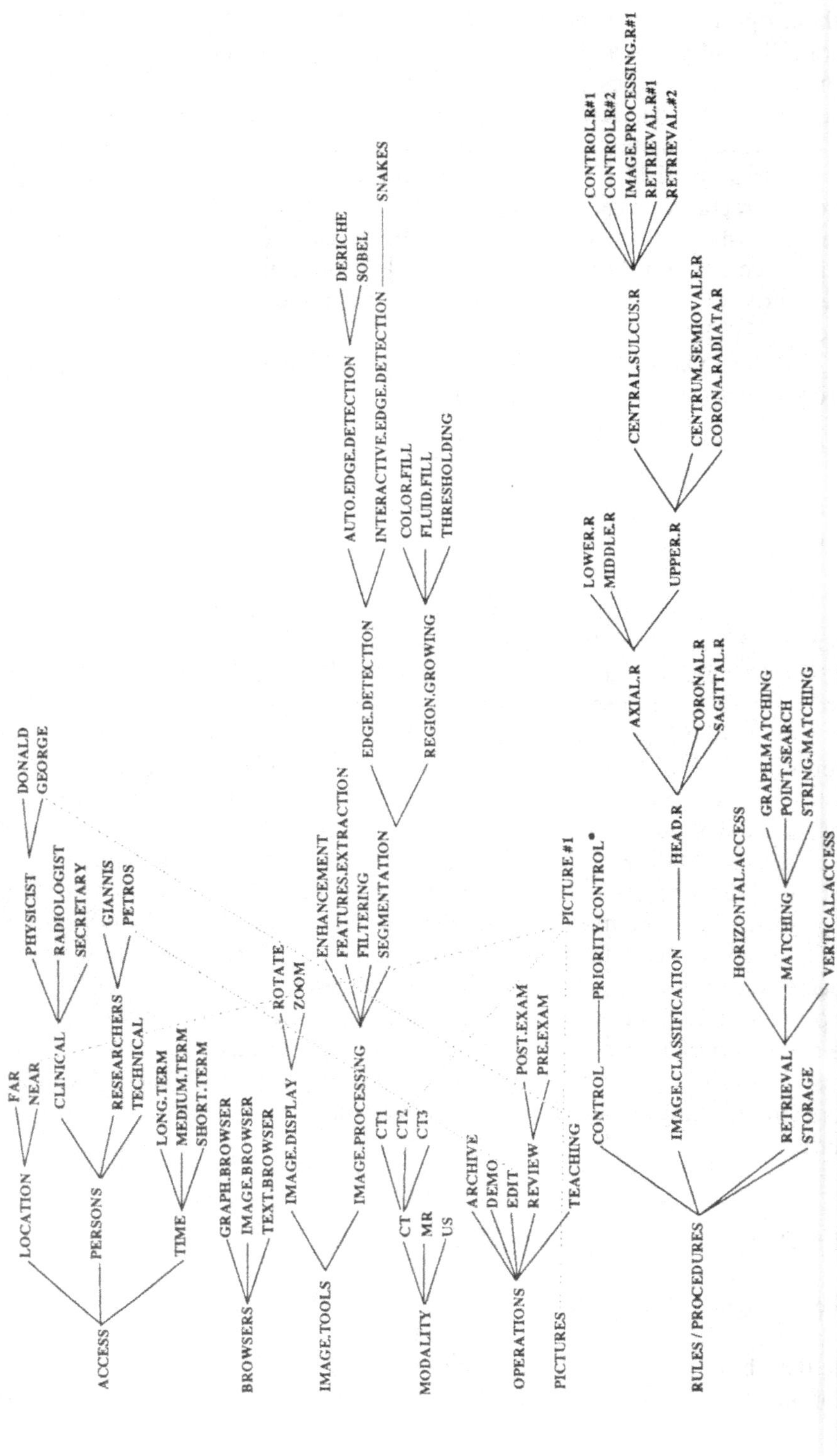

Fig. 7.31. Organization of the system

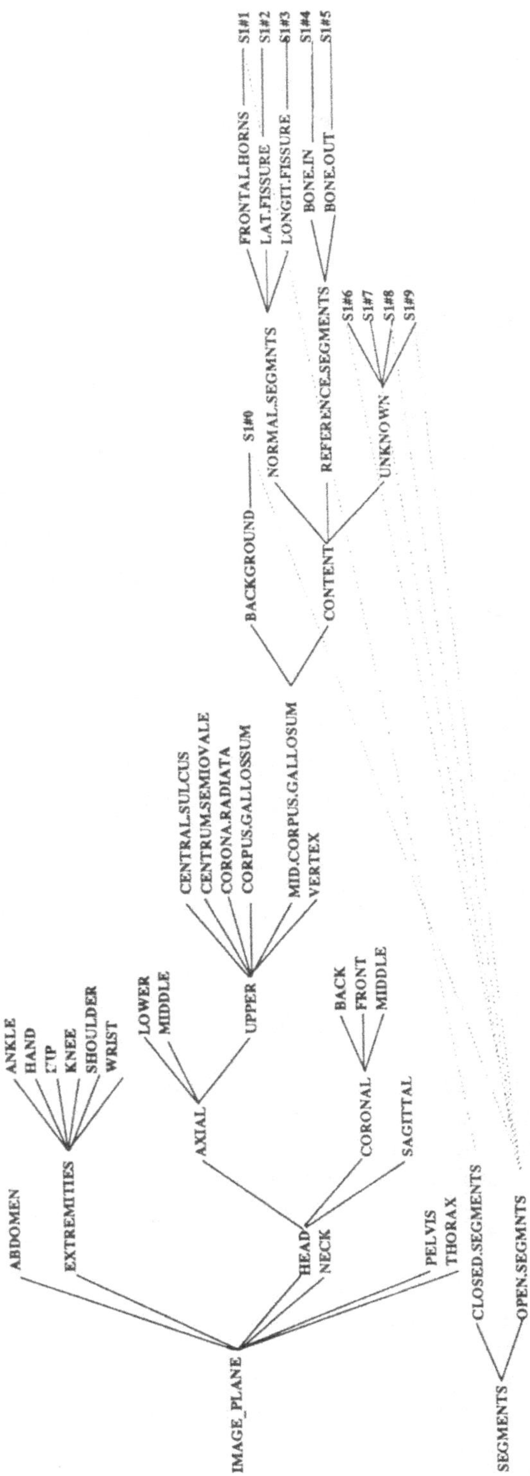

Fig. 7.32. Hierarchy of image and segment classes

objects at the top level. Figure 7.31 shows the organization of the system and Fig. 7.32 shows the hierarchy of image and segment classes. In Fig. 7.32 the high level of abstraction is on the left, and the low level of abstraction is on the right. For simplicity, at each level of the hierarchy only one class is expanded:

1. Hierarchy of segment classes (SEGMENTS). Imagine a complex object that describes the topology of a CT image of the brain. The topology can be represented as a complex object that is composed of other complex objects (directed tree graph). The lower level of abstraction consists of parts of segments and their attributes. Relationship objects indicate the different relationships between the different entities in the image. Some parts of the image (e.g., skull) are relatively stable (detected without ambiguity) and can belong to a special class of reference objects. These reference objects can have their own methods for the display, but also for the activation of special image analysis methods for the part of the image they enclose.
2. Hierarchy of image classes (IMAGE.PLANE). Image classes are defined depending on the part of the body and the image plane position and orientation (Christoforidis 1988). By creating classes based on the anatomical hierarchy, we organize the information efficiently and we partition the data base space for fast retrievals. In the same sense, we can create diagnostic classes in order to offer physicians support at different levels of abstraction and permit them to organize their data. For each class of images we add background knowledge in the form of procedures, rules, and parameters (for image processing and retrieval functions) that can be inherited to subclasses.
3. ACCESS. This defines the different classes of users, storage time and location organization, data, and procedures (e.g., methods and rules). Parameters (for display, processing, and retrieval) can be inherited by a specific class of image content.
4. IMAGE.TOOLS. Procedures for the display and processing (interactive and automatic) of images are considered as complex objects (methods + parameters + rules).
5. RULES/PROCEDURES (see Sect. 7.3.3.6). We build a hierarchy which is similar (same structure) to the images/segments hierarchy. Thus, for each class of images, we have specific operators and parameters for image processing and retrieval, for example.

7.3.5.2 User Interface

The system will be used by many different groups of users (e.g., radiologists, referring physicians, physicists, nurses, and technicians) with their own retrieval, processing, and user interface requirements (Wendler 1989). Object-oriented techniques facilitate the implementation of specific display and user interface methods for different classes of users and images; they

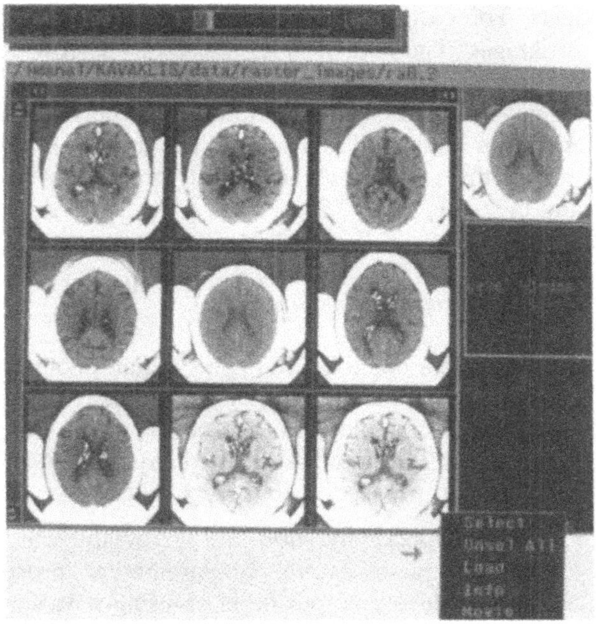

Fig. 7.33. An image browser

also support extensibility. This means that the system can support new devices and operations on the images stored in the data base. For example, a new color display device may be added to the system with relative ease if, at a high level of abstraction, the color display can be viewed as a more specialized presentation device rather than a more general display device already supported by the system.

The display subsystem can be built around a family of methods and messages; each method (routine) may consist of an iterative scheme for scanning and accessing the object using messages, and the code needed to display the object(s) on the screen(s). A small set of display functions can be used on a wide variety of objects. The use of virtual objects enhances and simplifies the display system. Rather than having options in the display routine, a virtual object can be created that captures the desired functionality. The different parameters of the display routines are stored in the database hierarchy.

Browsers are an interactive query mechanism for finding and exploring objects and relationships between objects. Browsers maximize the amount of information presented at one time and provide a means to interactively apply functions to select objects. Browsers are a valuable tool to formulate iterative queries because in most cases users do not know what they are looking for. When a user opens a document (object) using a browser, he can, for example, look at it at various levels of abstraction (resolution), examine iteratively lower levels of abstraction, and navigate to other objects. Three different types of browsers are used for the access and retrieval of images. The text browser is used to narrow down the number of images to browse with an image browser. The graph browser (see Fig. 7.35) displays objects and the relationships between these objects (e.g., parent and child links, and hierarchy). The image browser displays reduced resolution pictures of objects as well as providing functions such as pseudocolor and inversion (Fig. 7.33).

7.3.5.3 Retrieval Example

To illustrate a possible use of the system under development, consider a CT image of the brain (Fig. 7.24). Our objective is to find all images in the data base that are "similar" to this specific image (most complex type of query). Retrievals of images based on their content and using the system under development proceed in four steps (Fig. 7.34).

1. *Image subclass selection.* To narrow the search space by defining classes and subclasses as well as parameters, procedures, and rules that are applicable for a specific class using a variety of tools, image subclass selection is used. Tools which have been developed include direct input of image class (manual or text browser based), a browser based on a

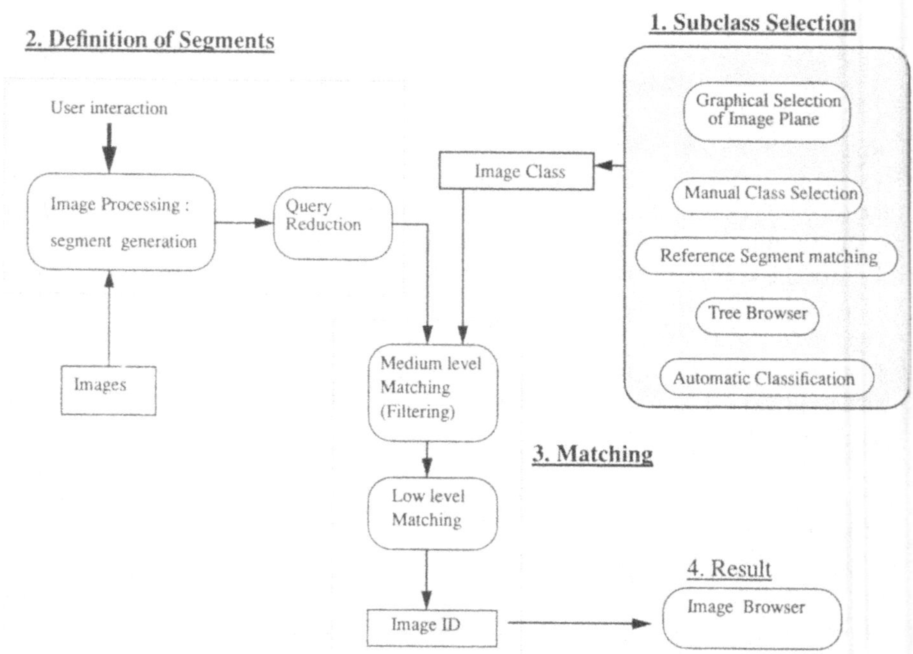

Fig. 7.34. Retrieval mechanism

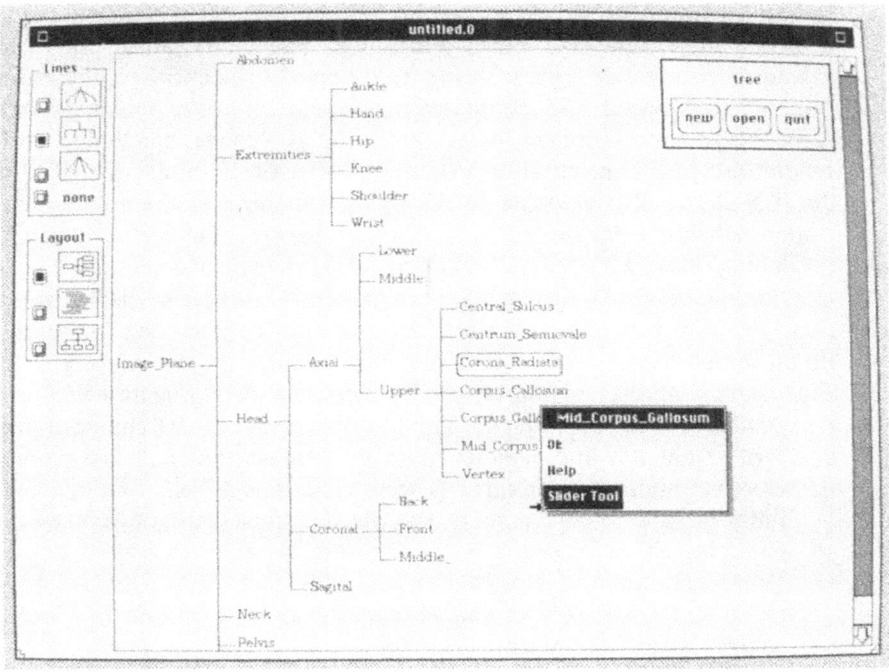

Fig. 7.35. Browser based on a hierarchy tree

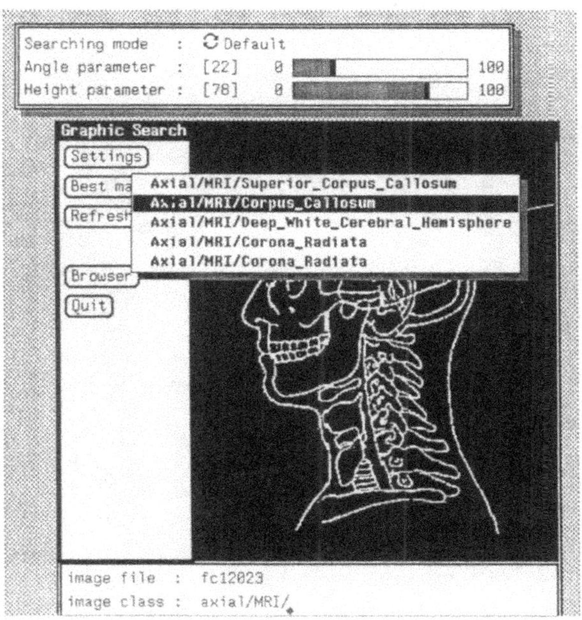

Fig. 7.36. Graphical definition of the image plane

hierarchy tree (Fig. 7.35) a graphical definition of the image plane position and orientation (level and angle; Fig. 7.36), automatic class selection (using machine learning techniques), selection of the most "likely" class based on a comparison of query reference segments with segments of representative images of each class (elastic matching), and, finally, use of the information from the header of the image file (SPI or ACR/NEMA), if it is available. Using one or more of the above mentioned subclass selection tools, the image becomes an instance of the predefined class MID.CORPUS.CALLOSUM, which is in turn a subclass of class HEAD, and it inherits image processing and display functions together with their parameters which can then be used for setting up an initial display and processing environment.

2. *Formulation of a query based on the definition of segments which are representative of image content.* The query image must be analyzed and a set of segments, and regions must be defined that will adequately describe its important structures. The procedure is as follows:
   - Filtering and enhancement, specific for this class of images, is automatically executed.
   - The specific methods/procedures for this class of images are triggered and a sequence of simple, robust, and fast (automatic) image analysis steps take place.
   - Using background knowledge (stored in the image hierarchy) or interactively, a reference segment (e.g., skull) or reference points are defined, and the normalized description of the image is calculated.
   - Using the results of the previous steps, a new environment with different graphic tools for interactive image analysis is activated in

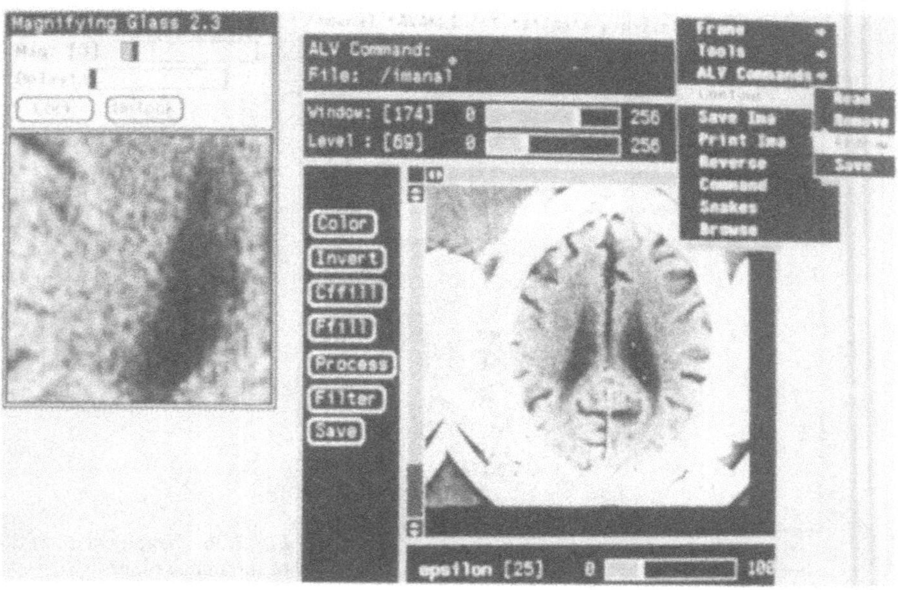

Fig. 7.37.

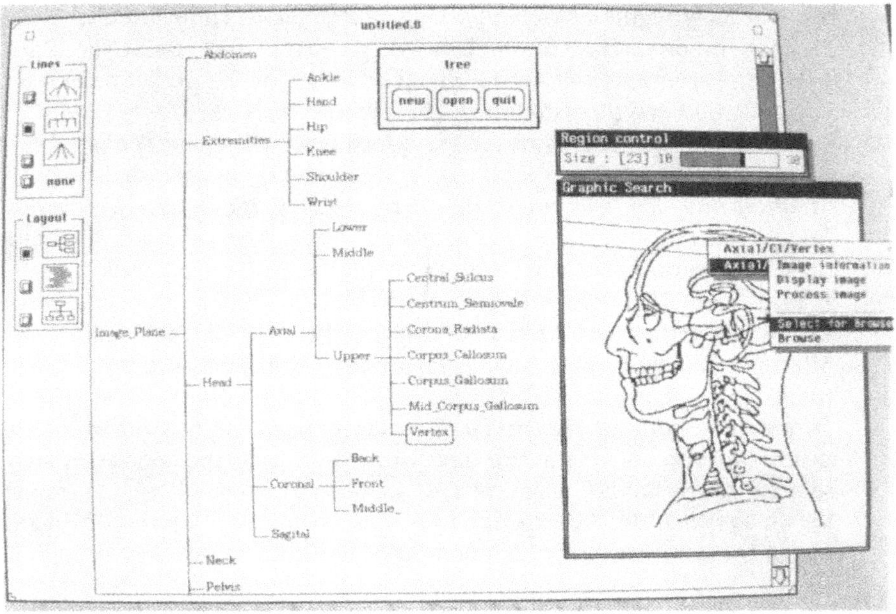

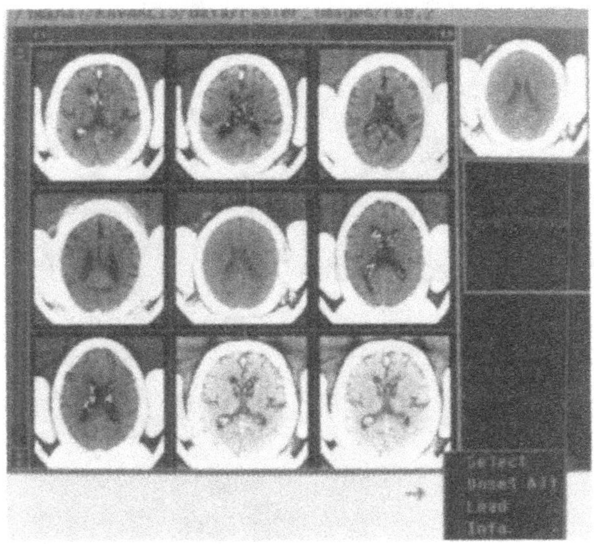

Fig. 7.37. Steps for retrieval: displays that appear sequentially

order to define the segments of interest and parts of the image that define the focus of attention. Using the mouse, specific functions can be activated at specific regions of the image. This is equivalent to model- and content-driven image processing, because at each location only a limited set of functions are available. If we click, for example, somewhere in the background, nothing will happen. If we click in the skull, only a fluid-fill function will be available.

- The new segments obtained from the previous steps are also classified in one of the known classes (e.g., FRONTAL.HORNS). Some of the segments will not be classified in any of the predefined classes and will become instances of the UNKNOWN class.
- Rules for the reduction of the query description are activated (see Sect. 7.3.4.1).

3. *Medium- and low-level matching to retrieve specific images by content.* Image retrieval strategies are activated. These are rules for the setup of search parameters, the evaluation of the results, and the possible readjustment of parameters for iterative search. The appropriate partition of the data base, linked to the specific class, is then loaded and filtering and low-level matching take place. This step is transparent to the user.
4. *Display or listing of retrieved images on a visual or text browser.* The results appear on a visual or text browser. Using the mouse, we can select a set of images of interest. If we are not satisfied, we can repeat the image analysis step to define a more complete description of our image for iterative query. As mentioned earlier, the system (through its

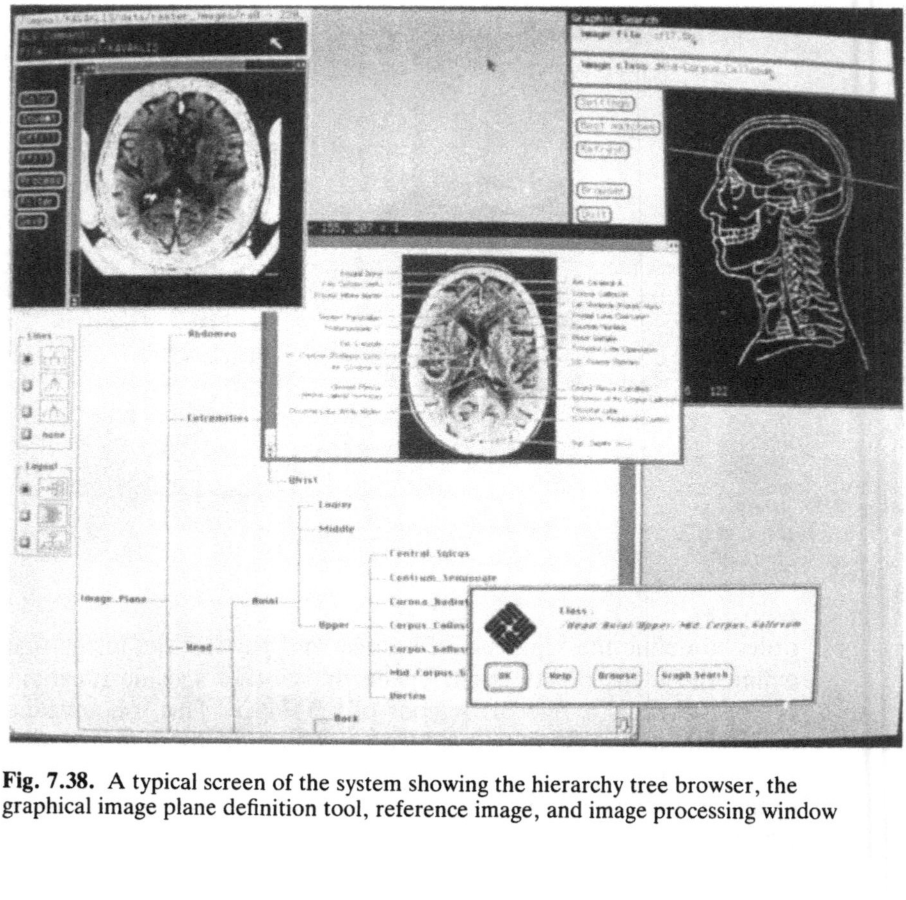

Fig. 7.38. A typical screen of the system showing the hierarchy tree browser, the graphical image plane definition tool, reference image, and image processing window

image processing module) also supports further interactive processing of retrieved images.

Figure 7.37 shows the steps used for image retrieval, i.e., the displays that appear sequentially on the screen. A typical screen of the system is shown in Fig. 7.38, including the tool for the graphical definition of the image plane and a browser based on the hierarchy tree.

7.3.5.4 Implementation

Programming constructs and environments for an image data base application have two conflicting requirements: they must be as general as possible, offering many levels of abstraction, and must also be efficient. Having a programming environment that satisfies the first requirement (e.g., KEE) maximizes the productivity and allows system implementation at a conceptual level without concern for efficiency. Object-oriented languages like C^{++} generate efficient code which is also portable on many machines. We are currently using two approaches in parallel: (a) Advanced tools like KEE (Intellicorp 1988) for the modeling and rapid prototyping; and (b) ET^{++} (Weinand et al. 1988) and C^{++} in order to implement efficiently what was modeled using KEE.

Modeling using KEE benefits from the rule based facilities of the system in order to implement the strategies, retrieval rules, and consistency check. It must be noted that these operations do not all need to be executed asynchronously and are sequential by nature. The rule-based approach facilitates the coding of knowledge. In the ET^{++} version, the reasoning is sequential and is implemented using C-shell scripts under UNIX. Some conditional tests (looping with parameter adjustment) on the results enable the implementation of model-based (specific to each class) procedures. The different external procedures were implemented using the UNIX command paradigm. Figure 7.39 shows the logical/physical implementation of the system.

In our system, we use a hybrid scheme that combines an object-oriented (long-term memory) and a data base system (short-term memory). The long-term memory contains descriptions of all permanent objects (e.g., definitions of classes, rules, and methods) and is the static part of the system. For efficiency reasons, it is resident in virtual memory. A specific hierarchy is loaded only when it is needed and stored back when it is no longer needed. A periodic automatic save of hierarchies can also be arranged. The object input/output facilities of ET^{++} (Weinand et al. 1988) are used to load/download an object structure of arbitrary complexity (to or from C^{++} streams). ET^{++} takes care of linearizing pointer structures automatically. The short-term memory includes the large number of objects that are instances of a class (leaves) and is the part of the system that changes dynamically. A RDBMS implementation (POSTGRES) is used.

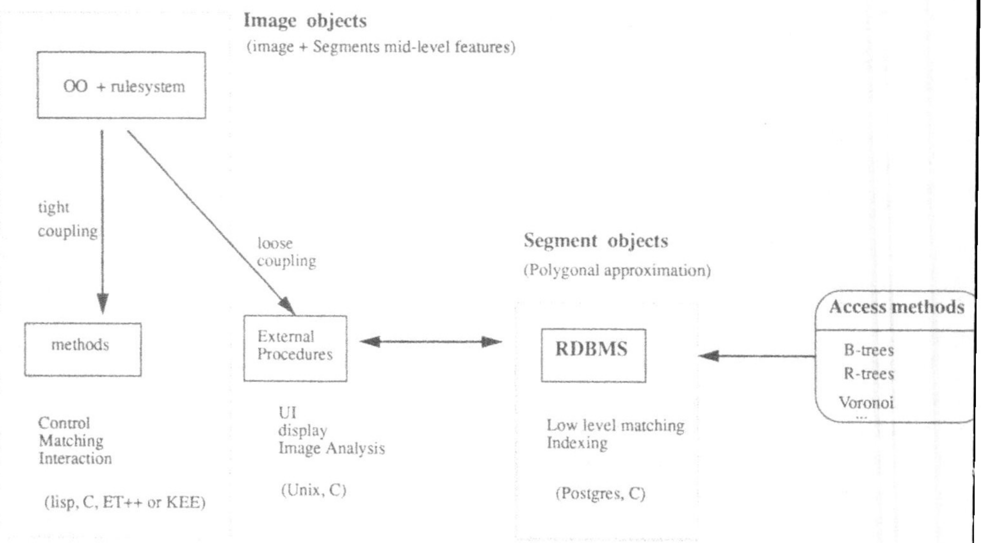

Fig. 7.39. Logical/physical implementation of the system

We use a simple control mechanism. In order to alleviate the overhead of many choices for the user, the system has a priority control that defines the most important functions that will appear on the menus or will be activated automatically. First the system reads the mouse position and creates a list of active objects that interact with the mouse. The priority control mechanism decides which processes will be activated and, after processing, active and passive objects are updated.

In order to implement our system, an object-oriented data base system could be used. Many systems are available today for this purpose, such as GemStone and Orion (Kim and Lochovsky 1989). We must point out that an object-oriented language (e.g., Smalltalk) or environment (e.g., KEE) is not a data base system. Data objects are resident in main memory only. GemStone (Servio Logic 1989) is a multiuser data management system that combines the functions of a DBMS, a file system, and an object-oriented programming language. ORION is a single-user, multitask data base system that runs in a workstation environment and is intended for applications in AI, multimedia document systems, and computer aided design (CAD). ORION has been implemented in Common Lisp. Advanced functions supported in ORION include versions and change modification, composite objects, dynamic schema change, transaction management, queries, and multimedia data management.

7.3.6 Evaluation

Many retrieval-by-content experiments with a data base consisting of about 400 CT and MRI images have demonstrated the efficiency of the system. Queries based on images obtained from the data base and subjected to a reasonable deformation (translation, rotation, scaling, and shearing) yielded only one correct answer. With similar images, the number of replies depends on how strictly our query was formulated. Queries formulated using many query segments and image features tend to give few answers. On the other hand, queries that are formulated using few query segments and image features tend to give many answers. The retrieval strategies and parameters will be studied for each class of images based on feedback from many users and classes of users. It has been found that most of the time is spent in the interactive formulation of the query. A strict evaluation methodology has to be defined in order to measure the performance of the system in terms of recall and precision (retrieval and rejection of relevant and irrelevant information respectively). Thus, one must define:

1. Different categories of retrieval tasks and operations.
2. Different categories of users.
3. Specific retrieval strategies for the categories mentioned in points 1 and 2. These strategies are to be evaluated using quantitative and qualitative measures.

   Strategies implemented and to be tested are:

- Strategies for the reduction of the query graph referred to in the retrieval example.
- Strategies for adjusting the parameters of the low-level search/matching step. In strategies geared for large retrievals, the system tries to obtain a lot of images by increasing the size of the search region. A main inconvenience is that the result of the query may contain too many images. Thus, a complementary query or specialization of the request is required. In strategies geared for precise retrievals, the system might yield very small image sets, thus missing important information.
- Strategies for rejecting some of the retrieved images before visualization. This refinement step may be activated depending on the number of retrieved images.

Quantitative evaluation will include statistics on the percentage of correct and rejected answers of the system, time required for each type of search and each retrieval strategy, time spent in each of the systems modules, and other system requirements (hardware and software).

The qualitative evaluation of different system components, such as the interactive image analysis module, was very satisfactory. Using the interactive image analysis tools, physicians were able to easily identify and define regions and segments of interest in order to formulate their query.

7.3.7 Possible Enhancements of the System

7.3.7.1 Use of Machine Learning

In order to achieve efficient retrieval, the organization of the data base should be such as to facilitate matching and retrieval operations. Specifically:

- The number of possible candidate images should be minimized as much as possible. Images which are similar should be clustered together. Documents should be classified according to a hierarchy (classes) at various levels of specificity in order to partition the image data base efficiently.
- The number of segments that would be checked for correspondence between the query image and the set of possible candidate images should be kept to a minimum. Thus, one should not try to match every segment in the image, but a limited subset of image segments (try to match differences). This means that one should not use segments that are characteristic of a specific class, since they would probably be present in most of the images in this class. The general description of a class can be used for the definition of retrieval strategies based on differential similarity. One can also limt the number of attributes for specific segments by using only relevant and discriminant attributes.

Machine learning can be used to support and enhance the above processes. Specifically, machine learning techniques can be used:

1. For the classification of segments for a specific class of images (e.g., tomographic images of the head). The objective is to obtain a decision tree or rules for the classification of segments (e.g., segments of ventricles). The attributes of a segment are in an unstructured form, thus symbolic (ID3, CN2) (Clark and Niblett 1989) or classical classification techniques can be used.
2. To derive automatically structural descriptions of complex image classes. The existence of relational and structural attributes requires the use of an inductive learning algorithm (INDUCE, AQ15) (Michalski et al. 1985) in order to obtain the characteristic and discriminant description of a limited number of image classes (some classes defined by the user, plus on UNKNOWN).
3. To automatically construct meaningful classifications of images, other than classes based on the anatomical hierarchy, using their content. Conceptual clustering techniques, used to generate classes together with their taxonomic descriptions, seem appropriate for this application.

As mentioned earlier, we use a *flat* description with no relationships, and inductive algorithms of the ID3 family can be used. In order to obtain robust and accurate descriptions, many "noise" images (negative examples) are used. The CN2 algorithm (Clark and Niblett 1989) was used as an induction algorithm that can handle real world data. It can be viewed as a generalization of the AQ algorithm and can elegantly cope with noisy domains. One of its primary features is that the dependence on specific training examples during search is removed, unlike AQ. The CN2 algorithm uses a set of training examples (attribute description) to induce an ordered list of classification rules of the form

if {complex expression} then predict {class}

7.3.7.2 Encoding and Selection of Attributes

In order to increase the speed of access and decrease the storage requirements, we need discrete data representation. The simplest way to go from numeric attributes to symbolic ones is to divide the continuous definition domain of each attribute into intervals that correspond to specific symbolic values (discretization). It is obvious that this kind of encoding is sensitive to noise. Connell and Brady (1987) use a representation adapted from the idea of Gray codes used in digital communications (Chambers 1985). Toggling a single bit in a Gray code only changes the value it represents by one (for example, 1 might be coded as 01, 2 as 11, and 3 as 10). In this way, semantic distance (the mathematical difference between encoded numbers) corresponds to (syntactic) Hamming distance. In digital communications, this property makes the effect of losing any one bit uniformly noncatastrophic.

An other interesting property of Gray coding is that it yields a uniform closeness metric. Gray coding can be extended to continuous intervals and data structures, allowing new data types to be added easily to the representation. Finer distinctions can be made by increasing the number of binary predicates used to Gray code the interval. First consider encoding intervals, which may be either discrete or continuous. For example, the representation maintains the discrete set *{flat, convex, concave, very convex, very concave}* of symbols for the curvature of a portion of a contour. However, it also maintains a continuum of numerical values for the curvature. Intervals and linear descriptors can be encoded by using overlapping ranges. Equivalently, we create a set of overlapping binary predicates whose ranges cover the interval. For each range, we have a Boolean variable which is true if the value being encoded falls in its range and false otherwise. Thus, a particular value is encoded by the set of intervals it is in. Counting can be used to determine how close two values are. The uniform closeness metric property of Gray coding guarantees that sets that differ by a small amount correspond to nearly equal values. This similarity metric can be used in clustering and inductive learning.

An additional property of Gray coding is that the resolution at which a quantity is represented can be increased (e.g., a finer discrimination in the curvature of an object is possible). Suppose we initially divide an interval into eight discrete ranges and create the corresponding Gray code predicates. If later we find that eight divisions are not enough, and that we really need 16 divisions, the granularity of the representation can be made finer by simply adding more predicates. Mechanisms that worked before continue to work on the refined representations. Gray coding can be extended to trees or any other data type.

Attributes may be of three types. Numerical attributes have real or integer value. Ordinal attributes have values which capture a true partial ordering. The third type is that of symbolic attributes. The values of symbolic attributes have no inherent partial ordering. We now consider the problem of reducing the initial set of attributes (image attributes generated by image analysis) needed for the classification processes. The determination of the relevant attributes, their proper encoding, representation, and structuring is a major problem. Various methods of attribute selection (Everitt 1986) such as factor analysis, multidimensional scaling, data standardization, and linear data transformation have been used to approach the problem of selecting the most relevant set of attributes to describe objects. These methods are most effective for numeric attributes when the size of the event set is statistically significant. When attributes are symbolic and the event set is small, these methods are not adequate. Novel methods exist which can handle the many-valued, nominal variables which often occur in classifications (Baim 1988).

7.3.7.3 Data Modeling for Three-Dimensional Applications

The modeling and representation of three-dimensional objects in an IDB is a challenge for the future. Instead of two-dimensional tomograms, we can have a set of adjacent slices and a three-dimensional representation of the body. Thus, we may have a three-dimensional model representing the human anatomy, instead of a large set of two-dimensional reference images.

The object-oriented system could support the modeling of such complex objects. These objects are seen and manipulated at different levels of abstraction. At higher levels they are treated as atomic units of data which are described by several attributes. At lower levels they reveal their internal structure. Their components may be complex objects or just primitive objects without internal structure. Different complex objects may share components. For instance, a three-dimensional object may share part of its surface (glued to) with another object, or a complex object may be composed of objects of the same type (recursive decomposition of a three-dimensional object into subparts). Complex objects are thus represented by a connected, directed, and acyclic graph as a subgraph of the data base schema. It is obvious that we have to cope with objects that change dynamically depending on the ctual view of the application (Mantyla 1988). For example, a boundary (surface) or a volume representation can be used for an object that represents a three-dimensional structure.

7.3.8 Conclusions

An object-oriented approach to the flexible design and incremental implementation of image data base systems has been presented. Using this approach, a system has been developed and implemented in which the user interface, the image data base, and the image retrieval modules are fully integrated. The object-oriented approach has permitted an implementation which is incremental in that, at first, only a hierarchy tree browser was implemented, and subsequently more features were added. These features include a reference image library and mechanisms for integrating knowledge for each image class (e.g., image processing parameters and operators, retrieval strategies and rules). The system, which is currently in the final stages of development and evaluation in our laboratory, is highly interactive and facilitates the quick and intelligent access of images based on their content. Finally, such a system can be seen as a stand-alone system as well as a layer of a PACS and offers image access tools that are not routinely available on a PACS.

References

Abul-Huda BAH, Bell DA (1988) An architecture for a distributed multi-media database system, KALEID. Proceedings of the Eurinfo Conference, Athens, Greece, (avalilable from the European Commission)

ACR-NEMA (1985) Digital imaging and communication. ACR-NEMA standards publication, Washington, DC

Alzner E, Arink G, Gitzwiller FW, Menke KC, Rissi MF (1984) A standard product interface for digital medical imaging equipment. In: Duerinckx A, Prewitt J, Lowe M (eds) Proc SPIE 515: 129–137

Asada H, Brady M (1986) The curvature primal sketch. IEEE Trans Pattern Recogn Mach Intell 8(1): 2–14

Assman K, Venema R, Riemer M, Hohne K-H (1984) The ISQL language. In: Duerinckx A, Prewitt J, Lowe M (eds) Proc SPIE 515: 42–45

Ayache N (1986) Efficient registration of stereo images by matching graph descriptions of edge segments. INRIA internal report, no. 559

Baim P (1988) A method for attribute selection in inductive learning systems. IEEE Trans Pattern Recogn Mach Intell 10(6)

Ballard DH, Brown CM (1982) Computer vision. Prentice-Hall, Englewood Cliffs

Banchillon F (1988) Object-oriented database systems. 7th Symposium on Principles of Database Systems, Austin, pp 152–162

Bell DA, Abul-Huda BAH (1987) Multi-media databases – present and future. Database Technol J 1: 26–29

Bell DA, Grimson JB, Ling DHO (1987a), "EDDS – a System to harmonise access to heterogeneous databases on distributed micros and mainframes, J Inform Software Technol 29: 362–370

Bell DA, Fernandez Mere Z, De Talens A, Gianotti N, Grimson J, Hutt A, O'Sullivan D, Turco G (1987b) Multi-star: a multidatabase for health information systems. Proc. 7th Int. Congr. on Medical Informatics Europe, Rome, pp 564–568, (available from the European Federation of Medical Information)

Bell DA, Ling DHO, McClean S (1989a) Pragmatic estimation of join sizes and attribute correlations. Proc IEEE Conf on Data Engineering, Los Angeles, 1989, (available from IEEE)

Bell DA, Ling DHO, Young IR (1989b) Medical image databases: state of the art. HIPACS internal report AIM-1008
Binford TO (1982) Survey of model based image analysis systems. Int J Robotics Res 1(1): 18–64
Boissonnat JD, Kofakis P (1985) Use of the Delaunay triangulation for the identification and the localization of objects. IEEE-CVPR'85, San Francisco, pp 398–401
Boursier P (1985) Image data bases: a status report. Proceedings of the IEEE Workshop on Computer Architecture for Pattern Analysis and Image Database Management, Florida, USA, pp 355–358, (available from IEEE)
Chang SK (1989) Principles of pictorial information systems design. Prentice-Hall, Englewood cliffs
Chang SK, Reuss J, McCormick BH (1977) An integrated relational database system for pictures. In: Proceedings of IEEE workshop on picture data description and management. IEEE Computer Society, pp 49–60
Chang SK, Shi QY, Yan CW (1987) Iconic indexing by 2-D strings. IEEE Trans Pattern Anal Mach Intell 9(3): 413–428
Chang, SK, Yan CW, Dimitroff DC, Arndt T (1988) An intelligent image database system. IEEE Trans Software Eng 14(5): 681
Chambers WG (1985) Basics of communications and coding. Clarendon, Oxford, pp 45–48
Chassignet P (1985) An image management kernel for the design of relational and pictorial data bases computer-generated images – state of the art. In: Magnenat-Thalmann N, Thalmann D (eds) Proceedings of Graphics Interface 1985, pp 478–484
Chin RT, Dyer CR (1986) Model-based recognition in robot vision. ACM Comput Surv 18(1): 67–108
Christodoulakis S (1987) Analysis of retrieval performance for records and objects using optical disk technology. ACM TODS 12
Christodoulakis S, Ho F, Theodoridou M (1986) The multimedia object presentation manager of MINOS: a symmetric approach. Proceedings of the ACM SIGMOD Conference, Washington, DC, USA, pp 295–310, (available from ACM)
Christoforidis AJ (1988) Atlas of axial, sagittal, and coronal anatomy with CT and MRI. Saunders Philadelphia
Clark P, Niblett T (1989) The CN2 induction algorithm. Mach Learning J 3: 261–283
Codd EF (1970) A relational model of data for large shared data banks. ACM Comm 13: 377–387
Connell J, Brady M (1987) Generating and generalizing models of visual objects. Artif Intell J 31: 159–183
Deriche R (1987) Separable recursive filtering for efficient multiscale edge detection. International Workshop on Machine Vision and Machine Intelligence, Tokyo, pp 18–23
Duda, RO, Hart PE (1972) Use of Hough tranform to detect lines and curves in pictures. ACM Commun 15(1): 36–38
Duda RO, Hart PE (1973) Pattern classification and scene analysis. Wiley, New York
Everitt B (1986) Cluster analysis. Halsted, Gower
Forsdick H, Thomas R, Robertson G (1984) Initial experience with multimedia document in diamond. IEEE Database Engin Q Bull 7: 159–176
Fox J, Walker S (1989) Knowledge-based interpretation of medical images. Springer, Berlin Heidelberg New York (NATO ASI Series, F, vol 39)
Giraudon G (1987) Chainage efficace de contour. INRIA Res Rep 605
Greene D (1989) An implementation and performance analysis of spatial data access methods. IEEE Conference on Data Engineering, Los Angeles, pp 606–615
IntelliCorp (1988) KEE software development system – user's manual. Intellicorp, Mountain View, CA, USA
Joseph T, Cardenas AF (1988) Picquery: a high level query language for pictorial database management. IEEE Trans Software Eng 14(5): 630
Kass M, Witkin A, Terzopoulos D (1987) Snakes: active contour models. 1st International Conference on Computer Vision, London, pp 259–268

Kim W, Lochovsky F (eds) (1989) Object-oriented concepts, databases, and applications. Addison-Wesley, Reading

Kleck J, Murphy J, et al. (1990) Design of a distributed image archival system. In: UCSC internal report, University of California, Santa Cruz

Kofakis P et al. (1990) Image archiving by content: an object-oriented approach. In: SPIE (ed) Medical imaging IV. SPIE, Newport Beach, pp 275–286

Lamdan Y, Wolfson HJ (1988) Geometric hashing: a general and efficient model-based recognition scheme. IEEE International Conference on Computer Vision, Tampa, pp 218–249

Lohman GM et al. (1983) Remotely sensed geophysical databases. Proceedings of the ACM SIGMOD Conference, Atlanta, (available from ACM)

Mantyla (1988) An introduction to solid modeling. Computer Science, Oxford

Meyer-Ebrecht D, Wendler T (1983) An architectural route through PACS. IEEE Computer 16(8): 19

Michalski RS, Garbonnell JG, Mitchell TM (eds) (1985) Machine learning – an A.I. approach. Tioga, Palo Alto

Mitschang M (1988) Towards a unified view of design data and knowledge representation. 2nd International Conference on Expert Database Systems, Sheraton Premiere at Tysons Corner, pp 33–49

Nagata M, Oonishi Y (1985) Video image manipulation in multi-media pictorial database management. IEEE computer architecture for pattern analysis and database management, pp 340–347, (available from IEEE)

Nguyen G, Rieu D (1988) Schema evolution in object-oriented database systems. INRIA Rese Rep 947

Orenstein JA, Manola FA (1988) Probe spatial data modeling and query processing in an image database application. IEEE Trans Software Eng 14(5): 611

Orphanoudakis S, Petrakis E, Kofakis P (1989) A medical image database system for tomographic images. In: Lemke HU, Rhodes ML, Zaffe CC, Felix R (eds) Proceedings of the 3rd International Symposium Computer Assisted Radiology – CAR '89. Springer, Berlin Heidelberg New York, pp 618–622

Preparata FP, Shamos MI (1985) Computational geometry: an introduction. Springer, Berlin Heidelberg New York

Rowe L. Stonebraker M (1987) The POSTGRES data model 13th VLDB Conference, Brighton, pp 83–94

Servio Logic (1989) GemStone: product overview. Servio Logic, Beaverton

Sloan KR, Lipman A (1982) Data bases of/about/with images. IEEE Int. Conf. on Data Engineering, pp 441–446, (available from IEEE)

Stonebraker M (1986) Object management in POSTGRES using procedures. International Workshop on Object-Oriented Database Systems, Asilomar, pp 66–71

Thonnat M, Clement V (1989) Handling knowledge on image processing libraries to build automatic systems. International Workshop on Industrial Applications of Machine Intelligence and Vision, Tokyo, pp 187–192

Tanaka M, Ichikawa T (1988) A visual user interface for map information retrieval based on semantic significance. IEEE Trans Software Eng 14(5): 666

Wendler T (1989) Co-operative human-machine interfaces for medical image workstations: a scenario. In: Lemke HU, Rhodes ML, Zaffe CC, Felix R (eds) Proceedings of the 3rd International Symposium Computer Assisted Radiology – CAR 89. Springer, Berlin Heidelberg New York, pp 775–779

Weinand A, Gamma E, Marty R (1988) ET^{++} an object-oriented application framework in C^{++}. OOPSLA' 88 Proceedings, pp 46–57

8 Standardization

R. Mattheus

8.1 Trends

8.1.1 The Information Technology Industry

The information technology industry is found worldwide and is rapidly becoming one of the most important industries. This industry provides the hardware, software, and services essential for managing information resources and for delivering this information in a form which people can use. The amount of information which now exists in electronic form highly exceeds that in print. The amount and variety of information available from outside and within organizations is continuously increasing. All this influences the technical developments and markets in health care.

8.1.2 The Need for Standards

Health care is an information intensive activity, and some 30% of operating costs are directly related to information handling which could benefit from electronic assistance. However, the communication patterns involve many people and a wide range of subjects. For example, a general practitioner (GP) may refer patients to many specialists, while each specialist receives referrals from many GPs. Each one also communicates with a variety of ancillary services, community care agencies, and administrative and funding bodies. The increasing specialization in medicine and influences in patient choice have led to fragmentation of care and hence to pressure for improved communication between those who provide care and services, both within health care organizations and between them. Clinicians use a wide variety of types of information such as patient records, forms and messages (e.g., test results), images such as computed tomography (CT), magnetic resonance imaging (MRI), ultrasound (US), digital radiology (DR), and X-rays, and signals such as electrocardiography, all of which may need to be communicated. These multimedia data form the kernel of the health care environment.

Although not widely recognized, a key problem is the provision of adequate interfaces between the numbers of heterogeneous systems and modules that are likely to be involved. Table 8.1 demonstrates the scale

Table 8.1. The number of links required to connect objects

No of objects (n)	1	2	10	100	1000
No of one-way links ($n^2 - n$)	–	2	90	9900	999000

of the problem. If two objects need to communicate, only two links are required (one each way), but if 1000 objects need to communicate, the number of links increases to 999000 (Table 8.1).

Furthermore, links between computers are not as straightforward as some users might imagine (Fig. 8.1a). A simple link (one-way) from A to B involves a message (information model) (Fig. 8.1b), which in turn requires some form of envelope (communication model) (Fig. 8.1c). The process of creating the message and its envelope requires one set of computer programs (AC), while the task of receiving the message requires another set of programs (BC) (computation) (Fig. 8.1d). Figure 1 shows the increase in complexity when moving from the user model, through the information and communication models and finally to the computation model.

Despite the need for a better use of resources if the delivery of quality health care is to be cost effective, the diffusion of information technology into the health care sector has fallen far behind that in other business sectors such as manufacturing and finance where it may exceed 10% of the operating costs. One of the primary impediments has been the lack of standards for communication between applications in a heterogeneous environment.

8.1.3 Open System Approach

In the past, most systems worked in closed environments. Systems probably came from the same supplier and were selected to be able to work together. An open approach becomes essential, not because everything needs to be open to everything else, but because a switch from closed to open systems is the only practical way forward in this revolution and evolution of hardware and software.

The range of technical aspects which have to be standardized is wide.

- Compatibility at the elementary level of plugs and signal voltages.
- Communication over each successive link in the whole series of links between transmitter and receiver.
- Determination of the addressing and routing of transmitted information.
- Dealing with deficiencies in the communication service.
- Coordination of the dialogue with the remote system.
- Coding of communication information in such a way that both systems can manage.
- Interaction with remote system to perform whatever task is the purpose of the communication.

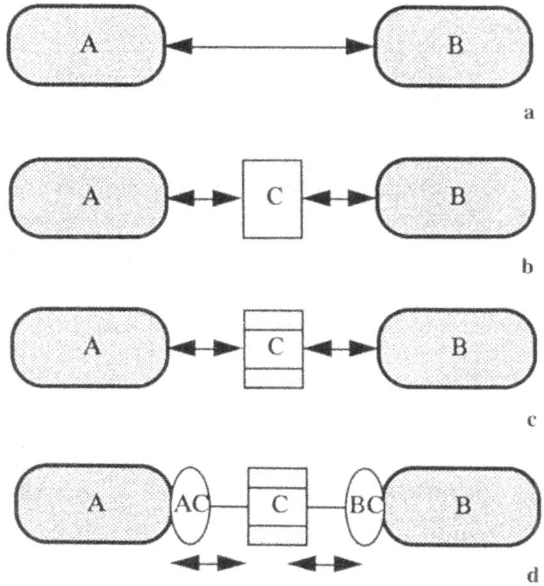

Fig. 8.1a–d. Simplified models for computer communication. **a** User model showing a one-way communication link between *A* and *B*. **b** Information model. The link between *A* and *B* is provided by message *C*. **c** Communication model. Message *C* comprises both information content and an envelope. **d** Computation model. *C* is created by process *AC* and is interpreted by process *BC*. *AC* and *BC* are computer programs which may include the OSI profiles

The set of standards called open system interconnection (OSI) standards provides the basic technical specifications for these aspects. The OSI reference model defines the framework within which the basic standards have been developed. Many of the terms associated with OSI come from the diagram used to represent the model, which is often called the seven-layer model (Table 8.2). One cannot have a single set of OSI standards with just one standard for each of the aspects. Multiple standards are needed to cope with variations such as:

– Different types of tasks (electronic mail, remote terminal operations)
– Different types of information (data, text, diagrams, images, voice, signals)
– Different types of networks (private/public, wide area/local area)
– Different types of environments (office, hospital, private practice, campus)

8.1.4 Functional Profiles

The term "functional standard" is shorthand for the definition: if you want to provide function X, then use standards A, B, C . . . in this way. In other words, a functional standard specifies how to use other standards (base standards) to archive a particular function.

The standards produced by the International Standards Organization (ISO) and the Comité Consultatif International Téléphonique et Télégraphique (CCITT) are usually referred to as "base standards" and

Table 8.2. ISO/OSI reference model

7	The application layer is that in which the actual service sought by the end user is provided	Application layer
6	The presentation layer provides a means of representing information in a data coded format in such a way that it preserves its meaning whilst resolving syntax differences	Presentation layer
5	The session layer provides the services required to establish a session connection between two presentation entities and support for orderly data exchange interactions	Session layer
4	The transport layer defines the rules for information exchange and manages end-to-end delivery of information within and between networks including error recovery and flow control	Transport layer
3	The network layer determines how data are transferred between computers and is mainly concerned with routing within and between individual networks	Network layer
2	The data link layer comprises procedures and protocols for operating the communication lines. It shapes the data into standard blocks and sets up "frames" to convey them. It also offers a means of detecting and correcting message errors	Data link layer
1	The physical layer provides the physical means of sending data over lines, i.e., the electrical, mechanical and functional control of the data circuits	Physical layer

often contain a large number of options. In an OSI environment, the principal requirement is that two implementations interwork. In order to achieve this, it is necessary for the same base standard to be implemented at each level of the reference model (for example, a system implementing multiple access collision detecting, CSMA/CD, cannot directly interwork with one implementing token ring). Even with this constraint, interworking is far from guaranteed and is usually necessary to select various options and to restrict the values of various parameters within the base standard. A set of base standards is restricted in this way.

8.1.5 Key Elements for Standardization

Standardization in the medical imaging field cannot be considered separately from the overall prospect of standardization in medical informatics. It has become clear that, for instance, the successful implementation of picture archiving and communication systems (PACS) depends on the integration of these systems in an overall hospital information system (HIS) and other departmental systems. Communication is the heart of a PACS environment. Communication takes place between systems, applications, and users. Standardization is needed on these different levels. This means that whatever standardization is decided on for medical imaging has to be compatible with any possible standard for a HIS system or departmental systems.

Several problems can then be identified. Firstly, the standards presently proposed in medical imaging, have been developed in isolation from their integration into HIS systems, e.g., the American College of Radiologists/ National Electrical Manufacturers Association (ACR/NEMA), European co-operation in the field of scientific and technical research (COST) project B2, and the Standard Product Interconnect (SPI). Secondly, a considerable user base of HIS systems has already been installed. These are all different and have been installed and/or developed on the basis of local needs with little if any consideration given to standardization and/or interconnection.

It has to be recognized that the ultimate aim of standardization is to facilitate the communication between multivendor systems and between different users. Hardware and software compatibility are needed. Standardization should concentrate on the decision of which data are essential and thus should be included in the design specification of medical imaging equipment interface systems. It is then up to the users and international standard organizations to ensure that manufacturers make this information available.

As the medical market is very small, the medical community has to base its applications on general communication standards. General standards, however, have often been developed with different profiles in mind. Elements related to standardization include:

- Problems of terminology and legal issues
- Communication hard- and software
  - User/display
  - Display/internal
  - Internal/external
- Technology assessment (requirements, quality, calibration)
- Image manipulation
  - Research tools
  - Education
- Security
- Introduction of equipment
- Life cycle of introduction of PACS systems
- Education

8.1.6 Decomposition of the Imaging Standard

There are several aspects of the imaging standard, namely:

1. The *on-line interface standard*, which is by far the most important standard. It has to be implemented in all imaging modalities (e.g., MRI, CT, DR), and US and in all PACS components.
2. The *off-line interface standard* is directed at the exchange of medical images on off-line media, e.g., optical disks in Write Once, Read Many (WORM) technology, magneto-optical disks (MOD), or optical cards. It is used for the exchange between imaging modalities and PACS

archives, in various health care institutions, or for image storage on personal disks/cards.
3. The *PACS – radiology information system (RIS) interface standards* is not an image interface, but related to the image interface standard. Data communication includes transfer of patient data, information on work flow, and administrative data. No fixed interface definition is possible. The interface depends on the respective PACS and RIS functionality. Harmonization with the other standards in the health care environment is required.
4. *Image processing standard* is not a standard on algorithms (several algorithms are suggested, as is compression), but a standard method to describe the algorithms used and coding for them.

8.2 Formal European Standardization Bodies

8.2.1 CEN/CENELEC

The Comité Européen de Normalisation (CEN), created in 1961, is the independent cooperative association of 18 Western European standards institutions that are, at the same time, members of ISO. CEN/CENELEC have central responsibility for the establishment of regional European standards through a structure of committees with member country representation. United States companies operating in the European Community can apply through the European national standards organizations to serve on CEN/CENELEC groups and subcommittees. The work of CEN is divided among a number of technical committees (TC) in different areas. Members of these TCs are elected by the national institutes as representatives. The work itself is done for a selected area in the scope of the TC by working groups (WGs). A WG consists of members selected by the national standardization institute, which may also contribute to the standard writing procedure. For fast action, a project team (PT) can be established for a specific objective.

8.2.1.1 CEN Standardization Aims

The standardization aims of the CEN include:

- Promoting the uniform implementation by its members of international standards prepared by ISO or the international electronics committee (IEC), when they exist.
- Harmonizing national standards.
- Preparing European standards when required, typically when no international standard exists.
- Implementing and promoting procedures towards mutual recognition of test results and certification systems.

- Co-operating with the European Community and European Free Trade Association (EFTA), and collaborating with European and international organizations, principally economic, scientific, and technical organizations.

8.2.1.2 Types of CEN Publications

An adopted European standard (EN) will be implemented in its entirety at national level by being given the status of a national standard, regardless of the way in which the individual member voted. The EN is implemented by the publication of a corresponding text. Conflicting standards are withdrawn.

A harmonization document (HD) is developed and adopted in the same way as an EN, but its application is more flexible so that the technical, historical, or legal circumstances pertaining to each country can be taken into account. The HD implemented by public announcement. Conflicting standards are withdrawn. The difference between a HD and an EN is that a HD gives some flexibility while there still is some divergence from national standards; it tries to harmonize the differences. The standardization body may announce a HD and prevent the publication of an identical standard.

A European Prestandard (V = *Vorausgabe*) (ENV) may be established as a prospective standard for provisional application in technical fields where the innovation level is high, or where an urgent need for guidance is wanted, and no aspects of safety for persons and goods are involved. The time required for its preparation is, therefore, reduced, as well as its lifetime, which is limited to 3 years. It is implemented by announcement, in the same way as EN/HD. Contradictory national standards may be kept in force. An ENV is not a draft standard in the sense that it is not yet adopted (prENV), but rathere an official European standard. It consists of provisional acceptances and represents a speedy way of realizing the drafting of a new standard. After its lifetime of 3 years, it must be reviewed, transformed, or withdrawn.

8.2.2 CEN TC 251: Medical Informatics

8.2.2.1 Scope of CEN TC 251: Medical Informatics

In order to respond to the challenge of integration and communication in the world of medical informatics, in June 1990 CEN founded a new TC, TC 251, in the area CEN TC 251 is responsible for the general coordination of all standardization activities in medical informatics in Europe (Fig. 8.2), and PTs prepare activities in the different fields. CEN/IT/PT001 has worked on an action plan which is being proposed to TC 251 for creating new WGs and starting new PTs on specific items.

CEN TC 251 deals with the organization, coordination, and monitoring of the development of standards, including testing standards, in health care

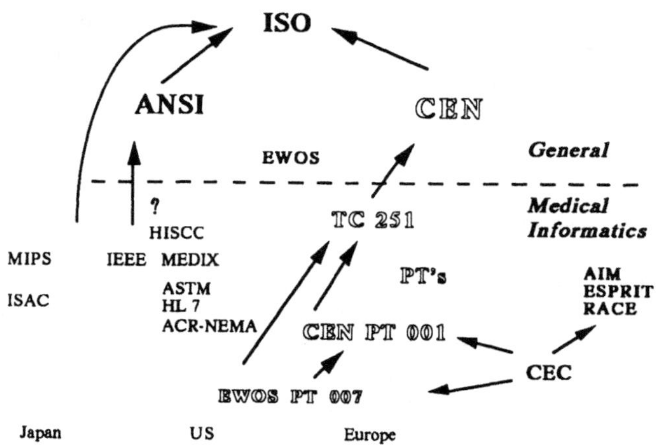

Fig. 8.2. Worldwide standardization efforts in medical informatics

informatics as well as the promulgation of these standards. The scope of the work is subdivided into the following domains:

- Methods and conceptual models (criteria, health care information model).
- Information systems for the Health sector (subsystems definitions, reference structures).
- Terminology (encoding systems, mapping or conversions between systems, data definition).
- Interface and communication (message syntaxes, transfer mechanisms).
- Quality, protection, and security (legal aspects).

8.2.2.2 CEN TC 251: Working Groups

By April 1991, the following WGs will have become active:

- Health care information modeling and medical records
- Health care terminology, semantics, and knowledge bases
- Health care communications and messages
- Medical imaging and Multimedia
- Medical devices
- Health care security and privacy, quality and safety
- Intermittently connected devices

8.2.2.3 CEN TC 251: WG Imaging and Multimedia

It is difficult to present here the real scope of activities being carried out by the WG on imaging and multimedia, but some topics which can be important are mentioned. If we want to exchange images, a standard format is necessary, which must consist of:

- Representation of complex image structure
- Related data
- Complex data

Imaging studies can be very complex, and involve many different types of data. Images come from various types of modalities and departments such as radiology, nuclear medicine, pathology, and radiation therapy. Moreover, if we want to interpret or process these images, additional image-related information is needed. Definitions of image-related data, i.e., patient and medical data, related to the study are particularly raried; some of them can be handled easily (e.g., patient name and age) and some by defining conventions (patient orientation), but many definitions and parameters remain complex, e.g., pulse sequence in MRI and parameters in SPECT. A specific image interchange transport profile is needed to meet performance requirements that exceed general medical interchange requirements due to image sizes (0.25–8 MB) and response time constraints. Subsets of the standard will be needed to match different performance requirements, and it is expected that emerging ISO/CCITT standards for fast local area networks (LANS) and wide area networks (WANS) will be adequate for this.

A standard command language must be defined to allow the interpreting and processing of instructions on other systems. Not all the systems are made for the same purpose and, therefore, have different processing possibilities.

In order not to interfere with the internal systems, a minimum set of instructions must be defined. On a CT image, complex multiple query is not necessary, but it probably is on storage devices. The introduction of image classes can be used in the future by a unified regulation to guarantee the medicolegal background of the use of image processing. The enormous amount of data produced by imaging devices calls for the implementation of highly advanced techniques of data compression to reduce transmission time and volumes undergoing archiving. It is important to know which compression algorithms are used and what the level of destruction is. An image must be identified uniquely world wide to allow communication in the IMAC world and outside the hospital (Tele-medicine). As with a telephone, a unique code is used worldwide.

Visualization needs to be common for each device in the department/hospital environment. To make this possible, software phantoms and material phantoms need to be standardized. Image generation devices like laser scanners need to be calibrated and made to conform with the display device. Common techniques to calibrate systems such as positron emission tomography (PET) and SPECT need to be developed. A better common documentation of equipment is needed in a multivendor world. Image quality and method of conformance testing of cathode ray tube (CRT) display for medical image presentation in PACS environment as well as

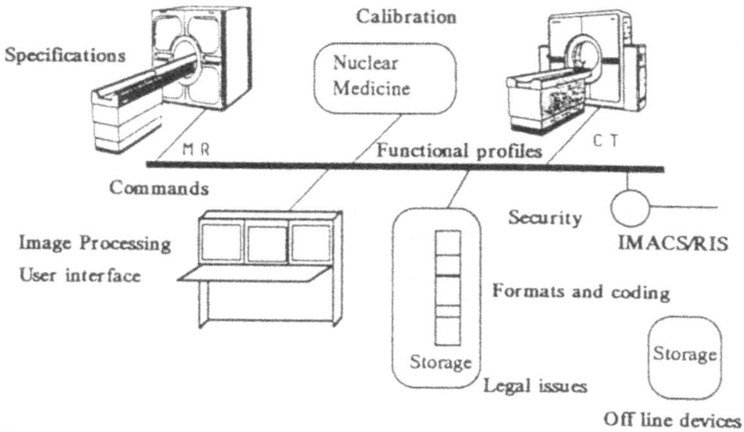

Fig. 8.3. Needs for standardization in the IMAC system. *Boldface* indicates aspects requiring standardization

spatial resolution, gray scale resolution, brightness and uniformity on the screen are items for standardization. Test patterns to check image quality need to be developed. Quality control and quality assurance should be established. The Harmonization of medicolegal information aspects need to be discussed, e.g., the length of time images need to be archived.

In order to allow for a consistent IMAC and HIS, data base command functions for minimal information exchange need to be standardized. Directory structures for off-line devices such as MODs need to be defined so that exchange is possible. In Fig. 8.3, an example of an IMAC system is reflected.

8.3 European Bodies Promoting Standardization

8.3.1 European Workshop for Open Systems

The European Workshop for Open Systems (EWOS) was created in 1987 by the most representative European federations of technology suppliers and users organizations (e.g., COSINE, ECMA, EMUG, OSITOP, RARE, and SPAG) in conjunction with the European standards institutions CEN and CENELEC. EWOS objectives are to serve as a truly open European platform for the development of OSI profiles and to define corresponding conformance testing specifications. The outcome of all the activities is fed into the formal standardization channels managed by the European and international standardization bodies CEN/CENELEC and ISO/IEC-JTC1. The EWOS infrastructure is small and flexible, and can, therefore, adapt itself easily to changing circumstances. The development process, however, is monitored as an industry-like project in which the delivery timing of results is set forward at the start.

8.3.2 X/Open

X/Open is a joint initiative by a large number of the world's major information system suppliers, supported by representatives of users, system integrators, and software development communities to make true open systems a practical reality. This is archived by establishing a comprehensive integrated common application environment, which ensures portability and connectivity of applications and allows users to move between systems.

- Portability of applications at the source code level.
- Connectivity of applications via portable networking services that are independent of underlying protocols, plus support for common protocol stacks to ensure that X/Open machines may be interconnected.
- A consistent approach to the user interface with the system.

8.3.3 European Community Framework Programme

The Third Framework Programme of research and technological development was approved by the European Community Council Decision of 23 April 1990. The main objective will be to contribute to strengthening the technological base for the development of standards in order to encourage the attainment of the single large market, thus making it possible for industry to invest in the design of products on the basis of common standards. Transfer of technology in order to encourage the use of new technologies will assume particular importance and will include certain demonstration projects with particular reference to the use of such standards. It was in the advanced informatics in medicine (AIM) framework that the hospital integrated PACS project was started and supported. This frame work is in close coordination with the work of CEN TC 251.

8.3.4 European Committee for Recommendations and Standards in Computer Aspects in Diagnostic Imaging

The board of EuroPACS, together with the European Association of Radiology has taken the initiative to form the equivalent of the American and Japanese structures for promotion of standards. The European Committee for Recommendations and Standards in Computer Aspects in Diagnostic Imaging (ECR/SCDI) was created at the beginning of 1991 and will organize contacts with European industry and the analogous American and Japanese organizations, and form working groups to tackle concrete problems. The line of actions of ECR/SCDI could be proposed as follows:

- Formation of dedicated working groups, open to interested members of the different organizations

- Collaboration with European industry
- Collaboration with the official standardization organs in order to avoid confusion

8.3.5 European Co-operation in the Field of Scientific and Technical Research

COST project B2 is a cooperative international activity which aims to set up a European procedure for quality assurance in nuclear medicine software ensuring:

- Standard protocol for exchange of nuclear medicine files
- Quality assurance of cardiac software
- Quality assurance and standardisation of kidney software
- Quality assurance of brain software
- Knowledge-based systems in nuclear medicine
- Quality assurance of bone phantoms data base
- Quality assurance of SPECT

8.4 Standardization Actions Related to Medical Informatics and Imaging

8.4.1 Food and Drug Administration

The Center for Devices and Radiological Health (CDRH) of the Food and Drug Administration (FDA) develops and implements national programs in the fields of medical devices and radiological health. These programs are intended to assure the safety, effectiveness, and proper labeling of medical devices; to control unnecessary human exposure to potentially hazardous ionizing and nonionizing radiation; and to ensure the safe exposure to potentially hazardous ionizing and nonionizing radiation and the safe and efficacious use of such radiation. The Center regulates medical devices intended for human use, including devices within the purview of medical informatics and conducts and otherwise participates in national and international voluntary and regulatory standards activities related to medical devices and radiological health.

8.4.2 American National Standardization Institute

The American National Standardization Institute (ANSI) coordinates the development of American national standards through a structure of distributed accredited organizations and committees. Recently, ANSI adopted a coordination committee for health care which will be the communication channel between Europe and the United States (CEN-ANSI).

8.4.3 Medical Data Interchange Committee

The IEEE P1157 Medical Data Interchange (MEDIX) committee sets out to define an architecture, an object-oriented data model, and OSI application layer services and protocols to support both interactive transactions and store and forward messages and documents involving health care data interchange.

8.4.4 American Society for Testing and Materials E31 Committee

A number of working groups have been set up under the American Society for Testing and Materials (ASTM) E31 (computerization) committee with the aim of developing standards that will enhance the ordered growth of computerization in medicine. The first standard produced was for the exchange of clinical laboratory data.

8.4.5 Health Level Seven Group

The Health Level Seven (HL7) group is a consortium of suppliers and users who are producing specifications for the format and protocol for the exchange of data among health care data processing systems, with particular emphasis on patient administration, orders, and results from services and financial information.

8.4.6 Open Document Architecture

Open Document Architecture (ODA) is a standard developed to facilitate the exchange of office documents. The ODA notion of a document is a structured amount of information intended for human perception that can be interchanged as a unit between users and/or systems. ODA requires documents to be defined by a logical structure which defines the logical relationship between the components, e.g. chapters, sections, and figures, of a document, and by the layout structure which defines how the components of a document should be laid out on the presentation medium.

8.4.7 EDIFACT

The EDIFACT Syntax Rules (ISO 9735, EN 29735) and the United Nations Trade Data Elements Directory have been adopted as European standards for electronic data interchange (EDI). In March 1990, a Pan-European EDIFACT user group known as the European Medical Electronic Data Interchange (EMEDI) group was established to support a common approach to EDI within the health services and health care industries. It will focus first on commercial interchanges such as ordering and paying for pharmaceuticals, but will also support the use of EDIFACT standards in administrative and medical data interchanges.

8.5 Standardization Actions for Medical Image Interchange

8.5.1 ACR/NEMA

8.5.1.1 Scope

The ACR and the NEMA recognized in 1983 the emerging need for a standard method for transferring images and started to define standards for the described area. The ACR/NEMA Committee was thus created as supervising board, and a number of WGs defining standards in the various subareas came into being:

- *WG I.* Hardware and protocols
- *WG II.* Data formats
- *WG III.* System and performance specifications

Currently, the following groups are active:

- *WG IV.* Compression standard
- *WG V.* Exchange media
- *WG VI.* Validation and further development
- *WG VIII.* RIS/HIS/PACS interface

The standard is intended to facilitate the development of PACS capability of interfacing with other HIS, and to allow the creation of diagnostic information database which can be interrogated by a variety of distributed devices. The ACR/NEMA standard specifies the hardware interface, a minimum set of software commands, and a consistent set of data formats for communication across an interface between an imaging device. The standard is not intended to be an overall PACS or network standard.

The ACR/NEMA standard has six layers; the network layer of the ISO/OSI model is not included. The standard was specified for point-to-point communication and, therefore, does not require the routing functions of the network layer. The physical layer is specified completely in hardware with a goal of supporting a 64 MB transfer rate.

8.5.1.2 ACR/NEMA Version 2.0

The standard of digital imaging and communications includes the data format, protocol, and hardware interface necessary for transmission of data between two pieces of medical imaging equipment. The location of the

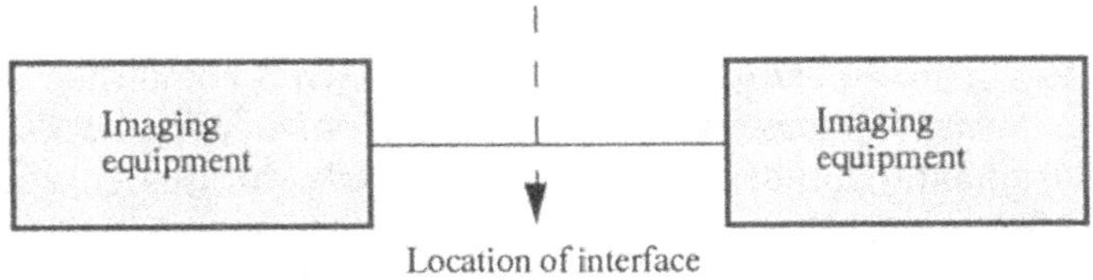

Fig. 8.4. ACR/NEMA interface for communication between imaging equipment

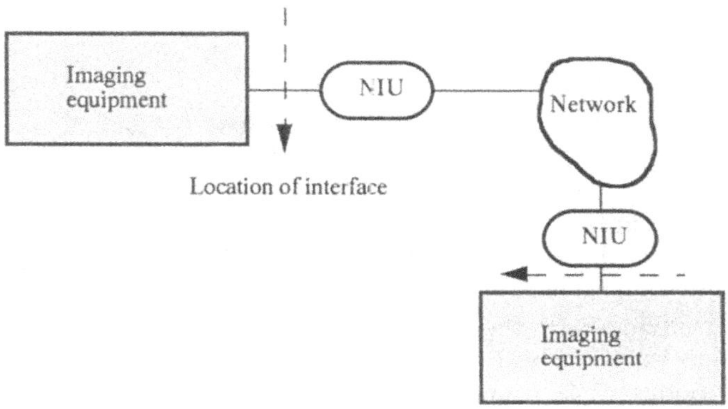

Fig. 8.5. ACR/NEMA interface for network communication (*NIU*, network interface)

interface is defined to be between the two devices (Fig. 8.4). It was not developed as a network standard, but a connection to a network is essential. In this case, the device on one side of the interface would be a network interface (Fig. 8.5). The network used will define the type of network interface. The design was based on the ISO layers, but without the transport network level which are combined. The medical image examination which is performed, the patient data, and image-related information form a set of data, these are further associated with commands, and the whole is called a message. The commands indicate certain operations on the data such as SEND, GET, and FIND.

8.5.2 Medical Image Processing System RC 109

The Medical Image Processing System (MIPS) organization was established in 1985 to undertake standardization activities in the field of medical imaging communications such as PACS. The core of the MIPS exist inside Japan Industries Association of Radiation Apparatus (JIRA) under the sponsorship of the sponsorship of the Japanese Ministry of International Trade and Industry (MITI). The aim of MIPS was to complete and carry out a standard of medical image communication. In March of 1990, the RC 109 committee (the new MIPS) in JIRA was started and took over the engineering or manufacturers' side of the old MIPS committee mentioned above.

The Japanese manufacturers and universities, supported by various governmental authorities, formed very early working groups to adapt the ACR/NEMA standard to Japanese needs. Two activities are to be mentioned within this context: The Japanese MIPS standard is compatible with the ACR/NEMA standard Version 2 and was published in April 1990 (MIPS Draft 89). For the representation of Japanese Kanjii characters two ASCII characters are employed. Moreover, a large working group is active to define a suitable directory format for MODs.

8.5.3 Image Save and Carry Committee

The Image Save and Carry (ISAC) committee was formed to propose standardization of use of the MOD in the medical field. It is composed of the Japanese Society of PACS (JPACS) and the Medical Information System Developing Center (MEDIS-DC). This committee continues its activities with the support of the MITI. The purposes of the committee are: to build an off-line system using a mobile, large-capacity medium such as optical disk; to maintain full exchangeability; and to have a filing system of medical information including images (Fig. 8.6). The proposed system will be applied to the medical information system within a hospital, the collaboration between hospital and general practitioners, the practical use of the personal health data system, and the highly information-oriented society for better medical care. The ISAC Committee is composed of:

- The Field test group
- Working group 1 for logical disk format
- Working group 2 for image data file format
- Working group 3 for system design
- Working group 4 for technical assessment

The committee is planning to make a proposal to ISO (from the SC-15 Committee, Japan), and to publish specifications. Furthermore, a field test will be conducted at a selected city with population of about 500 000, starting in April 1992.

8.5.4 Standard Product Interconnect

The two manufacturers, Siemens and Philips, joined forces and developed additions to the ACR/NEMA standard which is called the SPI standard. The SPI specifications were completed in November 1986, and in 1988 were submitted to ACR/NEMA WG VI for consideration in the further development of the standard. In the meantime, some of SPI concepts have been adopted by ACR/NEMA. In addition to the ACR/NEMA standard, SPI

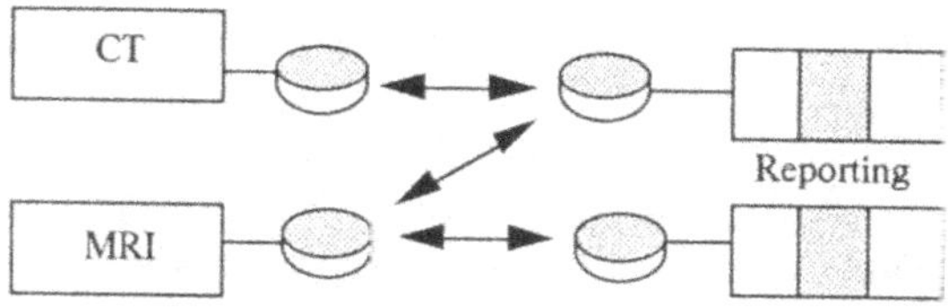

Fig. 8.6. Image storage and transmission

defines the directory format for optical disks, is based on a service concept, and has additional functionality on the application protocol level. The SPI has not really been implemented and accepted as a standard up to now, but a lot of good ideas are developed in the proposal.

8.6 Conclusion

For standardization, it is important that one should focus not only on images from radiology, but on the whole scope of images within the hospital, e.g., endoscopy, microscopy, nuclear medicine, and the health care frame work. Technology is moving very fast, and one could also say that on the medical side, a lot of additional knowledge has come from the medical doctors to add to the technology. This is important for standardization work, because from there we can define a lot of priorities, and also because the work items are focused from the application point of view. Everything which has to do with imaging can be translated to communication and integration. One needs communication between systems, between user and between different applications.

A special feature of images is that one is dealing with high amounts of information. One is not interested in one image but in a sequence of images, an examination, and a patient history, so information from various media is needed. This means that hundreds of megabytes will be needed and must be manipulated in seconds. This is also a multivendor world, which requires standardization in the direction of interconnections.

In order to ensure the compatibility of the various components within a PACS, definition and implementation of standards are required; this is even true for equipment produced by just one manufacturer. Often the PACS components installed in hospitals were produced by different manufacturers. In these instances, the need for standardization is even more evident. Areas where standardization is absolutely necessary or highly desirable are:

- Exchange of digital images between the various PACS components
- Management of medical images within the total PACS environment
- Integration of the PACS into the HIS

If a manufacturer's product is designed with only the manufacturer's own idea of the solution of a technical problem in mind, then incompatibility with equipment from other manufacturers is unavoidable. This leads to a limited scope for connecting the product and a short product life, because other solutions will come onto the market, bringing about a further delay in the development of a standard.

One of the most important considerations for the customer is to safeguard his investment. A scenario where medical apparatus from a certain manufacturer can only be connected to the PACS of the same manufacturer would place the customer in a very unfavorable position. Normally, equipment installed in a hospital is supplied by several manufacturers. The money spent in solving incompatibilities within a PACS project is not spent economically. Such a limiting scenario would not be helpful in marketing PACS. Alternatively, if the interconnection of equipment from various manufacturers is possible, an increased market acceptance for PACS is expected. ACR-NEMA, CENTC 251 and other activities are clearly making progress in the right direction, and we must try to support these activities. It is not realistic to reinvent the wheel again and again: we need standardization soon with imegration and harmonization paths worldwide.

References

Akisada M (1990) MIPS standard activities in Japan. Med Inform 15(1): 39–51

Horii S (1990) The ACR-NEMA standards: a tutorial on their structure and use. In: Arenson F (ed) Proceedings of SCAR. pp 405–422

Ohyama N (1990) Transportable image recording medium: a proposal of ISAC (Image Save and Carry) system. IEEE publication CH 2837–3/90/0000, pp 250–255

Tesche G (1988) SPI: a PACS interface specification. Med Inform 13(4): 281–288

9 Second Generation PACS Concept: A Global View

M. Osteaux, A.R. Bakker, D. Bell, P. Kofakis, R. Mattheus,
D. Meyer-Ebrecht, R. Van de Velde, and Th. Wendler

9.1 First Generation PACS: Reasons for Their Failure

The first generation of picture archiving and communications systems (PACS) implementations developed in the last decade were mostly technologically driven. Most proved technically quite successful and were important for gaining experience. It is, however, generally accepted that they failed to demonstrate any real use in the clinical environment and were not cost effective. As a consequence, PACS is not yet universally recognized as a useful medical system by all those responsible for the health care community.

The failure of the system was partially due to the lack of maturity of the technical tools such as storage network and digital radiology, the absence of recognized standards, and some misconceptions in the system itself. We will consider these three factors in more detail:

1. *Technological factors*. After the definition of the PACS acronym in 1982, further development was undertaken in different directions, and several tentative implementations performed. These implementations were immediately challenged by serious technical problems. First of all, very large archiving capacities were needed, and the conventional magnetic tape technology was definitely not adaptable. Better archiving only became possible with the introduction of the optical disk technology and more recently with optoelectronic, erasable disks and optical tapes. Further research in this field, however, is still necessary. Second, the bottlenecks moved towards the networking and data base environment, which proved totally insufficient to provide an acceptable access time for the images in the archive. The viability of these systems is rapidly improving with the development of modern technology based on fiber-optical multiplex networking in conjunction with specialized network management software. However, the problem cannot be considered totally solved: progress is still needed in the performance of the components as in the cost efficiency. Extensive research into network management is still necessary.

   PACS needs digital input. It is a fact that digital modalities such as ultrasound, computed tomography, magnetic resonance imaging, or digital subtraction angiography are being used more and more to produce images, and medical interest continues to increase. However, conventional radiology remains an important issue. Secondary digitalization from conventional radiology provides only a temporary and inefficient bridge between the analogue and the PACS world. It combines the poor dynamic range of conventional radiology with the relatively small spatial resolution of the digital modalities: the worst of the two worlds. It also adds the cost of both procedures together and, therefore, cannot be cost effective.

Replacement of the film as primary support for the acquisition of the information is already under development with digital fluoroscopy and phosphor plate technology, for example. However, further development is still needed (as well as diminution of the costs) before these technologies become largely available in the hospital environment. The full PACS concept (filmless option) will not be possible until these technologies are completely mature. On the other hand, it must also be said that digital radiology needs the PACS environment to exploit its advantages.

2. *Standards*. The absence of recognized standards such as image format transfer protocol and physical interface has been identified as one major problem with the first PACS realizations. Substantial efforts have been made and significant results achieved (see Chap. 8). However, the level of real implementation by the manufacturers upon the acquisition modalities is still rather low.

Until very recently, manufacturing companies saw the development of new products as an autonomous procedure; its integration into the PACS environment was not given such high priority. The philosophy is now changing in the research and development departments of the big companies of the radiological industry, although rather slowly. It can be foreseen that the absence of implementation of standards in the acquisition modalities will make fitting new PACS components into existing installations complex, expensive, and possibly clinically inefficient. Prospectively, PACS integrability must be built in during the conception of the modalities themselves, a factor will still seriously limit the implementation of the PACS technology in this decade.

3. *Conception*. The first generation PACS realization were mostly technologically driven. They did not take the functional needs of the medical community sufficiently into account. The systems were, namely, characterized by an inadequate architecture, e.g., centralized or with star network structure, and by the absence of intelligent routing of images. As a consequence, an unacceptable access time to the images was generated. This led to the rejection of the system by radiologists as a tool for primary reporting. The existence of a central and unique data base without prefetching and preloading strategies also contributed to difficulties in terms of access to the images (see Sect. 5.3).

Most first generation systems were inadequately integrated with the hospital or radiological information systems (HIS, RIS). This led to inconsistencies in patient data and difficulties and errors in retrieving the information. Experience also shows that the need for repetitive introduction of the patient data via the keyboard is a factor leading to complications, possible errors, and nonacceptance of the system in the clinical environment. Finally, the problems of the user interface were insufficiently researched and addressed. As previously stated, the needs of the different classes of users can be very different and specific. Those very diverse requirements cannot be addressed in a centralized architecture.

9.2 The New Generation: Medically Determined PACS Concept

A synthesis of the knowledge acquired from the first implementations, the progress of the available technologies, and the cooperative work undertaken by the partners in our research consortium has led to a general innovative concept of the future of PACS. It can be presented as an integrated, but decentralized structure, where small- or medium-sized units are specialized to the requirements of specific clusters of users in the hospital. They are linked together as a logical whole which remains transparent for the users. The characteristics of our PACS concept can be summarized as follows:

- Designed to suit the needs of the different cluster of users in a medical environment, namely, an adaptive user interface
- Options for modular architecture, i.e., (specialized small systems, integrated as a logical whole with a distributed network)
- "Open" architecture, i.e., multivendor environment, making use of recognized standards, and maximum use of digital interfaces
- Architecture allowing progressive and phased approach
- Upgradability
- Distributed data base (DDB) and/or multiple local temporary store with prefetching and preloading capability
- Integration with RIS and/or HIS including provision for prefetching and preloading strategies
- Knowledge-based networking, allowing an intelligent distribution of the image within a distributed network

These characteristics will be discussed in the following sections.

9.3 Adaptive User Interface

Diagnostic image workstations will provide the interface between fully digital PACS and their clinical users, both radiologists and clinicians. User-friendly, appropriate interfaces which meet the requirements of various user groups and which support the relevant diagnostic tasks will be of utmost importance for the success of PACS. The adaptive user interfaces relate their functioning to the context they work in. To achieve context sensitivity, system actions and reactions have to be based on knowledge about the specific requirements of users and tasks and about the general task domain. These explicit and formal user, task, and domain models may be pre-specified, e.g., using a priori knowledge of the medical diagnostic process, derived from interviews or questionnaires, or acquired and updated during the users' dialogues. The purpose of adaptation and the degree of adaptivity may be defined in wide limits.

User-friendliness is generally regarded as the result of a predominantly user-centered, cyclic, and interactive design process. User-centered design, however, often focuses on some kind of "average" user and assumes a number of general goals the user is interested in. Changing requirements arising from different kind of users and the diversity of goal oriented tasks and subtasks which users have to perform are rarely considered during system design, and almost never at system run-time. Most human–machine interfaces appear to be "static". They function uniformly, regardless of what kind of user is working with a system and with what task the user is immediately concerned. Adaptive user interfaces are, in contrast, dynamic.

Conceptually, adaptive user interfaces take into account that work-station users and their actual tasks are variable during run-time. In radiology, digital diagnostic display systems will be used by quite different stereotypic categories of users, e.g., radiologists, clinicians, and technicians, with diverse duties and information requirements. Even within a particular user group, personal perferences and styles can be observed, e.g., how to arrange images on a display screen. Analyzing the film-based diagnostic process, various categories of goal-oriented tasks can be distinguished, ranging from simple control actions, e.g., image quality check after an examination, to quite complex image handling and display procedures, such as preparing a demonstration session for referring clinicians.

Adaptive user interfaces are designed with the main objective of increasing usability and convenience. From the user's point of view, adaptive systems should appear to be supportive by acting in a co-operative manner. This has to be seen under the boundary condition that the consistency and predictivity of the interface will not be affected by the adaptation mechanisms. From the designer's point of view, user interfaces have to be based on formalized descriptions (models) of the requirements for different users and tasks. These models have to define major parts of the workstation's functionality at a high level of abstraction.

In recent years, interest in adaptive user interfaces has substantially increased. Extending the idea of user-centered design, these interfaces will use models of users and tasks not only during the design cycle, but also as part of the functioning of a system. As a result, models have to be explicit, formalized and represented in a computer executable way.

9.4 Distributed Data Base

In the 1980s, it became possible to develop image storage and retrieval systems. The enabling developments which underpin this advance have come from a variety of sources and include both hardware and software advances. On the data base front, there have been great enhancements of the functionality of data base management systems (DBMS). As data bases grow, they make heavy demands on storage capacity. Terabyte systems are likely to be needed in future large image data bases. A key problem in designing these systems is providing the required levels of performance. During the last few years, optical mass storage technology has matured to the stage where various standards have been developed for organizing different types of information on CD-ROM. In comparison with alternative mass storage systems, this technology has special features such as slow access to data.

The recent advances in very large scale integrated (VLSI) circuit logic, data communications networks and computer technology in general, coupled with the large volume of data and complexity of the application requirements, have led to the design of distributed computer architectures, where computer systems can be interconnected via telecommunications links. The availability of these hardware configurations supports the design of the software management systems needed to meet advanced application requirements. These hardware and software architectures triggered the emergence of the DDB era in about 1975. A distributed DBMS (DDBMS) allows data sharing among a community of users, while ensuring the integrity of the data over time and providing security against unauthorized access. It provides transparency of the location of data so that users need not be aware of the geographical location of data and the details of the underlying DBMS. The design of such a DDBMS is complex, and many of the pertinent issues are still under intensive research.

Multimedia data bases emerge as a natural evolution of the distributed data base systems (DDBS). The main aim of a multimedia data base system (MMDBS) is to provide uniform representation and manipulation of heterogeneous data on multiple media. The distributed aspects of such systems are clearly desirable in many application areas. In the real world, information is often communicated and exchanged among people by means of a variety of media. They communicate through speech, drawing diagrams and pictures, and write notes and point to things. Therefore, in addition to record-based information, people seek computer-based support for storing and managing data represented as voice, images, text, and for communicating using these media.

The stage has been reached when such generalized MMDBS capable of being applied to many diverse applications can now be contemplated. The innovations which have led to this are development of storage media, input/output media, communications (open systems interconnection, OSI), semantic data models, and continual requests to improve flexibility and productivity. Therefore, an MMDBS is a data base system that integrates data bases which are organized in many media, i.e., alphanumerical data, picture data, voice data, and video data. In order to accelerate the search of very large image data bases, data classification and/or cluster analysis techniques can be used to extract the attributes that are discriminating and efficient for image classification for the specific domain of application. Knowledge-based image classification/analysis techniques are investigated. It is possible to extend the capabilities of a medical image data base. The quality and efficiency of information retrieval highly depends on the indexing process.

9.5 Integrated PACS/HIS/RIS Environment

From the viewpoint of total medical information systems a PACS is not an autonomous system, but a logical extension from the HIS that is responsible for the delivery of patient information (administrative and medical) coupled with examination data from the RIS. Therefore, the interface between PACS and HIS/RIS is an essential part of the conception of PACS which forms the main objective of the work programme within the hospital integrated PACS (HIPACS) project. The implementation of a full-scale PACS, replacing all radiographic films throughout the whole hospital, can only be realized successfully if such a PACS is coupled with the HIS/RIS in that hospital, and this for different reasons. The images within the PACS need to be identified by means of patient data. To avoid re-typing and errors, patient identification data must be transferred to the PACS together with the images; in the PACS, the medical history and the radiodiagnostic reports of that patient residing in the HIS must also be available at the workstation. It should be possible to present both the image and the alphanumerical data from the same patient in a coherent way at the PACS workstation. In such a situation, part of the HIS/RIS functionality, e.g., report editing, should be available through the PACS workstation.

The memory and communication capacities of PACS systems are limited, even with leading-edge information technology. To obtain acceptable response times, it will be necessary to devise intelligent image management strategies, e.g., to send the images in advance from the central archive to the workstation where the user is going to require these images (prefetching). Such strategies for image migration can be based on data from the HIS such as patient location and patient medical history. The RIS/HIS/PACS model has to be considered as composed of three components:

1. An application model (application architecture)
2. A data model (data architecture)
3. A network model (network architecture)

9.6 Prefetching

Presently, it is expected that only the application of prefetching combined with high-speed networks and image compression can provide a response time that is acceptable for the user. A quick delivery of the images will be one of the main demands to be fulfilled by the second generation of PACS systems. One of the strategies for reducing the waiting time is to place those images for which the probability of retrieval is enhanced in a storage device near the workstations from which they can be presented quickly before they are expected to be retrieved. This strategy, uses knowledge rules about the images retrieval patterns, is called prefetching.

For the second generation of PACS, the following model has been proposed: a hierarchical layered storage structure, consisting of at least the following three layers: a huge but slow archive on optical disks, fast parallel transfer disks (or even random access memory) with limited storage capacity near the workstations and a central buffer of those disks with intermediate properties. The waiting times can be diminished if we succeed in a retrieval of a maximum percentage of images from fast storages instead of the slower ones, images which are more likely to be retrieved have to be placed beforehand in the faster storages. The rule-based system, called the prefetch algorithm, which evaluates this probability, is initiated by events occurring in the hospital. The following three processes in a chain have been distinguished from the moment of the encountering of an event up to the final image reallocation. The chain is activated by an event (data base transition) occurring in the HIS/RIS, e.g., an admission to be detected in an admission, discharge and transfer (ADT) subsystem. The first process evaluates the expected retrieval of the images of a patient's history according to medical rules, e.g., the medical preference of the most recent *n* images is high. The second process combines all these expectations for single images (of various patients) in a coherent logistic strategy to satisfy all HIPACS users. The final process takes care of the physical image transport in the HIPACS hardware, regardless of the medical contents of the images.

Because the events that initiate the prefetching algorithm occur in the HIS/RIS, and the final image reallocations occur in the PACS, it is clear that the HIS/RIS/PACS interface should include prefetching. Besides the definition of the events, the specification of the interface should include an accurate description of the process that caused the event and of the actions which should follow the event. The model described above can also be applied in the film-based situation. In the transition phase from the film situation to the HIPACS situation, the current film folder management system has to be integrated with its HIPACS counterpart.

As PACS has not yet been introduced on a large scale, the potential effectiveness can only be studied in the conventional film-based situation. A pilot study has been performed at Leiden University Hospital. Some main prerequisites for such a study are: the availability of the required data in an integrated HIS, the use of film folders per examination (instead of one film folder per patient), and the availability of an information system (embedded in the HIS) that supports the lending of these examination film folders. The first results of this pilot study are encouraging, suggesting that this research should be continued, although the results have to be translated in terms of real improvement in response time, which does not depent on prefetching only. Because prefetching makes use of knowledge of the image retrieval patterns, the response time offered to the user becomes related to his pattern of usage. A method of assessing the required response time in relation to the working procedures has to be (further) developed.

It can be expected that prefetching will be one of the prerequisites in offering a user acceptable response time. Its effectiveness may be limited by its complexity, by a too short period between event and image transfer, by the unavailability of necessary data and/or events, by an inappropriate interface between HIS/RIS and PACS, and the inability to recognize retrieval patterns. These patterns of image retrieval can only be observed in a reliable way if a lending system (embedded in a HIS/RIS) for examination film folder management is used. Moreover, the information required for the development of prefetching a lending system will improve the logistic process immediately. It is suggested that further research should focus on the retrieval patterns, on the definition of the response time requirements, and on the development of a standardized interface.

9.7 Intelligent Distribution of Images: Knowledge-Based Networking

Image data, which are characterized by an extremely large data set, require a very high transport speed to a communication network between different PACS image devices to allow an image exchange during normal work without long waiting periods for the images. Standard networks for data communication only make use of one physical data channel, the transfer capability of which is to be distributed to the number of active users. The effective transfer rate remaining for each user will be too low for this type of application.Communication networks are becoming more and more complex, and computer networks in particular are becoming more and more heterogeneous. Careful management of these networks becomes a crucial factor for maintaining efficient and reliable network operation and for increasing the performance of the network in terms of quality and quantity of the services provided to the end users. Since traditional methodologies for network management are not coping well enough with today's complex networks, new approaches are being investigated. Recently, research has started into the possibility of applying network management to artificial intelligence and expert systems.

A network management is needed in a PACS environment, the size of a data transfer being several orders of magnitude larger than a typical data transfer in a local area computer network. The existing local area network technology uses protocols which are not suited for image transport. Therefore, it is necessary to sequentialize the image traffic on the network explicitly, i.e., access conflicts are not left to be resolved by the transport layer but are arbitrated by a software module. In addition, the network traffic can be distributed over time because knowledge about patient, radiologist, and image flow is available. This knowledge can be exploited for careful planning and scheduling, e.g., for organizing prefetching of images from central archive to local store overnight.

Traffic management is a prime issue. To a certain point, traffic management can be static, taking into account the network configuration and knowledge on image flow, patient flow, and radiologist flow in a hospital environment. But beyond that point, decisions on which transfers should be served first must be made dynamically taking into account the current state of the network including pending request, and actual disk usage.

The next process takes the physical dimensions such as the number of storage layers, the access time of a layer, and the throughput of the network(s) into account. It will use rules dictating how to make optimal use of the PACS configuration. A change in the configuration, e.g., a workstation out of duty will be recorded in this data entity. The actual occupancy of the storages and the actual network traffic is recorded in the entity PACS network/storage. Somewhere the logical description has to be translated into a physical description. It is assumed that this takes place at the start of this process. After the physical routing of an image (move a certain image from storage x to storage y at a certain point in time) has been decided, the process continues with the physical transport: e.g., breaking the images down into transportable packets. The result is the transfer of an image to another storage (or the release of storage space occupied by an image).

9.8 Modular Architecture; Phased Approach

Modular network architectures, capable of reacting to growth and changes in traffic patterns are essential. Partitioning the network into subnets will reduce speed requirements and increase response time by distributing network traffic. A hierarchical decomposition will make it easier to use existing transmission techniques. As an additional benefit, this design strategy offers the possibility to start introduction of PACS into a given environment by establishing the local subsystem first. In subsequent steps, the integration of a complete PACS could be performed, accompanied by a step-by step training of personnel and a gradual change in work routines. In the future, new techniques for faster communication will be available, but there will always be an advantage in managing image distribution in a clinical environment.

There are several reasons why setting up a PACS environment must take place in different phases. The first reason is that the cost of a PACS environment in a hospital is very high. Also, we still have very little experience in building up such an environment. A PACS is mostly built with new equipment, and subsequently extended with interfaces to pre-existing equipment. It is obvious that one cannot shut down all activities in a hospital in order to perform a few PACS experiments. Last but not least, a gradual implementation will allow the medical community to adapt itself to the new technology and progressive change its work organization.

9.9 Conclusion

Within the next few years, a new PACS concept – HIPACS – will be developed within the clinical environment. Image digital management is a specialized part of the future prospect of global information all in digital form within the hospital environment, all of which will be integrated in the acquisition modality itself and in the HIS. This idea entails modification of the conception philosophy of the radiological systems, and of the structure of the informatics of the hospital. In has also consequences for the organization within and outside the department of radiology.

Regarding PACS technology as an appendage grafted onto existing and unchanged systems has failed in the past, and will fail in the future to produce acceptable clinical results. From this point of view, much research and development is still needed before the global PACS concept is realized, i.e., the filmless hospital. However, it must also be stated that partial solutions in a hybrid environment, i.e., coexistence of digital and analogue solutions, are already available and effective.

In any case the global potentialities and perspectives of PACS technology can no longer be questionned. The authors wish to encourage every hospital, especially the teaching hospitals, to invest some – perhaps limited – efforts and interests in order to progressively gain some technological and organizational experience.

www.ingramcontent.com/pod-product-compliance
Lightning Source LLC
Chambersburg PA
CBHW051150180926
51611CB00001B/12
* 9 7 8 3 6 4 2 7 6 9 6 5 8 *